Synergistic Stuttering Therapy

Butterworth–Heinemann Series in Communication Disorders
Charlena M. Seymour, Ph.D., Series Editor

Battle, D.E. *Communication Disorders in Multicultural Populations, Second Edition* (1998)

Bloom, C. & Cooperman, D.K. *Synergistic Stuttering Therapy: A Holistic Approach* (1999)

Billeaud, F.P. *Communication Disorders in Infants and Toddlers: Assessment and Intervention, Second Edition* (1998)

Huntley, R.A. & Helfer, K.S. *Communication in Later Life* (1995)

Kricos, P.B. & Lesner, S.A. *Hearing Care for the Older Adult: Audiologic Rehabilitation* (1995)

Maxon, A.B. & Brackett, D. *The Hearing-Impaired Child: Infancy Through High School Years* (1992)

Velleman, S.L. *Making Phonology Functional: What Do I Do First?* (1998)

Wall, L.G. *Hearing for the Speech-Language Pathologist and Health Care Professional* (1995)

Wallace, G.L. *Adult Aphasia Rehabilitation* (1996)

Synergistic Stuttering Therapy
A Holistic Approach

Sister Charleen Bloom, Ph.D., M.S.W.
Department of Communication Disorders,
The College of Saint Rose, Albany, New York

Donna K. Cooperman, D.A.
Department of Communication Disorders,
The College of Saint Rose, Albany, New York

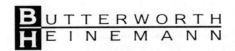

Boston   Oxford   Auckland   Johannesburg   Melbourne   New Delhi

Every effort has been made to ensure that the drug dosage schedules within this text are accurate and conform to standards accepted at time of publication. However, as treatment recommendations vary in the light of continuing research and clinical experience, the reader is advised to verify drug dosage schedules herein with information found on product information sheets. This is especially true in cases of new or infrequently used drugs.

 Recognizing the importance of preserving what has been written, Butterworth–Heinemann prints its books on acid-free paper whenever possible.

GLOBAL Butterworth–Heinemann supports the efforts of American Forests and the
RELEAF Global ReLeaf program in its campaign for the betterment of trees, forests,
2000 and our environment.

Library of Congress Cataloging-in-Publication Data
Bloom, Charleen.
    Synergistic stuttering therapy: a holistic approach / Charleen
Bloom, Donna K. Cooperman.
        p.   cm. — (Butterworth-Heinemann series in communication disorders)
    Includes bibliographical references and index.
    ISBN 0-7506-9527-7
    1. Stuttering—Treatment. 2. Stuttering—Psychological aspects.
I. Cooperman, Donna K. II. Title. III. Series: Butterworth-Heinemann
series in communications disorders.
    [DNLM: 1. Stuttering—therapy. 2. Speech Therapy—methods.
3. Stuttering—psychology. 4. Behavior Therapy—methods.   WM 475
B656s 1999]
RC424.B564   1999
616.85′5406—DC21
DNLM/DLC
for Library of Congress   98-50995
                                                                        CIP

British Library Cataloguing-in-Publication Data
A catalogue record for this book is available from the British Library.

The publisher offers special discounts on bulk orders of this book.
For information, please contact:

Manager of Special Sales
Butterworth-Heinemann
225 Wildwood Avenue
Woburn, MA 01801-2041
Tel: 781-904-2500
Fax: 781-904-2620

For information on all Butterworth–Heinemann publications available, contact our
World Wide Web home page at: http://www.bh.com

10 9 8 7 6 5 4 3 2 1

Printed in the United States of America

Contents

Preface

The fluency program at The College of Saint Rose has a long history. It was first developed by Sister Charleen Bloom during the early 1970s and evolved, much as a child does, through many developmental stages. But always, our program included an emphasis on effective, successful communication as a foundation for our teaching. The clients who came through the Saint Rose Fluency Program during the early years of our existence consistently had access to a support group, since we understood the value and importance of the community that people who stutter so firmly establish when provided the opportunity.

This view was not always as popular as it is today, when such support groups as the National Stuttering Project and Speakeasy International were so significant a force in stuttering treatment. This emphasis on support remains an integral part of our treatment model. As you read about our program and its focus on the synergistic interaction between the physiological, emotional, and environmental variables that impact people who stutter, you will no doubt recognize elements of both *fluency shaping* and *stuttering modification*. We view ours as an integrated program that utilizes the strengths of each of these schools of thought in order to individualize treatment in the most holistic way for people who stutter.

You will see that we do not just treat stuttering; rather, we treat people who happen to stutter, and our philosophy is rooted in the necessity of treating the whole person rather than just the speech mechanism attached to that person. The synergistic framework, from which our model has grown, does not attempt to explain why people stutter. We believe that different people may stutter for different reasons. But regardless of the etiology, we believe that people who stutter can be effective communicators who positively influence others. It is from this starting place that we have come, and which we always seem to return.

Acknowledgments

A work such as this is always the product of the input of many scholars. We have been influenced in our philosophy of treatment by the writings, lectures, workshops, and the conversations we have shared with many of our friends and colleagues. We are especially indebted to the work of Woody Starkweather, Meryl Wall, Ronald Webster, Barry Guitar, Hugo Gregory, Rebekah Pindzola, Martin Schwartz, Kenneth St. Louis, Oliver Bloodstein, Eugene Cooper, and Ed Conture. Their influences can be seen throughout this text. We thank Charlena Seymour for inviting us to contribute to Butterworth–Heinemann's Series in Communication Disorders.

Carol Prutting, many years ago, proposed synergy as an apt description of our philosophy of stuttering treatment. She would have enjoyed sharing the pleasure of publishing this work with us. We miss her clear and insightful thinking almost as much as we miss her wonderful wit and humor.

Our graduate students and clients in the Council of Fluency at the College of St. Rose and all other clients have been our teachers, our support, and the tangible inspiration behind our research. They have taught us, firsthand, about the work that must be done as we all journey toward self-empowerment and independence. We truly appreciate their partnership and willingness to explore their needs as they grow evermore assertive, effective, and confident. In particular, we thank Joy Emery who has participated for five years as a voluntary team instructor in the Graduate Fluency classes. Her experience and courage in facing and overcoming her fear of stuttering have taught all of us more than any textbook could ever capture.

Our graduate assistants have worked faithfully and diligently in the years since we began this journey. Although there have been many students who contributed to this process, we especially wish to thank Chris Wilber and Tina Lika for their perseverance during the final stages of manuscript preparation. Sandy Rivenburg of the Department of Technology at the College of Saint Rose has our sincere gratitude for sharing so generously of her wisdom, advice, and time in helping us to understand what the computer can do to help us in our work.

And, finally, we thank those who have supported us daily throughout the writing of this manuscript: the Sisters of St. Joseph of Carondelet, who made Sister Charleen's education in this field possible; Sister Charleen's local CSJ community, Mary, Veronica, Marlene, and Gar; the Cooperman family; the CMD department members; the administrators at the College of Saint Rose; and all our friends whose encouragement enabled us to continue.

1

Introduction

The purpose of this book is to present a stuttering treatment program that integrates the principles of normal speech production with the socioemotional aspects of communication. It is our hope that speech-language clinicians will return to clinical problem solving with people who stutter and their families. In order to do this, it is our belief that an integrative approach is essential.

However, before we begin to examine what is entailed by such an approach, we feel that it is necessary to summarize the stuttering behavior that we will be considering clinically. We also think it important to examine the multiple approaches to this disorder that have been used in the past; this historical perspective is crucial to understanding the integrative rehabilitative process that we will propose. Finally, in this introduction, we would like to present the rationale for and outline of a "synergistic approach to stuttering."

DEFINITIONS

After years of research and clinical practice, both clinicians and researchers agree that stuttering is a complex, multifaceted phenomenon. This is not surprising, since we understand that speech itself is such a dynamic, patterned, coordinated skill. There are many possibilities for interference with this process of normal speech production. Throughout the years, the attempt to find one all-inclusive, acceptable definition of stuttering has been difficult. This is due, in part, to the fact that early research itself was unidimensional. Researchers and clinicians alike believed that stuttering was the result of a single cause. Most now agree that such a unitary view was too narrow. Yet, researchers continue the debate over which aspects of the disorder are essential to the definition. As developments of technology increase, and our knowledge of neuroanatomy grows, our definition continues to expand.

Conture[1] compared the definition of stuttering to that of the common cold. He pointed out that some define both as catchall terms for a number of related but different problems. Conversely, others support the idea that they have a single cause. He stated that

it is our hunch, that the speech and related behaviors of stutterers are sub-
tly different and the reasons for their problems are also different . . . some
of the things we label and react to as stuttering may have different etiologies and courses of development and may in turn be more or less responsive
to different therapeutic approaches.[1]

If these hunches are accurate, and we are inclined to agree that they are, it is
our belief that the definition of stuttering that drives our therapeutic approach
must be broad and allow for both integration and individualization.

In defining stuttering, we think it also necessary to remember that both
people who stutter and those who don't have variability in their speech. All
speakers exhibit normal dysfluencies at times and those who stutter have many
periods of fluency. Thus, although the theory and definition of stuttering must be
broad, they must not become a label to easily identify the person who exhibits
the behavior. It is also important to recognize that all individuals who stutter
know more about their problem than anyone else. It is important to include the
people who stutter in the attempt to define their problem.

Given these disclaimers, we would like to briefly consider some of the basic
definitions that have influenced an integrative, synergistic approach to remediation of stuttering.

FLUENCY

Ultimately, we believe that the best therapy for dealing with any disordered
speech production is one that is based on the principles of normal speech production. As speech-language pathologists, our research and clinical practice are
grounded in the principles of respiration, phonation, articulation, and resonance. These are the bases for our assessments and remediations. When dealing
with a person who stutters, another aspect of normal speech production is highlighted—namely, fluency. Often, stuttering is simply defined as a disorder of fluency. Thus, it is important to understand the components of fluency that have
been identified.

The term *fluency* is derived from the Latin word *fluere*—to flow. When
identifying a person who is fluent in speech, we generally think of one whose
speech is easy and that flows from word to word without effort. In recent years,
we realized that before we can define what a person does who is dysfluent, we
must have a better understanding of fluency itself. Starkweather[2,3] has made considerable contributions to further understanding of fluency and has identified
three basic elements in speech fluency: rate, continuity, and effort. These components of fluency are important and merit further consideration.

Rate

The rate of an utterance is usually measured in syllables or words per minute. Starkweather[3,4] also suggested that the rate of information flow, not just
sound flow, is an important consideration in understanding fluency. It is clear

that multiple variables affect the rate of our speech. Ham[5] has stated: "Overall rate will be affected by the length of words used, by word familiarity, message significance, situational concerns, and other factors. Other affecting factors include physiological considerations, the sound or sound sequence being produced, coarticulation effects within units, duration of utterance and prosodic stress points."

Continuity

Continuity is seen in the smooth movement from phoneme to phoneme, across words, and from phrase to phrase. Hesitation is the disrupter of continuity.[5] However, Golddiamond-Eisler[6] helped us understand that normal speech is filled with hesitations. Starkweather[3] stated that these hesitations, or pauses, may occur for a variety of reasons:

(a) As a planned or practiced pause to create a dramatic effect
(b) As a tactic to allow time to formulate the cognitive and/or linguistic content and sequence of the next utterance
(c) As a method of preplanning the neuromotor production sequence of speech sounds
(d) As an avoidance to delay the onset of utterance where problems in production, content acceptability, or auditor reaction are anticipated

Clearly, one can see the complexity and breadth of this concept.

Effort

Effort is the cognitive or physical ease of production. Many utterances are produced easily and without effort. Little cognitive attention or awareness is necessary. Darley, Aronson, and Brown[7] pointed out that effort can then be neuromuscular in the timing and coordination of respiration, phonation, and articulation, using the formula of 14 phonemes per second multiplied by 100 muscles involved in sound production, multiplied by 100 motor units per muscle!

One can see how important physical, psychological, linguistic, and social elements are as contributing components of fluency. While there is still much to understand about the parameters of fluency, it is clear that the concepts of rate, continuity, and ease of production are elemental to an understanding of dysfluency or stuttering. Fluency connotes a continuous, forward-flowing, coordinated manner of speech.[8] Dysfluency is a disruption in these elements. Because of the complexities of the interactions, fluency must be understood on multiple levels if we are to become more aware of how the interactions affect each other. It is this awareness that a synergistic approach will address.

STUTTERING AND DYSFLUENCY

Because stuttering is such a multidimensional phenomenon it is extremely difficult to define. An additional difficulty in formulating a definition of stuttering is the variability of the problem for each person who stutters. Every person who stutters reports that their stuttering characteristically differs in certain situations and at certain times. Most people who stutter state that they experience fluency in many situations. It is for these reasons that we will be encouraging clinicians to increase their individual approach to the disorder. All people who stutter will have their own combination of interactions responsible for perpetuating their dysfluency. Therefore, a definition of stuttering must be both broad enough to be inclusive and limited enough to be discriminating. This is difficult to accomplish. Conture[1] believed that it is very hard, if not impossible, to develop an absolute definition of stuttering. At best, our definitions will be relative and capture the essentials of *what* stuttering is and *who* a person who stutters is. With this in mind, we would like to present some of the definitions of stuttering that have been frequently discussed and conclude with our own definition.

"Stuttering occurs when the forward flow of speech is interrupted by a motorically disrupted sound, syllable, or word, or by the speaker's reaction thereto."[9] It is difficult to capture the complexity of stuttering in a concise definition; however, the essence of a definition of stuttering consists of anomalies in the flow or rate of speech that are minimally distinguished by involuntary repetitions and prolongations, particularly of units of utterances smaller than a word. Wingate[10] referred to the audible and silent repetitions and prolongations as the universal and distinctive features of stuttering:

> The term "stuttering" means: I. (A) Disruption in fluency of verbal expression, which is (B) characterized by involuntary, audible or silent, repetitions or prolongations in the utterance of short speech elements, namely: sounds, syllables, and words of one syllable. These disruptions (C) usually occur frequently or are marked in character and (D) are not readily controllable. II. Sometimes the disruptions are (E) accompanied by accessory activities involving the speech apparatus, related or unrelated body structures, or stereotyped speech utterances. These activities give the appearance of being speech-related struggle. III. Also, there are not infrequently (F) indications or report of the presence of an emotional state, ranging from a general condition of "excitement" or "tension" to more specific emotions of a negative nature such as fear, embarrassment, irritation, or the like (G). The immediate source of stuttering is some incoordination expressed in the peripheral speech mechanism; the ultimate cause is presently unknown and may be complex or compound.[10,11]

Other definitions of stuttering, with different emphases, are as follows:

> Differences have been found in the laryngeal and articulatory dynamics of stutterers. Differences have been found in their sequencing, timing and temporal programming abilities, genetic and familial tendencies, central nervous system characteristics, linguistic abilities, environmental influences and psychological characteristics and attitudes.[12]

Stuttering is characterized by an abnormally high frequency and/or duration of stoppages in the forward flow of speech. These stoppages usually take the form of (A) repetitions of sound, syllables, or one-syllable words, (B) prolongations of sounds, or (C) "blocks" of airflow and/or voicing in speech. Individuals who stutter are usually aware of their stuttering and are often embarrassed by it. Moreover, they often use abnormal physical and mental effort to speak. Children who are just beginning to stutter may not always be highly conscious of it, but they usually show signs of tension and increased speech rate, which suggests they are at least minimally aware of their difficulty.[13]

Fluency is deviant when speech is produced with effort, when speech is more discontinuous than normal, or when the discontinuities are immature, when the rhythm of speech is atypical, or when it is not serving the speaker by making the speech production easier.[14]

Finally, the summary by Van Riper[15] of what he had learned about stuttering after 85 years of research can also be considered a definition:

- Stuttering is essentially a neuromuscular disorder whose core consists of tiny lags and disruptions in the timing of the complicated movements required for speech.
- The usual response to these lags is an automatic part word repetition or prolongation.
- Some children, because of heredity or as yet unknown brain pathology, have more of these than others do.
- Most children who begin to stutter become fluent perhaps because of maturation or because they do not react to their lags, repetitions, or prolongations by struggle or avoidance.
- Those who do struggle or avoid because of frustration or penalties will probably continue to stutter all the rest of their lives no matter what kind of therapy they receive.
- These struggle and avoidance behaviors are learned and can be modified and unlearned though the lags cannot.
- The goal of therapy for the confirmed stutterer should not be a reduction in the number of dysfluencies or zero stuttering. Fluency-enhancing procedures can easily result in stutter-free speech temporarily but maintaining it is almost impossible. The stutterer already knows how to be fluent. What he doesn't know is how to stutter. He can be taught to stutter so easily and briefly that he can have very adequate communication skills. Moreover, when he discovers he can stutter without struggle or avoidance most of his frustration and other negative emotion will subside.

Clearly, the definitions that have been given for stuttering are as individual as both the people who stutter and the therapy that is provided for them. It is our belief, however, that each clinician who does therapy with people who stutter must sift through the research and reports of past experience of those who have worked with both children and adults who stutter. The next step is to formulate one's own beliefs about stuttering, bringing together the known research and one's personal clinical experience. Clinicians who develop a working definition of stuttering in this way—tying together research, clinical experience, and therapeutic approach—properly earn the confidence placed in them as therapist by the children, parents, adults, and families with whom they work.

For too long, our lack of agreement on an all-inclusive, single definition of stuttering has produced clinicians who have a corresponding lack of confidence. Not having a generally agreed-upon definition or theory to provide solid footing, clinicians have been hesitant to develop their own diagnostic and therapeutic techniques. Moreover, lacking a framework for what they do, clinicians have often become slaves to someone else's program for people who stutter. As a consequence, individualizing the therapeutic approach is not encouraged, as the variability in both the stuttering behavior and the individuals who stutter is ignored. St. Louis[16] has reported that this lack of confidence begins in the training program. Few people have specialized in working with people who stutter and students all too often leave their Master's program without the necessary understanding or experience with this population. We encourage our readers to draw on the experience of those presented here and to formulate your own definition of stuttering or to choose the persons theory that coheres with your own theoretical understanding of speech and language disorders.

In drawing together the results of our own experiences and research in the field of fluency, our definition of stuttering builds on the research of others that we have found to be important and expands their theories to accommodate our present understanding of disfluency. We are conscious, however, that any proposed definition of this complex phenomenon will change as our understanding grows.

We believe that these basic components of stuttering are included in the synergistic processes of normal speech-language production. Our definition is: The synergistic process of normal speech production includes the interaction of physical, psychological, linguistic, and psychosocial components. We believe that each individual who stutters has developed individual and learned attitudinal and behavioral responses to the underlying neurologic disorder. These responses include the production of audible or silent-sound repetition, part-word repetition, whole-word repetition, prolongations, blockages, or secondary behaviors (i.e., patterned bodily reactions suggesting speech-related struggle). We also believe that the complex synergistic interactions exist individually within the attitudes and behaviors of persons who stutter and in their interactions with their environment. Therefore, any evaluation and therapeutic process of remediation must include the examination of the individual person who stutters' physical, psychological, linguistic, and psychosocial patterns.

HISTORY OF STUTTERING TREATMENT APPROACHES

Our belief that a personal definition of stuttering is essential for clinicians who wish to work with individuals who stutter is not new. From the earliest days, stuttering treatment has flowed from a persons theory of what caused the person to stutter. The Romans believed that people who stuttered were filled with evil spirits. Naturally, exorcism was employed. In the seventeenth century, Sir Francis Bacon attributed stuttering to a dryness of the tongue and prescribed drinking wine in moderation because "It Heateth." In the eighteenth century, the Oracle of Delphi, a surgeon, believed that people who stuttered were more dysfluent in familiar surroundings. Therefore, their treatment was to be banished from their homes forever. In 1795, Dieffenbach noted that the tongue of a person who stuttered cleaved to the roof of his mouth. Accordingly, he cut a triangular wedge from the tongue. It is clear, therefore, that the theory of what causes stuttering historically has directly influenced the therapy to treat it.

However, even a serious student of the disorder of stuttering can find it difficult to sort out the many theories of stuttering that have been proposed from the earliest days to the present. Because of this, many present-day clinicians are groping for both a theory and a therapy that will apply to the variety of behaviors evidenced in their clients who stutter. In a recent book by Bloodstein,[17] he pointed out the wide range of factors that have been suggested as the cause of stuttering: enforced right-handedness, conflicts over oral-erotic gratification, being tongue-tied, talking faster than one can think, labeling a child a person who stutters, parental overprotection, brain abnormality, communicative pressures, and high fetal levels of the male hormone testosterone. Bloodstein[17] also stated:

> Like theories of the cause of stuttering, assumptions about the treatment have vacillated between widely divergent views. Relaxation, suggestion, psychotherapy, hypnosis, drugs, operant conditioning, and many other forms of therapy have been tried. But reduced to its simplest essentials, our attempt to aid stutterers has veered back and forth between methods that teach them to talk differently and methods that teach them to stutter differently.

We are in agreement with Bloodstein's assessment of the vacillating nature of the treatments that have emerged from the earliest theories of the cause of stuttering. We believe many of these theories and treatment approaches were lacking in effectiveness because they continued to look for the "seductive unitary cause" of stuttering. We now know that a single cause of the disorder of stuttering will never be isolated because stuttering is a complex, multidimensional disorder. It may be that most of the wide variety of theories and therapies reported in the literature each have their own validity, in that they embody a partial truth and can find their place in a rationale that integrates the various theories in a broad heterogeneous scheme.

With this prospect in mind, research was undertaken to reduce theories and therapies to their "simplest essentials" and to integrate these essentials. Guitar and Peters[13,18] and Bloom[19] have described treatment programs based on such an integrated framework. The essential components that have been integrated summarize years of stuttering therapy and are entitled "stuttering modification therapy" and "fluency shaping therapy." Gregory[20] focused these therapies into two approaches and named them the "Stutter More Fluently Approach" and the "Speak More Fluently Approach." Curlee and Perkins[21] have grouped these two approaches to therapy and called them: "Those That Manage Stuttering" and "Those That Manage Fluency." Each of these therapies summarizes major approaches to therapy throughout the years, and some familiarity with these approaches is essential to the understanding of a synergistic model of treatment. Guitar and Peters[13,22] helped to bridge the gap between these two approaches and have provided us with the categories of "stuttering modification therapy" and "fluency shaping therapy."

Stuttering Modification Therapy

Stuttering modification therapy has been defined as "[r]educing avoidance behaviors, speech related fears and negative attitudes toward speech. It also includes helping the person who stutters learn to modify the form of his/her stuttering."[13] Since the person who stutters carries an accumulation of fears, anxieties, hesitations, and other emotions, this attitudinal aspect of stuttering has been the object of a great deal of speculation and attention. We consider this an integral part of dealing with the person who stutters. In addition to working with the attitudinal components of stuttering, advocates of this approach teach the person to work with the moment of stuttering. The client is taught how to modify the stuttering by reducing its tension and rate—that is, by stuttering in an easy, relaxed manner. This particular aspect of treatment has been used throughout the years by some of the greatest contributors in our field. Although the list of these therapists is extensive, we will be highlighting the works of Van Riper,[23] Sheehan,[24] Bloodstein,[25,26] Conture,[1] Cooper,[27,28] and Williams.[29,30]

Fluency Shaping Therapy

Fluency shaping therapy has been defined as "[t]herapy which is based on operant conditioning and programming principles, i.e.: successive approximations of antecedent stimulus events, use of reinforcement of appropriate responses and so on. In a fluency shaping therapy program some form of fluency is first established in a controlled stimulus situation. This fluency is reinforced and gradually modified to approximate normal conversational speech in the clinical setting."[13] The goal of fluency shaping is not to work with the moment of stuttering but to systematically increase the fluent utterances of the client until they replace the stuttering behavior. In addition to increasing the focus on fluency, one of the greatest contributions of this approach has been to systematize therapy for fluency. Frequency of stuttering behavior began to be counted and tracked, and we believe that overall accountability for stuttering therapy was increased. Fluency shaping clinicians emphasize accurate data collecting and reporting, as well as establishing behavioral objectives and targeting specific behaviors to be changed. It must be noted, however, that the majority of fluency shaping proponents do not work with the attitudes and feelings of the person who stutters. Some of the principal contributors to this approach are Boberg,[31] Costello,[32,33] Webster,[34,35] Ryan,[36,37] and Ingham.[38] Each of these researchers has influenced the development of our synergistic approach.

Integration of Approaches

For many years the controversy between the stuttering modification approach and the fluency modification approach was greatly divisive. Therapists who practiced one of the therapies were strongly opposed to the techniques of the other. However, it is our sense that even the strongest advocates of each approach are now more willing to be open and to integrate some aspects of each approach in their therapy. Although the goals for the two approaches are different, they are not incompatible. Techniques for each approach apply to a different aspect of the problem of stuttering. Bloom[19] supported the integration approach presented by Guitar and Peters.[13] Both agreed that clients benefit from combining the two approaches. They found that fluency shaping therapy is more efficient than stuttering modification for changing speech patterns but that stuttering modification therapy is more effective in reducing a client's speech fears and improving speech attitudes when needed. In our definition of stuttering, we included our belief that each person who stutters has developed individual and learned attitudinal and behavioral responses to the underlying neurological disorder. It is therefore important to us to integrate both of these approaches.

Integration of Service Delivery

Another aspect of stuttering that some clinicians have integrated is the service delivery model. Therapy traditionally has been given once or twice a week. Limitations were found with this approach, which sometimes yielded unsatisfactory results. Consequently, in the 1970s and 1980s, programs were initiated[31,35] that offered intensive therapy.[31,35] These are usually three-week programs and can bring about dramatic changes in a person's speech. We have found that a period of intensive therapy is necessary but is not sufficient to bring about long-term change in a person's fluency. While the short-term, intensive therapy has brought excellent results, maintenance requires long-term therapy. Bloom[19] described a group program that integrated short-term intensive therapy with long-term maintenance therapy. Turnbaugh and Guitar[39] presented the results of a single subject's treatment that combined short-term intensive therapy with long-term therapy, which they offered as an alternative approach for use in public schools. Both reported favorable results. We believe this integration is essential for a synergistic approach to fluency therapy.

As researchers began to look more at the interactive effects of the components of stuttering, two principal investigators influenced an integrative approach to both theory and practice—namely, Wall and Myers.[40] In 1984, they wrote:

> Stuttering results from a lack of synergism or coordination between several major factors. Reflecting our broadly based and eclectic view of childhood stuttering, and to organize information about the topic, we propose a model consisting of three interlocking circles. The model represents three factors and their respective variables, which are pertinent to the clinical management of childhood stuttering. These three factors consist of the psychosocial, physiological, and psycholinguistic characteristics and possible etiological variables of stuttering.[40]

Wall and Myers helped to point out that the intersection of factors was an important aspect of the disorder of stuttering. In addition, Guitar and Peters[13,18] and Wall and Myers[40] were leaders in the area of integration of theories and therapies that led to the synergistic view of stuttering. The works of Gregory,[20,41] Starkweather et al.,[3,14] and St. Louis and Meyers[42] were also important.

Synergistic Approach

Synergistic psychology was proposed by Smoluchas[43] as a metatheory for synthesizing different psychological theories into an explanation of how social, cognitive, and biological factors interact in human behavior. He stated: "Synergism refers to the mutually cooperating action of separate substances which taken together produce an effect greater than that of any component taken alone. Synergistic psychology provides a neutral vantage point for synthesizing other theories that is not inherently biased toward one or the other theory."

It is our belief that the complex, multidimensional disorder of stuttering must be analyzed and treated from a synergistic perspective. That is, we must isolate the individual social, cognitive, and biological factors that interact in the lives of each person who stutters, and be aware of the effect of the interaction of these factors. To do this, we must be well trained in the synergistic framework of stuttering and the possibility of co-existing dysynchronies. Myers and St. Louis,[44] when writing about cluttering, noted that when there is a multidimensional disorder with co-existing problems it may be fruitful to consider the associated symptoms from a systems approach. A systems approach is one that views the speech and language functions of communication not as independent but as interrelated. It is just such a systems approach that we present as the synergistic approach to treating stuttering, noting the interaction of the physiological, psychological, linguistic, and social components.

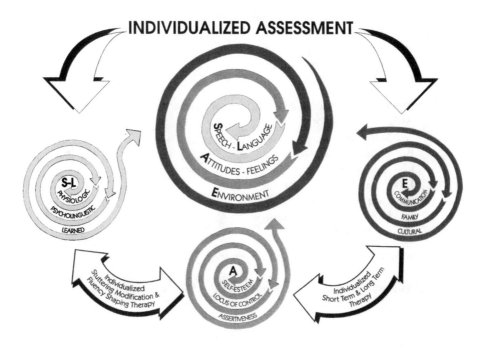

Figure 1.1 A synergistic approach to fluency therapy by C. Bloom and D. Cooperman.

We have illustrated the components of a synergistic approach to fluency therapy in Figure 1.1. It can be seen that the primary interrelating factors are (1) speech-language factors, (2) attitudinal factors, and (3) environmental factors. Each of these operates in an interactive, interrelated mode as is depicted by the movement of the arrows.

Each of these primary factors is made up of several interrelated layers. We have separated these layers for purposes of identification and treatment. However, the circular arrows are used to depict movement and interaction on all levels. The synergistic character of the entire process is meant to be depicted by the use of open-ended arrows. The delivery of the individualized assessment of the synergistic components is through both individualized short-term and long-term therapy and individualized stuttering modification and fluency shaping components.

The synergistic approach to fluency therapy consists of the components of therapy that we believe can be identified as having an important role in the continuance of the stuttering behavior and, therefore, in the treatment for fluency. It comprises the areas to be included in the assessment and the treatment, as well as the method of delivery. This approach can be outlined as follows:

I. Components of Fluency Shaping Therapy
   1. Speech-Language Factors
      A. Physiological Factors
      B. Psycholinguistic Factors
      C. Behavioral Factors

II. Components of Stuttering Modification Therapy
   1. Attitudinal Factors
      A. Self-esteem
      B. Locus of Control
      C. Assertiveness
   2. Environmental Factors
      A. Communication Factors
      B. Family Therapy Factors
      C. Multicultural Factors

III. Individualized Long-term and Short-term Therapy

It is these factors that we will expand on in the following chapters.

REFERENCES

1. Conture EG. *Stuttering* (2nd ed). Englewood Cliffs, NJ: Prentice Hall, 1990.
2. Starkweather CW. Speech fluency and development in normal children. In NJ Lass (ed), *Speech and Language: Advances in Basic Research and Practice*. New York: Academic Press, 1979.
3. Starkweather CW. *Fluency and Stuttering*. Englewood Cliffs, NJ: Prentice Hall, 1987.
4. Starkweather CW. A multiprocess behavioral approach to stuttering therapy. *Semin Speech Lang Hear* 1980;1:327–337.
5. Ham RE. *Therapy of Stuttering*. Englewood Cliffs, NJ: Prentice Hall, 1990.
6. Golddiamond-Eisler F. *Psycholinguistics Experiments in Spontaneous Speech*. New York: Academic Press, 1968.
7. Darley FL, Aronson AE, Brown JR. *Motor Speech Disorders*. Philadelphia: W. B. Saunders, 1975.
8. Adams M. Fluency, nonfluency and stuttering in children. *J Fluency Disord* 1982;7: 171–185.
9. Van Riper C. *The Nature of Stuttering* (2nd ed). Englewood Cliffs, NJ: Prentice Hall, 1982.
10. Wingate ME. *Stuttering Theory and Treatment*. New York: Irvington, 1976.
11. Wingate ME. A standard definition of stuttering. *J Speech Hear Disord* 1964;29: 484–489.
12. American Speech Language-Hearing Association. Historic treatments of stuttering. *ASHA* 1988:31–37.
13. Guitar B, Peters TJ. *Stuttering: An Integration of Contemporary Theories*. Memphis, TN: Speech Foundation, 1980.
14. Starkweather CW, Gottwald CR, Halfond MM, et al. *Stuttering Prevention: A Clinical Method*. Englewood Cliffs, NJ: Prentice Hall, 1990.

15. Van Riper C. Final thoughts about stuttering. *J Fluency Disord* 1990;15:317–318.
16. St. Louis KO. Linguistic and motor aspects of stuttering. In NJ Lass (ed), *Speech and Language: Advances in Basic Research and Practice*. New York: Academic Press, 1979.
17. Bloodstein O. *Stuttering: The Search for a New Cause and Cure*. Boston: Allyn and Bacon, 1993.
18. Guitar B, Peters J. *Stuttering: An Integrated Approach to Its Nature and Treatment*. Baltimore: Williams and Wilkins, 1991.
19. Bloom C. *Stuttering Therapy*. In R Daniloff (ed), *Articulation Assessment*. San Diego: College-Hill Press, 1985.
20. Gregory HH. Controversial issues: Statement and review of the literature. In HH Gregory (ed), *Controversies About Stuttering Therapy*. Baltimore: University Park Press, 1979.
21. Curlee RJ, Perkins WH. *Nature and Treatment of Stuttering: New Directions*. San Diego: College-Hill Press, 1984.
22. Guitar, B. *Stuttering: An Integrated Approach to Its Nature and Treatment*. Baltimore: Williams and Wilkins, 1998.
23. Van Riper C. *The Treatment of Stuttering*. Englewood Cliffs, NJ: Prentice Hall, 1973.
24. Sheehan JG. *Stuttering: Research and Therapy*. New York: Harper and Row, 1970.
25. Bloodstein O. Stuttering as tension and fragmentation. In J Eisenson (ed), *Stuttering as a Second Symptom*. New York: Harper and Row, 1970.
26. Bloodstein O. *A Handbook on Stuttering* (4th ed). Chicago: National Easter Seal Society, 1987.
27. Cooper E. Intervention procedures for the young stutterer. In H Gregory (ed), *Controversies About Stuttering Therapy*. Baltimore: University Park Press, 1979.
28. Cooper E. Treatment of disfluency: Future trends. *J Fluency Disord* 1986;11:317–327.
29. Williams DE. Stuttering therapy for children. In LE Travis (ed), *Handbook of Speech Pathology*. New York: Appleton-Century-Crofts, 1971.
30. Williams DE. A perspective on approaches to stuttering therapy. In HH Gregory (ed), *Controversies About Stuttering Therapy*. Baltimore: University Park Press, 1979.
31. Boberg E. Intensive adult/teen therapy program. In WH Perkins (ed), *Stuttering Disorders*. New York: Thieme-Stratton, 1984.
32. Costello J. Operant conditioning and treatment of stuttering. *Semin Speech Lang Hear* 1980;1:311–325.
33. Costello J. Current behavioral treatment for children. In D Prins, R Ingham (eds), *Treatment of Stuttering in Early Childhood: Methods and Issues*. San Diego: College-Hill Press, 1983.
34. Webster RL. Empirical considerations regarding stuttering therapy. In HH Gregory (ed), *Controversies About Stuttering Therapy*. Baltimore: University Park Press, 1979.
35. Webster RL. Evolution of a target-bases behavioral therapy for stuttering. *J Fluency Disord* 1980;5:303–320.
36. Ryan BP. *Programmed Therapy for Stuttering Children and Adults*. Springfield, IL: Charles C. Thomas, 1974.
37. Ryan BP. Postscript: Operant therapy for stuttering children and adults. In GH Shames, H Rudin (eds), *Stuttering: Then and Now*. Columbus: Charles E. Merrill, 1986.
38. Ingham R. *Stuttering and Behavioral Therapy*. San Diego: College-Hill Press, 1984.

39. Turnbaugh K, Guitar B. Short-term intensive stuttering treatment in a public school setting. *Lang Speech Hear Servs Schools* 1981;VII:107–114.
40. Wall MJ, Myers F. *Clinical Management of Childhood Stuttering.* Baltimore: University Park Press, 1984.
41. Gregory HH. *Stuttering: Differential Evaluation and Therapy.* Austin: Pro Ed., 1986.
42. St. Louis K, Myers F. Management of stuttering and related fluency disorders. In RF Curlee, GM Siegel (eds), *Nature and Treatment of Stuttering: New Directions* (2nd ed). Needham Heights, MA: Allyn and Bacon, 1997.
43. Smoluchas L. Synergistic psychology applied to artistic creativity. 10th International Colloquium of Empirical Aesthetics. Barcelona, Spain, Oct. 15, 1988.
44. Myers F, St. Louis K. *Cluttering: A Clinical Perspective.* Great Britain: Far Communications Ltd., 1992.

2

Components of a Synergistic Model Theory

Because we believe that good therapy flows from a strong theoretical basis, it is important to review the research out of which this book grew. It is upon these concepts that both our diagnostics and therapy procedures will be based. It is from these components that therapy will be derived for the preschool, school-aged, and adult clients that we will meet.

SPEECH-LANGUAGE COMPONENTS OF FLUENCY SHAPING THEORY

Clearly, research into the disorder of stuttering contains some of the most pertinent data for our purposes. Wall and Myers[1] noted that references to the physiologic and organic factors in stuttering date back to Aristotle. Since then, every aspect of stuttering has been examined and re-examined. As technology and sophistication in researching the speech and language aspects of stuttering increase, so does our understanding of it. And while it is not our purpose to discuss all of the theoretical reports about the causes of stuttering that have influenced our thinking and practice, we will attempt to highlight some of the most salient.

Our belief is that the "normal processes" of speech and language should be the goals of treatment for fluency. Therefore, a clinician must know both what the normal processes of speech and language are and how the behavior of stuttering is interfering with these normal processes. There is a recent trend to interpret the disruption of the normal processes of speech and language as caused by the interaction of neurologic, linguistic, and learned behaviors. Guitar and Peters[2] wrote:

Recently . . . new explanations have appeared, reflecting a new trend of thought about stuttering. It has been suggested that reduced stuttering is associated with conditions in which the neuro-physiological demands of speech motor control and language formulation are reduced. Thus, the ear-

15

lier view of stuttering as a neuro-physiological disorder has not been forgotten. It has reappeared with a new sophistication that acknowledges a learning component and incorporates some understandings of speech and language production.

It is this interaction of the physical, psycholinguistic, and learned behaviors that interact synergistically to compose the layers of the speech-language component of our model. We will examine each of these separately.

Physical Factors

The major physical factors that interact to interfere with the normal speech process will be discussed under the headings of genetics, central nervous system, and peripheral nervous system. It is important to restate that these layers not only interact with each other, but they also interact with the attitudinal and environmental aspects of the program.

Genetics

One of the known facts about stuttering is that it runs in families.[3] For years, researchers in communication disorders have tried to unravel the "nature or nurture" controversy so that they might better understand whether people stutter because of their environment or because of heredity. Conclusive evidence for one or the other would have a dramatic effect on therapeutic approaches. Whenever a trait is observed to run in families, however, genetic involvement is immediately suggested. One of the primary researchers in this area is Kenneth Kidd.[4–7] Kidd's analysis of family data related to the transmission of stuttering has yielded the following:

1. Significantly more males stutter than females.
2. If at least one parent ever stuttered, the familial risk is also significantly increased.
3. There is a lower overall incidence of relatives of females who stutter. However, there is a higher incidence of affected relatives of females who stutter, suggesting that more factors promoting stuttering are necessary for a female to stutter and females have these factors since they have more affected members.
4. An inherited genetic susceptibility, possibly necessary but certainly not sufficient, is a major factor in stuttering.
5. Females are more resistant than males to an inherited susceptibility to stutter.

In addition to Kidd's research, twins have been studied for decades in order to determine genetic factors in behavior. Howie's[8,9] research on twins indicated that if one twin from a single ovum (monozygotic) stuttered, then the chances were 77 percent that the other twin would stutter. When twins came from separate ova (dyzygotic), the probability of their both stuttering was 32 percent.

While Kidd's and Howie's studies have helped to confirm the fact that genetics plays a role in the transmission of stuttering, they have also demonstrated that genetics alone is not responsible. Once again, we are conscious of the fact that genetics interacts with other factors in perpetuating stuttering. If there is a susceptibility to stuttering, we must seek some of the identifying characteristics of that susceptibility, and we must try to understand the effects that environmental pressures, birth trauma, and nutrition (among others) have on the development of stuttering. Hamm[10] noted that we must accept that some or many of those who stutter have a predisposition or susceptibility to stutter. We do not know how strong this predisposition may be, if there is a continuum of susceptibility, or if there are genetic subgroups yet to be described further. We would add that we must also seek to learn the interactive triggers of this susceptibility. Yairi, Ambrose, and Cox[11] support this view when they write that future studies may want to examine subgroups of people who stutter, the influence of inheritance on recovery, characteristics of family members who don't stutter, and environmental factors that may interact with genetics.

Summary   All of the genetic studies, although limited, offer strong support for the presence of a physiologic predisposition to stutter as well as for further exploration of the interactive, synergistic dimensions of the disorder. While genetics has been generally accepted as a factor in the development of stuttering,[1,3,10] more research is needed to reveal the specifics of the interactive processes. The data that we have now, however, can help us in assessing and treating fluency disorders. The person who has a strong genetic history of stuttering in their family will have special counseling needs. A person who has not only a genetic history but also unfavorable environmental conditions will present a different therapeutic challenge.

Central Nervous System

It has been known for years that choral reading, rhythmic speaking, singing, adaptation, delayed auditory feedback and masking are fluency-inducing measures for those who stutter. Early attempts to interpret these findings as indicators of central nervous system disorder[12,13] were dismissed. In recent years, however, there has been increased interest and research in this area, which has led to a growing understanding of the role that the central nervous system plays in fluency disorders. There are many and varied hypothesis that have been proposed; we will integrate some of them in an attempt to explain this multifaceted area. Although the past research was published separately, we feel that the possibility of a unified understanding is possible using a synergistic approach.

Initially, research that renewed our interest in the central nervous system and its relationship to stuttering behavior was reported by Moore and Lorendo,[14-16] who pointed out the compelling evidence of asymmetries in the cerebral hemispheres. While they did not support an absolute dichotomy of left-linguistic, right-nonlinguistic processing, they did verify a qualitatively distinct nature of processing in the two hemispheres: the left hemisphere is uniquely suited for processing time-dependent, segmental, auditory stimuli and the right hemisphere specializes in time-independent, nonsegmental information. They also stated that the right hemisphere is capable of processing linguistic information but does so differently than the left hemisphere.

For people who stutter, Moore and Lorendo[15] proposed that there was considerable evidence for a dependency on right hemispheric processing of meaningful linguistic stimuli. This was demonstrated by showing an increase of frequency by stutterers on the same words of initial segments of long sentences compared to short sentences; on low-frequency words compared to high-frequency words; from base structure to transformation; at clause boundaries compared to internal position of clauses; and when voicing adjustments are required. Moore and Lorendo[16] wrote:

> Observations of the occurrence of dysfluencies in stutterers' language reveal greater fluency breakdowns associated with linguistic variables that are not typically processed by the right hemisphere. These observations may have clinical and assessment implications for the management of dysfluent verbal behaviors. One might predict that the greater the severity of stuttering, the greater a stutterer's dependency on right hemispheric processing. The research reviewed supports this prediction and suggests that we evaluate not only stutterers' verbal behaviors, but also their primary modes of hemispheric processing.

Geschwind and Galaburda[17] reported findings that indicate that many disorders such as stuttering, dyslexia, and autism are the result of a delay in left hemisphere growth during fetal development. They believe that the cause of this male-related happening may be the result of excess secretion of the hormone testosterone with the result that the right hemisphere receives cells suited for speech and language that cannot develop in the delayed left hemisphere.

Fox, Ingham, and Ingham[18] supported this view when they reported greater activation of speech-motor and language-processing areas during fluent and stuttered speech:

> When speech and language structures are delayed in development or damaged, a range of localization of speech and language functions can occur. Depending on when the delay or damage occurs and how much occurs, three outcomes are possible. Speech and language functions may develop in the damaged or delayed left hemisphere, they may develop in the right hemisphere, or they may develop in both hemispheres. These additions to the localization view of stuttering allow for different etiologies to result in somewhat similar problems.[17]

Although the research in this area is not complete, nor is it universally accepted, we agree with Guitar and Peters that this integrated interpretation of the cerebral dominance theory provides one possible understanding of the underlying central nervous system's involvement in stuttering behavior. There remain many unanswered questions and researchers continue to study the hemispheric differences in adults who stutter as well as in children.[19] Nevertheless, we believe that expanding the possible outcomes of the delay or damage to the left hemisphere provides a useful framework for understanding individual differences, which are an integral part of the synergistic model. Although no one factor appears to be the *sole* reason for stuttering, the *interaction* of *all* factors must be examined.

Many researchers have attempted to further delineate the central nervous system's involvement in stuttering. One explanation that we feel is important to include in our understanding of the synergistic model concerns the issue of timing. Raymond Kent[20] has proposed a detailed explanation of how the central nervous system is involved in stuttering. He asserts that the central disturbance in stuttering involves a reduced ability to generate temporal patterns. Fluency-inducing conditions that reduce rate and temporal uncertainty (choral reading, rhythmic speaking, singing, adaptation) or allow more time for the preparation of temporal programs (slowed speech, speaking with rhythmic movement, and delayed auditory feedback) are explainable by this model. Kent also adheres to Geschwind's[17] theory and has stated:

> The peculiar weakness that underlies stuttering (and perhaps other disorders such as developmental dysphasia or dyslexia) is a reduced capacity to generate fine temporal programs that are necessary for motor regulation, for efficient auditory perception, and for language expression. Males are more at risk for developmental speech disorders because they as a population are less adept than females at tasks of auditory sequencing and fine motor control. They may be more at risk because testosterone slows the growth of the left hemisphere to process rapid auditory patterns and intricate motor sequences.[20]

We agree with Kent that the generation of temporal programs is influenced by affective input. He has stated that the vulnerability of both males and females to environmental conditions during development is the explanation for the combination of genetic predisposition and a host of social and psychological forces. Guitar[21] summarizes the research by noting that the brain imaging studies demonstrate clear differences in the brain functioning of those who stutter and those who don't. People who don't stutter activate left hemisphere brain structures, and those who stutter show less left hemisphere activity and more activity in the same areas of the right hemisphere.

Summary   In our review of central nervous system research, we are once again confirmed in our belief that stuttering is best viewed from a synergistic framework. Recall our proposition that synergism occurs when two or more separate components interact to produce an effect greater than that of either component alone. Clearly, research has demonstrated that although there is central nervous system involvement in stuttering, it is not a sufficient explanation. It is in combination with environmental and other factors that stuttering happens. However, as Guitar[21] writes, this is essentially an "interim report." As researchers continue to examine the interaction of these factors, we will gather new data and understand more clearly the effects of the central nervous system's role in stuttering.

Peripheral Nervous System

Research has demonstrated the complexity of involvement of the peripheral nervous system in motor speech tasks. To separate these complex interactions is to necessarily oversimplify. For the purpose of this book, however, we will briefly consider how the factors of respiration, phonation, and articulation are related to the behavior of stuttering.

Respiration   A great deal of literature on stuttering focuses on the irregularities of respiration in stuttering. Wall and Myers[1] and St. Louis[22] asserted that there is no evidence that disorders of respiration cause stuttering nor can stuttering be explained in terms of known breathing abnormalities alone. However, abnormalities in the breathing pattern have been identified as part of the symptomatology of stuttering. Hill[23] concluded that one of the most common breathing irregularities of a person who stutters is a sharp inspiratory gasp prior to or during stuttered words. Other characteristics of irregular breathing that he mentioned were thoracic-abdominal oppositions, lack of precise synchrony between the thorax and the abdomen, and shallow breathing. Hill compared these reactions to similar reactions of normal speakers under conditions of shock, startle, or surprise, and concluded that stutterers are not physiologically different from normal speakers.

Wall and Myers[1] found a variety of speech-related respiratory differences in 17 people who stuttered. These subjects displayed a greater relative increase in breathing rate prior to stuttering compared to fluent utterances when responding to questions, but a similar relative increase when repeating prerecorded words. Although these findings were not statistically significant, they are of interest to us because of the great variety of individual reactions the subjects displayed. The conclusion that respiratory cycles may be disrupted in a variety of ways, and probably on a highly individual basis, is in strong support of our synergistic approach to fluency.

Phonation   Historically, there have been times when the larynx was considered the primary contributor to the disorder of stuttering. Then, like so many other factors, it was reported that there were no differences in the phonotory ability of those who stutter and those who didn't. In recent years, there has been a return to the consideration of laryngeal influences on stuttering behavior, in part because of new and more sophisticated measuring devices. The areas that have primarily been investigated are (1) stutterers' voice onset (VOT), voice intonation (VIT), and speech initiation (SIT) times; (2) electromyographic investigations of stutterers' laryngeal muscle activity; and (3) fiberoptic studies in which it is possible to view the larynx during moments of stuttering.[24]

Although it may seem that VOT, VIT, and SIT are the same, they are not. VOT is a measure of the timing of the onset of voice in relation to the movement of the articulators for the release of a consonant. The boundaries of VOT are defined by an articulatory event and a phonatory event. It is within syllable measurement. The researcher measures the time that elapses from the release of the consonant burst to the onset of the glottal vibration for the vowel. VIT is the time lapse between the appearance of some external stimulus (for example, a pure tone or flash of light) and a subject's initiation of glottal vibration for phonation. SIT is yet another variation of measurement. It is when a subject responds with one word or more, beginning with a voiced sound, and the initiation time is measured. Comprehensive studies have reported on the results of VOT, VIT, and SIT times.[3,24–27] All of these researchers agree that the VOT, VIT, and SIT times of people who stutter are slower than those of people who are fluent.

Guitar and Peters[2] cited researchers who have pointed out that even when people who stutter are fluent they have longer vowel durations, slower transitions between consonants and vowels, and delayed onsets of voicing after voiceless consonants. Despite the awareness of the reported laryngeal findings, researchers continue to interpret with caution. Adams[28] noted that exceptions do exist. Research generally reports an average, and we cannot make a blanket statement about phonation and stuttering. Hamm[10] cited Starkweather's comment that present information led him to support the concept that the larynx is involved in stuttering, as are respiration and articulation, but that there is minimal support for the idea that the larynx is the primary or causative agent in stuttering.

An increasing number of researchers are beginning to examine the laryngeal differences in terms of the aerodynamic irregularities that can be described by the control of air pressure and airflow during speech. St. Louis[22] believes that when aerodynamic influences of the glottis are considered, a more comprehensive and understandable picture of the laryngeal function emerges. Stuttering can be understood in terms of deficits of precise timing or respiration and phonation, which in turn generate the complex supraglottal articulatory symptoms. He quoted Bell:

> Rational analysis, clinical investigation, and systematic research are lending support to an old suspicion: many of the abnormal dysfluencies judged as stuttering involve problems of smooth coordination of phonation with articulation and respiration.[22]

We believe that this research supports the premise of a synergistic approach to understanding the disorder of stuttering.

Articulation Many researchers have investigated the pattern of articulation in stutterers. Zimmerman[29-32] has reported unexpected differences between the movement patterns in perceptually fluent utterances of those who stutter and those who do not. He pointed out that there were slower onsets, slower achievements of peak velocities, and a synchrony of the articulators in fluent speech. Starkweather and Myers[33] found that people who stutter have slower transitions into and out of the fricative /s/ in fluent speech. Van Riper[34] reported a breakdown in the co-articulatory events in the production of syllables. He hypothesized that people who stutter were deficient in their ability to time or integrate motor sequences. However, again, researchers have come to realize that we cannot separate the system of articulation from that of respiration and phonation. Perkins et al.[35,36] have proposed a discoordination hypothesis that understands stuttering as a discoordination of phonation with articulation and respiration. He emphasized that for smooth, integrated speech production to occur, the entire vocal tract must function as a synergistic whole. Indeed, this is in agreement with our proposed model and encourages both an integrated and an individual approach to fluency disorders. In addition to recognizing that there are interactive factors within the phonatory system itself, we must remember that a synergistic approach recognizes additional components. We agree with Zimmerman[32] when he wrote:

> While many descriptions of differences between stutterers and non-stutterers may be useful and while many explanations may be offered, all such explanations should be interfaced with knowledge and theories of perceptual-motor control. Recognizing that speech breakdowns, or any behavioral breakdowns for that matter, are often contextually (environmentally) conditioned, it is apparent that the effect of the environment, or how the speaker/actor perceives the environment plays a crucial role in achieving or maintaining stability in the production process. From this point of view the perceptual aspects of interactions are probably critical to a full account of speech breakdowns or the behaviors associated with stuttering. The evaluation and modification of these speaker-environment interactions (perception, attitudes, etc.) warrant a great deal of discussion and research.

Summary It can be seen that the physiologic components of respiration, phonation, and articulation are each individually and synergistically involved in the behavior of stuttering. Each of these behaviors must be included in the assessment and rehabilitative process for people who stutter. Continued research is also necessary. While we have come a long way in understanding the physiologic components of people who stutter, the majority of this research has been carried out with adults. Caruso, Conture, and Colton[37] reported that there is no significant difference in the temporal aspects of speech production in children indicating that young people who stutter are not appreciably different from their nonfluent peers. Conture[38] reported that integrity of children's speech mechanisms remain intact during stuttering behavior and, at least for perceptually fluent speech production, children who stutter are similar to normally fluent children in terms of temporal onsets, offsets, and duration of speech production events. This would suggest caution before applying the findings of adults who stutter to children. It also encourages us to pursue further interactive and individual factors that may be involved in the development of stuttering, which brings us to the next level of the synergistic approach: psycholinguistic factors.

Psycholinguistic Factors

Traditionally, researchers have recognized some relationship between dysfluency and language. Early studies were carried out at the University of Iowa in the 1930s. A leading researcher in this area was Spencer Brown.[39-41] Brown attempted to identify the speech and language characteristics that would account for the locus of stuttering in the speech sequence. His research led him to conclude that "most stuttering [was] associated with linguistic variables that were conspicuous, prominent, or meaningful to the speaker."[41] He interpreted these findings, which were based on adults performing oral reading tasks, as further indications of the Johnsonian understanding of the cause of stuttering. That is, a person stutters when he or she perceives that stuttering will happen.

Brown's identification of the focal points of stuttering provided a framework for future research. The general linguistic components that he identified as important are the grammatical class of the word, its position in the sentence, the sound the word begins with, and the length of the word. Specifically, Brown[41] pointed out that stuttering seems to occur more on content words (nouns, verbs, adjectives, and adverbs) than on function words such as articles, prepositions, and conjunctions. He found that stuttering is on words that begin with consonants more than on words that begin with vowels, more on words that are at the beginning of a syllable or a sentence, and more on words that are five letters long or longer. Brown[40] also reported that stuttering tends to occur more on stressed syllables of words. Wingate,[42-44] however, attributed the grammatical changes noted as due to the substantial changes in stress or prosody. He believes that prosody is not only a linguistic but also a physiologic change and notes that many of the old (and new) methods of therapy incorporate techniques that involve prosodic manipulation.

While these early studies were of great importance in tracing the outlines of the relationship between linguistic factors and fluency disorders, our recent understanding of this interactive influence has been dramatically informed by the contributions of developmental psycholinguistics. Wall and Meyers[1] have provided a helpful summary of the growth of the field of psycholinguistics from the pre-Chomsky to the post-Chomsky era. We recommend that our readers review their text, since the overview it provides is too detailed to include here. In addition, both Bloom[45] and Cooperman, the authors of this book, have been clinically involved with exploring the psycholinguistic influences on fluency disorders. Specifically, we believe that the psycholinguistic revolution has helped us understand language as a synergistic system that integrates the linguistic components of phonology, morphology, syntax, semantics, and pragmatics, and simultaneously, has provided an additional framework for identification and remediation of fluency disorders. Although there is no universal conclusion about the specifics of language that are impaired in those that stutter, our clinical observations and research support the view that stuttering is more likely to occur when more advanced forms of speech and language are used. In addition, a researcher's and clinician's knowledge of language development and of the multiple levels of linguistic interaction will influence their clinician's choice of assessment techniques and therapy approaches.

In fact, more researchers today are assessing this complex interaction of linguistic levels. Crystal[46] pointed out that the demands made by one level of language production (for example, syntax) may deplete resources for other levels (for example, prosody or phonology), which results in a breakdown in fluency. He concluded that the more complex the syntax and semantics used by a child, the more stuttering will occur. Further evidence of the synergistic interaction of the linguistic demands placed on the developing child's fluency has been verified by Bloodstein,[47] Logan and Conture,[48] and Brundage and Bernstein Rotner.[49,50] These findings support Starkweather's[41] demands and capacities model of stuttering. Starkweather has demonstrated that both the production of speech and the formulation of language place significant demands on a young person's fluency. If the demands of either are excessive, performance in fluency may be reduced.

Wall and Myers[1] proposed guidelines, listed below, for integrating the psycholinguistic component into fluency research and clinical procedures. We believe these are important for implementation of our synergistic model. Although Myers and Wall were writing only about stuttering in children, their guidelines are adapted to include adults where appropriate.

1. Be sensitive to the interplay between the various aspects of language on the fluency behavior of the client. Variations in the syntactic-semantic structure in a client's utterance may have a significant impact on the types and extent of the dysfluency the client exhibits.
2. Be mindful of the client's individual threshold of tolerance for linguistic complexity. Thresholds vary from person to person and, at least during therapy for stuttering, one must be careful not to overstretch the client's linguistic limits, which might result in a greater degree of dysfluency.
3. Be mindful of the influence of pragmatic contexts on the client's stuttering. Some communication situations carry greater stress for the client than others. Moreover, the particular pragmatic intention of a communication act can also have profound influence on the client's stuttering. The contexts of utterances and their influences on a client's subsequent communication, including the fluency of his or her speech, are of particular interest in the current trend of using language samples as a primary means of communication assessment.

4. If using high structured, standardized tests for language assessment, be cognizant of the author's perspective on language and the validity and reliability of the test.

5. Be mindful of individual differences in the kinds of patterns of fluency and language behaviors exhibited across clients.

6. In addition to examining psycholinguistics variables, one is encouraged to consider the contributions to fluency of various psychosocial and physiological factors that are likely to co-occur with psycholinguistic variables. For example, production of a longer, more complex sentence may also require a more sustained and complex level of motor coordination.

Summary   It can be seen that within the component of psycholinguistics there are additional levels operating synergistically—phonology, morphology, syntax, semantics, and pragmatics. These components interact in both children who stutter and those who do not. Therefore, our theory demands that each of these synergistic components be considered on an individual basis. As we gain more information in this area, a clinician's own theoretical background in language development will be important for both the assessment and rehabilitation of fluency disorders.

BEHAVIORAL FACTORS AND LEARNED FACTORS

Learning Theory, which was first developed in the field of psychology, is concerned with the conditioning of behavioral responses, The application of this theory to fluency disorders has been developing since the 1930s, when researchers at the University of Iowa initiated a dramatic departure from the way stuttering had until that time been viewed. Instead of thinking of stuttering as a disorder that was caused by physiologic, psychological, or linguistic factors, these theorists proposed that stuttering was a behavior that a person learned. Wendell Johnson[52] was one of the first to expand this idea. His Diagnosogenic Theory stated that stuttering develops after diagnosis, or labeling, of the child who stutters. Johnson pointed out the parent is usually the first person to identify the problem. He believed that what parents called stuttering was not any different from normal childhood dysfluency and that the true stuttering behavior developed not before the parent's diagnosis but after. For many years, Johnson's theory was held by the majority of speech-language pathologists in the United States. Although we now have a much broader understanding of the development of stuttering, we have learned a great deal about stuttering from the work of Johnson and his colleagues at Iowa. Bloodstein,[53] in pointing out one of the main contributions of Johnson, wrote that "[s]ome theories that turn out to be wrong are nevertheless very fruitful because they stimulate research and lead to new points of view. In that sense, the Diagnosogenic Theory was an exceptionally productive one. A great deal of what we know about stuttering today was learned as a result of attempts to verify this theory."

Some of the theorists who departed from Johnson's view, and who have added greatly to our developing understanding of the role that learning plays in stuttering behaviors, are Bloodstein,[54,55] Sheehan,[56] and Van Riper.[3] Each of these researchers has provided valuable data, which will be considered as part of our analysis of stuttering modification therapy. For present purposes, it is important to recognize that this research was for many years the driving force behind the therapy carried out by speech-language pathologists. People who stutter were taught to modify or change the way that they stuttered. In addition to gaining a new, easier way of speaking, they were encouraged to accept themselves as people who would always stutter. Although they knew that they could unlearn many aspects of their speech behaviors, they did not consider fluency a goal to be incorporated into their therapy programs. But while this research supported the fact that stuttering was a learned behavior, rather than a physiologic or psychological one, there were many unanswered questions as to how this behavior came to be learned.

In the 1950s and 1960s, many theorists turned to the principles of Learning Theory to answer these questions and to explain the etiology and the development of stuttering. Initially, they drew from the work of B. F. Skinner,[57] who demonstrated that speech was an operant behavior. Skinner had analyzed verbal behavior—including reading, writing, talking, and thinking—and concluded that speech was an operant behavior that was controlled by the consequences provided by the listener. The research became overwhelmed with possible applications of this principle to the behavior of stuttering. Goldiamond,[58,59] Martin and Siegel,[60] Azrin,[61] and Shames and Egolf[62] were some of the major contributors. Shames and Rubin[63] have summarized much of this research in their book *Stuttering: Then and Now*. All these contributions to our field have been significant and extremely helpful for further developing therapy. Although the specifics are too detailed to be included in this text, we would like to highlight the works of Brutten and Shoemaker,[64] Costello,[65,66] and Ingham,[67] whose applications of the principles of Learning Theory have influenced our synergistic approach to treatment.

Brutten and Shoemaker

Brutten and Shoemaker[64] helped clarify some of the conflicting research results of stuttering behavior by seeking to integrate the previously dichotomous positions of genetic (physical) and learned etiologies of stuttering. Their Two-Factor Theory, which stressed the understanding of stuttering as a multidimensional problem, postulated that while there was an underlying neurologic predisposition to stutter, stuttering occurs when two different types of conditioning interact. The first is classical conditioning and the second is instrumental conditioning. Brutten and Shoemaker believed that classical conditioning can be discerned in people who stutter when dysfluencies are associated with negative emotional responses. Initially neural stimuli come, through experience, to evoke negative emotions—for example, a certain word, a particular sound, words that begin a sentence, or words that are longer than usual. These stimuli make such people anxious, and physiologically they experience heart pounding, breathing abnormalities, and, usually, fluency failure. Thus, the stuttering behavior itself is one of learned negative emotion. It is an involuntary, reflexive reaction to a learned stimuli. In order to escape from this negative stimulation, each person who stutters learns individual, voluntary methods of struggle and avoidance. These learned behaviors are instrumentally conditioned according to the individual characteristics of each person's experience and environment.

Van Riper[3] found that the Two-Factor Theory was valuable, although it does not completely explain the onset of stuttering. And while Brutten and Shoemaker[68] themselves have recognized that there are shortcomings to their theory, they have nevertheless highlighted a basic premise of their theory that we believe underlies the synergistic theory. It was their research that first enabled us to move from the unidimensional research of the 1960s and 1970s. Brutten and Shoemaker[68] wrote

> Basic to the Two-Factor position is the assumption that genetic and environmental factors interactively determine the behaviors of stutterers. This stance is clearly at odds with the purely environmental explanations of stuttering that have dominated the scene until recently. It differs sharply from the positions that look with considerable skepticism at genetic risk, predisposition, and condition ability (Johnson, 1967). It reflects the view that stuttering is a response pattern that is acquired as the result of only environmental consequences (Shames and Sherrick, 1963; Siegel, 1970). The Two-Factor position has always maintained that both heredity and environment contributed to the determination of stuttering behavior.

Although we have expanded the number of components that interact, certainly this premise of interaction that pervades the Two-Factor Theory is essential to an understanding of the synergistic approach to fluency. In addition, we believe that Brutten and Shoemaker's explanation of individual, learned responses is important to understand and include in both assessment and remediation of fluency disorders.

The Inghams

Considerable contributions to understanding how theories of learning can be applied to the field of disfluency have been made by Roger Ingham[67] and Janis Costello Ingham.[65,66] In Roger Ingham's book *Stuttering and Behavior Therapy,* one can find strong support and credible documentation for the need to recognize the principles of Learning Theory and behavioral treatment in the therapy for people who stutter. Indeed, Ingham's book served to introduce an alternative treatment orientation to stuttering: a behavioral paradigm. It is our belief that the principles presented by the Inghams are essential for any therapy program. They have helped us to recognize the need to demonstrate clinical validity of both our assessment and our therapy procedures. The results of their research have greatly influenced our own approach and have helped form a structure for our integrative treatment. Their behavioral treatment was summarized by Ingham[67] as follows:

> Let us now try to put together all the pieces of our therapy assessment puzzle. It begins with a series of diagnostic sessions designed to establish the subject's suitability for therapy. This is followed by a base-rate period, containing repeated within and beyond-clinic recorded assessments conducted once weekly over at least four weeks. These assessments continue at this frequency throughout the maintenance phase. The maintenance phase may include decreasingly frequent assessments that might be tied to the treatment process. The pattern of maintenance assessment should continue until they occur at three-month intervals over a year. The overt assessment procedure should be supplemented by at least four unobtrusive or covert assessments made during the treatment and transfer phases, plus another four during the immediate posttreatment phase. In addition, perhaps covert assessments (of one form or another) should be made at regular intervals over the maintenance and follow-up periods. The content of the overt assessments should include representative speech samples from the speaker's natural environment, oral readings, monologues, and telephone conversations within the clinic. The minimum data should be syllable or articulation rate and percentage of words or syllables stuttered. These data should be supplemented by ratings of speech quality. Finally, the posttreatment phase of therapy should be supplemented by a questionnaire reporting the subject's estimate of his or her speech performance.

The Inghams hoped that their suggested therapy format would be accepted by other therapists and could become a means of shifting stuttering therapy towards a common pattern of assessment and rehabilitation, which would allow for the collection of a common data base of information about the disorder of stuttering. This needed data base would be of great value in measuring the strengths and weaknesses of various treatment approaches as they are carried out in the clinical arena. However, it was not until later that researchers saw that these behavioral components could be integrated with aspects of attitudes and feelings. We, now, believe that they cannot be separated.

Summary   The results of the research on the learned components of stuttering is compelling evidence that our clinical approach to stuttering must address both the multidimensional and synergistically learned elements that are found in the behavior of stuttering. This thinking can provide both a breadth and a depth of structure to our assessment and therapy. It calls us to a greater level of accountability and demands that we test all our assumptions about our assessment and treatment procedures. Because of the contributions of these theorists, we believe that therapy can become more focused and specific. However, it is clear to us that operant theory and therapy based upon it are limited. That is to say, learning is but one piece of the multidimensional puzzle of stuttering. Indeed, many of the "basics" of therapy are addressed in operant approaches. Even Janis Costello[66] has noted that "additives" may be necessary: reduced speaking rate, initiating utterances with a gentle voice onset, simplifying linguistic complexity of utterances, and modifying attitudes. These components are not perceived by us to be "additives." Rather, they comprise some of the essential components of a synergistic approach to dysfluency. They include not only the learned components of the fluency shaping therapy, but also the physiologic factors (rate and gentle onset) and the psycholinguistic aspects of linguistic complexity of utterance. In addition, she also adds a part of the stuttering modification aspect (attitude). Janis Costello[66] supports our present approach with the statement that "perhaps, sometime in the future, a combination of stuttering and fluency management procedures, as Guitar and Peters propose will provide a more effective framework for guiding stutterers to fluent speech." Clearly, this shift in thinking by proponents of the operant model was another step toward greater integration of fluency approaches.

Having summarized the background of the important research underlying the fluency shaping components of the synergistic theory, we now turn to a consideration of the important aspects of the stuttering modification approach.

COMPONENTS OF STUTTERING MODIFICATION THERAPY: ATTITUDINAL AND ENVIRONMENTAL FACTORS

In Chapter 1 we defined stuttering modification therapy[69] as an approach to stuttering that is based on the theory that most of the problems related to the behavior of stuttering are connected to the fears, avoidances, and attitudes of people who stutter. Therapists who follow the stuttering modification approach place a great deal of emphasis on reducing the fears of stuttering and changing the avoidance behaviors. Stuttering modification therapy encourages one to develop positive attitudes toward speaking and those who stutter are urged to seek out speaking situations that have formerly been avoided. Therapists who follow this approach are hoping to assist in an overall adjustment of the person. Attitude change is a primary component of the goals of this therapy.

However, the inclusion of attitude change as a goal in therapy has been an ongoing controversy among clinicians. Supporters of the fluency shaping therapy approach do not generally support working directly on attitudes.[63] Nevertheless, these therapists agree that attitudes are affected by successful therapy. They believe that changing the speech behavior of the person who stutters is all that is necessary, because the attitude change will follow.

We agree with the proponents of the stuttering modification therapy approach that it is important to directly work with the attitudes of people who stutter. The components of the stuttering modification theory should be integrated with fluency shaping techniques. After learning specific fluency behaviors, a person who stutters may find that he or she speaks fluently within the clinical setting and increasingly in the nonclinical setting as graduated transfer and maintenance activities are built into the program. However, we find that the transfer of fluency is more effective when we deal directly with the fears and avoidance behaviors central to the problem of stuttering throughout the therapy process.

Guitar and Peters[69] expressed our own thinking when they stated that advanced stuttering includes chronic frustration, embarrassment, and fear. If these feelings become too intense, the person who stutters will have excessive muscular tension in the speech musculature. Under this condition, the person's motor control will break down and speech production cannot occur as planned. They feel that less work on attitudes, however, is necessary with the intermediate level of stuttering.

In addition to working on the fears and avoidances associated with stuttering, we have isolated several components that we believe to be critical in understanding and working with people who stutter. We have called these "attitudinal factors" and "environmental factors." A synergistic approach to therapy includes direct attention to these factors in either a proactive stance or a remedial approach. Therefore, all levels of therapy will include aspects of the components. We will briefly consider them now, but expand our analysis in Chapter 7.

Self-Esteem

A necessity for everyone's healthy development is the building block of self-esteem. Nathanial Branden[70] expressed the conviction held by many people that self-esteem is the key to success or failure in a person's life:

Apart from problems that are biological in origin, I cannot think of a single psychological difficulty—from anxiety and depression, to fear of intimacy or of success, to alcohol or drug abuse, to under achievement at school or at work, to spouse battering or child molestation, to sexual dysfunctions or emotional immaturity, to suicide or crimes or violence—that is not traceable to poor self-esteem. Of all the judgments we pass, none is as important as the one we pass on ourselves. Positive self-esteem is a cardinal requirement for fulfilling life.

We believe that many people who stutter suffer from low self-esteem. Curlee[71] found in his experience that many adults who stutter have reported feelings, attitudes, and beliefs that (1) seem to interfere with their ability to cope satisfactorily with many of life's experiences that involve interpersonal communication, (2) can result in their substantial and unnecessary subjective discomfort, and (3) may foster self-defeating behavior.

Each of these feelings, attitudes, and beliefs is often related to low self-esteem, which will therefore be the first of the attitudinal factors we will consider in our synergistic approach. The issue of self-esteem may also be important in our field for a different reason: the majority of clinicians are women and it has often been reported that low self-esteem primarily affects females.[72] This may be extraneous to our primary interest, since most people who stutter are male. What is not clear at present is how low self-esteem of the clinician might affect the therapeutic outcome. Unfortunately, the research in this area is limited. It is our goal to continue to explore, assess, and apply current research in self-esteem to the synergistic approach to fluency disorders.

We often use the term *self-esteem* interchangeably with self-concept, self-respect, or self-love. However, Sanford and Donovan[72] pointed out that these terms are not synonymous. Self-concept or self-image is the set of beliefs and images we all have and hold to be true about ourselves. By contrast, our level of self-esteem (or self-respect, self-love, or self-worth) is the measure of how much we like and approve of our self-concept. Or, as it is sometimes put, self-esteem is the reputation you have with yourself.

In defining self-esteem, Steinem[73] gave the official definition of a California task force which had the goal of promoting personal and social responsibility: appreciating my own worth and importance and having the character to be accountable for myself and to act responsibly toward others. She further cited the *Oxford English Dictionary*'s primary definition as a "favorable appreciation or opinion of oneself." Thesaurus synonyms are self-reliance, assurance, pride, or self-sufficiency.

Branden[70] pointed out that self-esteem has two components: a feeling of personal competence and a feeling of personal worth. He believes that self-esteem is the sum of self-confidence and self-respect. "It is what I think and feel about myself, not what someone else thinks and feels about me." As children, however, our self-confidence and self-respect can be nurtured or undermined by adults—depending on whether we are respected, loved, valued, or encouraged to trust ourselves. Nevertheless, self-esteem is ultimately our own evaluation of ourselves.

I can be loved by my family, my mate, and my friends, and yet not love myself. I can be admired by my associates and yet regard myself as worthless. I can project an image of assurance and poise that fools virtually everyone and yet secretly tremble with a sense of my inadequacy. I can fulfill the expectations of others and yet fail my own. I can win every honor and yet feel that I have accomplished nothing. I can be adored by millions and yet wake up each morning with a sickening sense of fraudulence and emptiness. To attain "success" without attaining positive self-esteem is to be condemned to feeling like an impostor anxiously awaiting exposure.[70]

How can a person be so esteemed by others and yet not hold that same esteem for themselves? There is not a simple answer. However, it is believed that a person with low self-esteem has incorporated negative thoughts of self into his or her self-concept to perpetuate and drive the person's low self-esteem. Rosenberg[74] wrote about intelligent students who are poor spellers. In almost every case further tutoring fails, despite the students' ability. The reason for this failure is that in the past these individuals incorporated into their self-concepts the negative self-understanding that they cannot spell and they resist any evidence that would force them to change that view.

Similarly, many people who stutter have incorporated the negative self-understanding related to being a stutterer into their self-concept. They have identified themselves as "Stutterers" rather than people who happen to also stutter. In formulating any therapy program for people who stutter, it is important to design a plan for each individual that will help them become aware of the negative components in their self-concept and of how they influence low self-esteem. Deliberate steps to change the self-concept and to increase self-esteem are built into our synergistic program. Joseph Sheehan[75] addressed this issue when he said that a person may have lived with stuttering so long that functioning without it would involve a radical change in self-concept which must be gradual. To put it another way, fluency may have become ego-alien. In the later stages of treatment the stutterer must learn to accept his new role with its fluency, just as in the early stages he needed to accept his old role with its stuttering.

Increased awareness, understanding, and application of the principles underlying the development of both self-concept and self-esteem can enrich a therapeutic program for those who are dysfluent. We believe that growth in these areas is an important factor in addressing the issues of rehabilitation and maintenance that confront our therapy programs. These concepts are further considered in Chapter 5.

Locus of Control

Locus of control has been defined by Rotter[76] as a generalized expectancy that one's outcome is either more under personal control (internal locus of control) or more under the control of external forces such as luck, fate, or powerful other people (external locus of control). A person with internal control will believe that an event is contingent upon their own behavior or upon their own relatively permanent characteristics. Those with an external locus of control believe that events are under the control of luck, chance, good days, bad days, or powerful others rather than under their own personal control.

Rotter's scale of locus of control has been applied to many areas of health care: diabetes, tuberculosis (TB), epilepsy, alcoholism, hypertension, dentistry, smoking, and aging.[77-80] Three studies have applied it to stuttering.[81-83] We believe that an understanding of the concept of locus of control can be used effectively in the diagnosis and treatment of people who stutter. Therefore, a brief summary of some of the salient aspects of the research studies follows.

Rotter[76] reported that a general finding of the earliest research characterized "internals" as potent, assertive, and effective persons, whereas "externals" were characterized as more retiring, less competent, and dependent. Seeman and Seeman[84] found that in relation to health, internal locus of control leads to an active approach to life and is significantly correlated with a positive and active role in health-related behaviors such as taking medication. We belief that an increased and active role in a person's speech behavior (internal control) would assist them in changing their stuttering behavior. Therefore, it seems important to explore the developmental aspects of achieving an internal locus of control.

Development in Children

Developmental studies demonstrate that the family is integral to a child's development of internal control. Stephens[85] found that greater warmth, attentiveness, "relaxedness," and a broadly good parent–child relationship are characteristic of mothers of children who have internal rather than external perceptions. Mothers whose children displayed more internal beliefs had displayed more overt affection, given more help and nurturing, been more protective, and more frequently used praise and approval. Mothers of children who have acquired internal perceptions have also reported that they early on engaged in independence training and were less likely to have encouraged dependence behaviors. Observations made in test contexts indicate that mothers of children who hold internal perceptions are attentive and offer suggestions. They do, however, give fewer overt directions and are less likely to impose help or participate directly in the child's task.

Wischner and Nowicki[86] reported that in addition to being more affectionate and attentive, parents of internals allowed their children greater independence at an earlier age. However, this varied with the gender of the child; females were given less independence. This greater freedom given internals when they were children perhaps allowed them to explore more varied situations and to learn about the consequences of their behavior. In addition to having greater freedom to act, internal as opposed to external children received less punishment, especially physical punishment.[87]

In summary, with the exception of protectiveness, relatively consistent parental warmth, involvement, and supportiveness seems to function as a major determinant of children's growth and internal perceptions. Consistency of discipline and independence training also appears to influence internal development in children. These findings are not necessarily conclusive, however, and future research must continue to refine them in the context of the following child development issues:

- The degree to which a consistent upbringing is related to internals
- The role of over-protectiveness in locus of control development
- Sex differences in internal control/home environment relationships
- The relative influence of mothers' and fathers' behaviors on the control expectancies of children

What is presently known about locus of control development in children is important for families of children who stutter, and is further discussed in Chapter 5.

Development in Adolescence

The process of adolescence is separation, individuation, and autonomy.[88] Developmentally, autonomy refers to the gradual diminishing of parental influence and the increase in self-reliance and self-governance. Autonomy in adolescence is not a single concept but contains a number of distinct dimensions. Two of the most important are the freedom to choose how to behave and the lessening need for parental approval.[89] Both of these concepts are an integral part of a person's gaining an internal locus of control.

During the time of adolescence, significant advances in self-reliance are achieved, and the influence of parents wanes as adolescents first attach themselves to peers and later move out of their parent's home. Both parents and adolescents seek to find a balance between separation and attachment—between too great a degree of individuation and too little psychologic differentiation. Finding the middle ground, which is acceptable to both parents and adolescents, is no easy task.[89] However, establishing this independence is essential for assuming control over one's own life and achieving internality.

In researching adolescents' locus of control development, Crandell and Crandell[90] found that both males and females who later developed internal perceptions had engaged in greater peer contact. For females, this contact consisted of more physical aggression, more social play, more nurturing and help to peers, and a greater number of siblings in the household. For internal males, peer contact consisted of nonphysical as well as physical aggression, attempts to dominate peers, and more seeking affection from and giving affection to peers. For the sexes combined, a somewhat higher incidence of dating behavior was also correlated with higher internal scores. These findings are important for speech-language pathologists to remember when working with adolescents in fluency therapy. Achieving these developmental milestones may be more difficult for those who stutter, since interaction and communication with peers is sometimes difficult.

Development in Adults

Adulthood finds the individual continuing to develop toward self-individuation and self-actualization. Maslow understood self-actualization as a positive process that was beneficial to society, leading people to identify their abilities, to strive to develop them, and to feel good as they become themselves.[91] Many people never become self-actualized, and it would seem reasonable that a person's perception of his or her own power and control would have a great influence on their progress toward self-actualization.

Although there is much research to support the view that a more internal locus of control is related to better social functioning while a more external locus of control is related to anxiety, we will briefly review only the findings related to health-related behaviors. This will provide further data that are applicable to working with individuals who stutter.

Hayes and Rose[92] have written that a person who is concerned about health will take action only if he or she also perceives that the action will work. A person's behavior depends whether there is an expectation that one's actions determine outcomes (internal locus of control). People with internal locus of control or sense of personal mastery believe they are in control of their lives and that their decisions and actions shape outcomes. Such people believe they can avoid illness by taking care of themselves and that ill health results in part, for example, from not eating right or not getting enough exercise. People with an external locus of control, on the other hand, believe that powerful others and external forces shape their destiny. In regard to health, they believe that there is nothing they can do to prevent illness and that people who do not get sick are just plain lucky.

Seeman and Seeman[84] found that an internal locus of control is significantly associated with a positive and active role in health-related behaviors. Internal control leads to better health as a result of this active involvement in health-promoting behavior. They noted the many health problems that are caused or compounded by behaviors that could be under a person's control: smoking, not exercising, overeating, or eating an unbalanced diet. People who feel that they control their health are more likely to practice healthy behaviors and avoid behaviors that increase the risk of disease (and thus be in better health) than those that think that health results from chance. Furthermore, good health habits learned as a child may affect later beliefs regarding controllability of health. Since a common remark of those who stutter is that "something is happening" to them, it seems to us that knowledge of the research related to internal locus of control provides essential elements to be incorporated into a rehabilitation program in fluency.

EXPANSION MODEL

Paulhus and Christie[93] felt that previous studies on control neglected the notion that an individual may have different expectancies of control in different behavioral spheres. They therefore expanded Rotter's model of the locus of control to comprise three primary spheres: achievement, interpersonal, and sociopolitical (Figure 2.1).

First, the individual vies for control with the nonsocial environment in situations of personal achievement such as solving crossword puzzles, building bookcases, and climbing mountains. Perceived control in this sphere may be termed "personal efficiency." Second, the individual interacts with others in dyads and group situations by defending his or her position on an issue at meetings, attempting to develop personal relationships, or maintaining harmony in the family. In this sphere, the control is appropriately understood as "interpersonal." Third, because an individual's goals often conflict with those of the political and social system of which they are a part, the person assumes control by such actions as taking part in a demonstration, boycotting a particular product in order to bring down the price, and writing letters to a member of Congress. Perceived control in this sphere is termed "sociopolitical control." A fourth possible level of control conflict involves the individual against himself or herself. These conflicts may be in self-discipline and/or self-actualization.

Although little research has been done using this model, it seems to us that this expansion model is directly applicable to a synergistic approach to fluency. Germain[94] has presented some preliminary research on an "integrated locus of control concept." He believes that by systematically balancing the interactions among their own control, that of powerful others, and chance, people can more

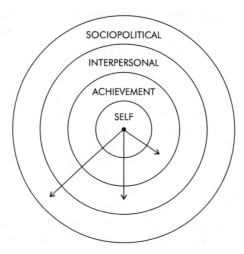

Figure 2.1 Sphere of control. (Reprinted with permission from Paulus D, Christie R. Sphere of control: an interactivist approach to assessment of perceived control. In H Lefcourt (ed), *Research with the Locus of Control Construct* (Vol. 2). New York: Academic Press, 1983, p. 23.)

effectively direct their time and energy to have the kind of impact they desire. It would seem that the interactive aspects of these spheres could also be taken into account in this process. Certainly, we know that people who stutter have a hierarchy of behavioral spheres that relate to increased or decreased frequency of dysfluencies. The areas of achievement and interpersonal and sociopolitical interactions seem important to research further.

Locus of Control and Stuttering

Preliminary research by Craig and Howie[95] using Rotter's scale found a minimal relation between pretreatment locus of control and pretreatment frequency of stuttering. However, they did find that pretreatment to 18 months posttreatment change in locus of control had a significant relationship to improvement in stuttering frequency.

Craig, Franklin, and Andrews[81] felt that the scales that had been developed did not adequately measure the locus of control over a behavioral problem such as stuttering. Both Rotter[96] and Lefcourt[78,79] had emphasized the need to develop a locus of control scale to measure special aspects of behavior. Therefore, Craig, Franklin, and Andrews[81] devised a 17-item Likert-type scale to measure locus of control over stuttering (LCB Scale). They reported that their LCB Scale was shown to have satisfactory internal reliability, to be test-retest reliable in the absence of treatment, to be independent of age, sex, and social desirability, and to distinguish clinical disorder from normal nonclinical subjects. In addition, their data confirmed that people who stutter chronically, as well as individuals with agoraphobia, scored higher on the LCB Scale, that is to say, they were more external than the normal nonclinical population. Based on this finding that the LCB Scale could predict people who stutter, the researchers hypothesized that as a result of behavioral treatment, the clinicians would see not only a reduction of the disorder but also LCB scores more indicative of internal control. They believed that such a reduction would imply that the patient's perception of personal control over their own behavior had been enhanced. They also showed that a change in locus of control during a short-term, three-week program was associated with a better long-term outcome. The LCB Scale also proved to be a more powerful predictor of relapse than Rotter's scale.[76] This research was a significant contribution to the field of fluency. However, it was based only on short-term fluency shaping programs. More data was necessary to confirm the usefulness of the locus of control concept as it was applied to fluency disorders.

McDonough and Quesal[82] authored a study to determine the validity of a speech locus of control scale (SP-LOC Scale) that measures the differences between those who stutter and those who do not. They believed that in many instances people who stutter do not differ from others in "general" personality measures, yet speech-specific measures do show a difference between the two groups. Their scale is comprised of eight items. A higher SP-LOC score indicates a more external speech locus of control. The results of McDonough's and Quesal's study provided preliminary evidence of their scale's validity. They wrote:

> Based on this, if the SP-LOC Scale is used clinically, an individual who ranked on the internal end of the scale may very well need different therapy strategies than the individual who ranked on the external end of the scale. In order to achieve success in therapy and ultimately transfer and maintain fluent behavior, a stutterer must possess an internal locus of control and be able to assume responsibility for his/her own behavior. The client should not rely on the clinician or "devices" used to establish fluency.[82]

McDonough and Quesal[82] also noted the possibility of interactive factors that might influence the SP-LOC score. Specifically, they cited length of time in a synergistic program, combined length of prior treatment, gender, internal and external locus of control, and frequency of stuttering. Results of the multiple regression analysis in this study demonstrated that only time in the synergistic program correlated with decreased frequency of dysfluency with a multiple R of .5261, significant at .0137 level of confidence.

Ingham[97] has argued that most treatment techniques have not enjoyed long-term maintenance benefits. However, Bloom's[83] preliminary study demonstrated that when synergistic therapy is maintained with a follow-up therapy program, the mean scores over time for both frequency of dysfluency and external locus of control are lowered. Results confirm that continuation in a maintenance program for five years shows significant relationship to gaining a stronger internal locus of control and a correspondingly decreased frequency of dysfluency. We therefore strongly believe that locus of control is an important concept for clinicians to both understand and incorporate into their therapy programs. When this is done, clients may obtain more long-term benefits.

Conture and Wolk[98] have encouraged the assessment of locus of control, even while recognizing the difficulty of making this assessment. But they added a valuable precaution to clinicians: "We may need to begin addressing the question of whether we, as clinicians, may perpetuate the stutterer's feeling of helplessness (external control) by making him or her feel dependent on a particular procedural technique and/or the clinician."[98] Clinicians who heed this warning must necessarily be aware of their role in the stutterer's locus of control, which requires clinicians' attention to growth in their own self-understanding. This is in agreement with what we have written in *The Clinical Interview: A Guide for Speech-Language Pathologists and Audiologists*[83]:

> We believe that before speech-language pathologists or audiologists can understand the concerns of clients, parents, or family members, they must try to have an objective understanding of themselves. Clinicians must be able to recognize their own strengths and limitations. They must be in touch with the choices they have made in their personal and professional lives and be aware of the freedom they have to make new choices. They must be aware of the struggle and pain involved in changing their own thoughts, feelings, and actions if they hope to help clients change theirs. If clinicians want to promote change and growth in the lives of their clients, they must be willing to promote the same in themselves.

Therefore, a clinician who hopes to help a client gain an internal locus of control must have identified her own dependence on outside reinforcements and be aware of how her own needs may be interfering in the therapy process. This concept is expanded in Chapter 9.

Summary   Measurement of internal and external locus of control can provide clinicians with valuable information for both diagnosis and treatment. If an individual is found to rank high on the internal end of a speech locus of control scale, the intervention strategies will be different than if that person is more externally controlled. In addition, it is important to examine the interacting spheres of control in a person's daily life.

Most importantly, we believe that locus of control is synergistically interconnected with self-esteem. As a person grows in awareness of one's ability to control the outcomes of one's own life, that person's self-esteem is increased. Conversely, activities that increase one's self-esteem are usually related to behaviors that increase one's mastery and competence. Both of these skills lead to an increased perception of one's control over everyday life. In turn, this leads to more assertive behavior. Each of these synergistic elements is important to fluency therapy and will be expanded on in Chapter 7.

Assertiveness

People who stutter ordinarily have speech-associated fears that result in a pattern of avoiding certain social and professional situations. Brutten and Shoemaker[68] stated that there is little question but that when forced to perform in provoking situations, stuttering magnifies interpersonal difficulties. Coming to appreciate the nature of assertive, nonassertive, and aggressive behavior will help us better understand those who stutter and develop more effective treatment for them. We have found that there is among people who stutter a fear of speaking that has led them to nonassertive behavior. Within our synergistic approach, we propose that this nonassertive behavior interacts with a low self-esteem and an external locus of control. It is important to recognize this interactive behavior. It is difficult to separate their mutual influences.

The following definitions by Jakubowski-Spector[99] summarize the behavior we believe is important to both our assessment of and remedial procedures for people who stutter:

- ASSERTIVE BEHAVIOR. That type of interpersonal behavior in which a person stands up for his or her legitimate rights in such a way that the rights of others are not violated. It is an honest, direct, and appropriate type of behavior conveying respect for the other person, although not necessarily for that person's ideas or behaviors.
- NONASSERTIVE BEHAVIOR. That type of behavior that enables the person's rights to be violated by another. Such behavior inhibits honesty, spontaneous reactions, and often leaves the nonassertive person feeling hurt, anxious, and angry.
- AGGRESSIVE BEHAVIOR. That type of behavior in which a person stands up for his or her legitimate rights in such a way that the rights of others are violated. The behavior is often viewed as an attack on the other person rather than the other person's ideas or behaviors.

We have found that increasing a person's fluency has brought about increased self-esteem. In addition, increased fluency and self-esteem have enabled our clients to break the nonassertive behavior patterns that previously dominated their lives. However, it has also been our observation that a significant number of clients move from nonassertive behavior to aggressive behavior. This feedback has been reported to us by our fluency clients as well as their families. Therefore, it seems important to us to understand the components of assertiveness well enough to incorporate assertion training into our remedial procedures. In this way, perhaps the aggressive behavior that has been reported by family members of our fluent clients can be eliminated.

Pamela Butler[100] has defined assertion as "[t]he freedom to state your feelings and opinions without anxiety or embarrassment, while at the same time allowing other people to have their own feelings and opinions." She highlighted four areas in which assertion plays an important role: positive feelings, negative feelings, setting limits, and self-initiation.

First, the expression of positive feelings includes more than just standing up for one's self. It involves expressing feelings of warmth, affection, and love. The expression of positive feelings may range from thanking someone for a small favor to telling someone that you love them. A person who stutters may have trouble expressing the affective areas. Many males find the expression of these feelings difficult, even if they don't stutter. Since stuttering is primarily a male disorder (incidence ratio of 4:1), stuttering just compounds this aspect of assertiveness.[100]

According to Butler there are four important aspects of assertion:

1. "[p]ositive feelings are the oil that keeps relationships running smoothly. In marital counseling, I have never seen a couple with the complaint, 'All I ever get is positive feedback.'"[100] Ease in expressing positive feelings is a strength that adds to a person's freedom, enjoyment, and success in life. For a person who stutters, growth in this area will have positive personal and social results.

2. The *expression of negative feelings* runs the gamut form "I feel uncomfortable" to "I am annoyed," "I am upset," "I feel irritated," or "I am angry" to "I am furious." In other words, the whole range of negative feelings from discomfort to fury can be expressed assertively.[100] People who stutter have strong feelings related to their stuttering. Rieber and Wollock[101] have noted that negative emotions of anxiety, shame, guilt, anger, fear, hostility, and aggression have been linked to stuttering for more than 2,000 years. Negative feelings do not just go away. It has been demonstrated that until negative feelings are expressed, there is little room for positive feelings. The people who stutter who have found support and strength in our group process are relieved to be able to express the negative feelings they have had for years. It is important for our clients that they express past feelings as well as learn techniques for expressing the present day feelings assertively.

3. By *setting limits* we let others know "this is where I draw the line." It involves saying "no" to the demands of other people when these demands go against our own internal needs. Limits must often be set in matters concerning time, privacy, energy, and money. When a person sets limits they teach other people how to treat them. Many people who stutter report that others laugh at them, they belittle them verbally or nonverbally. A person who can set limits can express their feelings to demand the respect they are due. For example, if someone were to laugh at a stutterer and say, "Ha! What do you know? you can't even speak," an assertive person who could set limits might respond, "Excuse me, I object to your connecting my knowledge of sports to my speech. My speech doesn't affect my awareness of the National League statistics, and I would appreciate your not saying that again." In our experience, those who suffer from stuttering have en-

dured mockery and insults since childhood. It is important to help them learn positive ways of self-protection.[100]

Setting limits is not only related to the expression of negative feelings. There are situations where limits must be set in which one's feelings about others and the particular occasion are positive. All people must learn to say "no" to the demands of others when their requests interfere with one's own personal needs. This is not always easy to do. As a person grows in self-esteem and internal locus of control, he or she is better able to respect their own personal needs and set the necessary limits for positive interaction with others.

4. The fourth important aspect of assertion is *self-initiation*. "Whereas through limit setting we learn to say 'no,' through self-initiation we say 'yes.' By self-initiation, a person expresses what one does want to do."[100] This area of assertion involves taking risks and initiating those actions that are important to personal growth. People who stutter have sometimes developed the habit of taking the path of least resistance. Their fear of stuttering has led them to opt for what appears "safe"—that is, where speaking will not be required. Often, their choices are not those that they really desire or those that they might be well suited for. The failure to act on what they really want to do decreases the probability that they will ever achieve their full potential. It is a goal of fluency therapy that this area of assertiveness be incorporated into programs for those who could benefit from increased self-initiation.

A person who is nonassertive in any of these four areas is not fully in touch with their own power or their own potential. In particular, the lives of many people who stutter would be more rewarding if they could practice assertion in these important areas. We will expand upon this theme in Chapter 7.

Summary   We have highlighted attitudinal components that interact with the speech-language aspects and environmental aspects of fluency disorders. These are self-esteem, locus of control, and assertiveness. In addition to interacting synergistically with the above-mentioned major areas, we also believe that they interact with each other. A person's self-esteem influences how much control they believe they have with others. A person's sense of self-worth will also determine how readily they will assert their ideas and opinions, especially if these differ from the thoughts of others. Likewise, it is difficult for a person to set limits in interacting with others if one is dependent on others for reinforcements rather than on one's self.

We encourage clinicians to continue to develop their own personal awareness and growth in each of the areas of self-esteem, locus of control, and assertiveness, and to include them in both the assessment and treatment of fluency clients. Most of our statements are based on our observations of those who stutter, and we urge clinicians to join us in researching these areas.

ENVIRONMENT

The last area of our synergistic approach to be considered is the environment. In giving our definition of stuttering in Chapter 1, we stated our belief that each person who stutters has developed individual and learned attitudinal and behavioral responses to the underlying neurologic disorder. We also believe that the complex synergistic interactions exist individually, both within the person who stutters and without, in their interactions with their environment. Therefore, the environment of the person who stutters assumes a very important role in the rehabilitative process.

Shames and Egolf[102] have written that "[o]ur concerns with stuttering should include those factors that appear to evoke stuttering as well as those factors that appear to maintain stuttering. This is not a problem merely of dealing with the people and events that affect the stutterer." And Gregory[103] observed: "As I began writing, I looked over 20 books on stuttering dating back to the 1930s. All of these books hold environmental influences as important in the development and maintenance of stuttering as well as effective prevention and therapy."

The Demands and Capacities Model of stuttering states that fluency breaks down when speech/language expectations surpass the stutter's ability to produce fluent speech. That is, when environmental and/or self-imposed demands exceed a child's cognitive, linguistic, motoric, or emotional capacities for responding, the child will stutter. According to Adams,[28] this model was first proposed by Andrews and Harris and later expanded by Starkweather. Some of the environmental demands that have been identified[104] are the following:

1. Time pressure—when listeners expect a rapid rate of speech
2. Demand speech—when a child is frequently questioned or requested to recount events
3. Very rushed households
4. Interruptions
5. Loss of security because of any of the following:
   Separation from parents
   Birth of sibling
   Illness of parent
   Change in day care setting
   Tense emotional atmosphere in the home
6. Parents' negative reactions
   Punishment
   Nonverbal movements
   Silence about stuttering

In order to help someone deal with environmental demands, one must not only know the effect they have on the person's stuttering but also understand the dynamics of the environment that produces these demands. We have identified three such areas that are important for clinicians to understand and include in their treatment of people who stutter: (1) communication skills, (2) family patterns of interaction, and (3) cultural influences.

Communication Skills

A clinician who works with persons who stutter must be knowledgeable and skilled in the area of communication. Communication skills are also clinically important for the persons who stutter. Ultimately, the driving goal is to assist clients in becoming effective communicators in their respective environments. This includes client's ability to monitor dysfluencies as well as to engage in meaningful communication.

Recently, the Stuttering Committee of the American Speech and Hearing Association (ASHA) Special Interest Division 4 (Fluency and Fluency Disorders) issued Guidelines for Practice in Stuttering Treatment.[105] One of the management goals is particularly applicable here:

> The clinician will help the person who stutters make therapeutic (e.g., adaptive) decisions about how to handle speech and social situations in everyday living. This would apply to clients who let others talk for them, or helping a client learn not to use behaviors that avoid, rather than confront, specific social situations such as using the telephone, ordering in a restaurant, or helping the client learn that changing words costs something in personal self-esteem. This also includes teaching the client how to politely influence listener's behavior so that the client's fluency can be improved.

In order to carry out this goal, we believe that a clinician must be skilled in the dynamics of communication. These skills are integrated with the specifics of linguistic intervention, particularly pragmatics. In an earlier work,[83] we discussed communication skills that assist the clinician in the interview process and throughout the entire therapeutic process as well. Some of these skills are attending, exploration, listening and empathetic responses, summarizing, and the use of "I-statements." We will briefly define these skills here and discuss them more fully in Chapter 8.

Attending   Physical attending is a basic skill that conveys caring, understanding, and respect. Attending means that you are really "tuned in" to all the signals that can be received from the other person. Attending takes time and a great deal of energy. Bolton[106] called it "listening with the whole body." Some of the behaviors that indicate that a person is attending is that they face the person with whom they are communicating, lean slightly forward, maintain eye contact (in our culture), and have an open, relaxed position. Attending also requires one to be fully present, that is, to maintain moment-to-moment contact with the other person through disciplined attention.

Exploration   An important principle behind the concept of exploration is to understand where the other person is. We often have our own idea of what another person's problem is. When using the skill of exploration, one puts one's own ideas aside and encourages the other person "to tell their story." In the clinical setting, the interview is the primary tool for exploration. The person exploring needs to attend to the other person's immediate concerns and emotional states, listening for both physiologic and psychological components of the situation. It is important to listen and to explore the content of the situation being talked about as well as the feelings the person has about that situation. This skill is used throughout the therapeutic process.

Listening and Empathetic Responses   The art of good listening involves paying attention to what the other person is saying, both verbally and nonverbally. Listening on all levels of response requires stepping into the shoes of the other person. The listener must try to perceive the world of the client. This understanding of the other person is both demonstrated and extended with empathetic listening responses. Empathetic responding involves reflecting back to the client both the content and the feeling level that the client first expressed. Hepworth and Larson[107] defined empathetic responding in this way

> Empathetic responding involves understanding the other person's feelings and experiences without taking that person's position (e.g. "I sense that you're feeling . . ." or "You seem to be saying . . ."). Thus, the clinician retains separateness and objectivity—a critical dimension in the helping process, for when clinicians take on the client's feelings and positions, they lose not only vital perspective but the ability to be helpful as well. What does happen, when the clinician remains separate, yet reflects on the client's experiences and feelings, is that the clinician provides a mirror for the clients to both hear what they have said and to get in touch with how they are feeling about it. In this process of both being mirrored and being understood, the client comes to a greater understanding of the problem and a clearer awareness of what he has to do for a solution.

Summarizing   When a topic has been completed, a session ended, or the initial assessment completed, clinicians can use the skill of summarizing to provide closure. In summarizing their perceptions, clinicians may highlight something of importance that emerged in the session: "From what you have said so far, your stuttering has affected all your relationships." A summary may also be a general statement of what has taken place: "To sum up, you seem very anxious to stop stuttering, but you don't feel as if you can spend the time or money required."

Summaries are also used to provide focus when a conversation seems to be going nowhere. An effective summary will bring together the relevant information that has been presented and leave out extraneous comments.

Use of "I" Statements   A final skill for clinicians to develop relates to the use of "I" statements. It must be remembered that one can only speak for one's self.

We believe that each of these skills is essential when working with both clients and parents of children who stutter. Many books have been published on the importance of attaining these skills and on the techniques for applying them.[107-109] However, one must both understand the principles behind these skills and practice them before they can be successfully used in the clinical situation.

Family

The complexity of the stuttering behavior that we have described demands that the family of the person who stutters be both understood and included in therapy. We agree with Mallard,[110] who wrote that "the problem of stuttering is much too complex to conduct therapy on an individual basis only (clinician and child). We must involve the people responsible for the child's communication environment from the beginning of therapy if the child is going to use what is learned in a meaningful way." This reasoning extends to the families of adults. Thus, not only have we found it important to include as part of therapy parents of children who stutter but also, in the case of adult clients, their spouses and significant others. However, much less has been written about families of adults who stutter.

Historically, when researching family involvement in the behavior of stuttering, the attempt has been to gain an understanding of the communication patterns and the attitudes of parents with their children. The primary area of interest has been the interactive communication patterns of the family members of children who stutter. Myers and Freeman[111-113] found that mothers of children who stutter have more rapid speech rates and are more likely to interrupt dysfluent speech rather than fluent speech. Riley and Riley[114] also found that 53 percent of parents of children who stutter had a similar effect on children's speech. They found that parents used a rapid speech rate, interrupted children as they spoke, and appeared impatient. Conture and Caruso[115] have reported that it is common to find parents of children who stutter talking in excess of 190 to 200 words per minute. In contrast, they cite Fairbrooks,[116] who reported that the median adult speaking rate is 170 words per minute.

This research highlights the role of the family members and demonstrates the synergistic, interactive importance of the first two areas of the environment that we have addressed: communication and family. The communication skills of family members are as important as those of the client and the clinician. In particular, as Ramig[117] has stated, "[p]arents have to be taught the specifics of how to slow down, give more turn-taking time, interrupt less, and positively reinforce the child. This is a difficult task that will require serious clinical effort."

Continued research in this area will provide more valuable information about the communicative interaction patterns of families. We also believe these interactional patterns are related to attitudinal issues of self-esteem and locus of control. When working with parents, it is important to discuss this relationship. Gregory and Hill[118] pointed out that it is important for parents to avoid frequent corrections of a child's verbal and nonverbal behavior in order to promote communicative interactions that may promote fluency. We agree and believe that the positive interactions promoted will increase fluency, self-esteem, and an internal locus of control. As will be discussed in Chapter 8, more research is needed to expand our understanding of the interactive aspects of adult clients and their families.

Additional studies have focused on parental attitudes. Moore and Nystul[119] found that the fathers of those who stutter were more conventional and rigid and less tolerant of fighting among children. Fathers and mothers of children who stutter were also less likely to allow expressions of curiosity about sexual matters. However, mothers were found to be generally more democratic and protective. They concluded that, in general, the families of children who stutter are more rigid and stereotyped in their behaviors. Riley[120] reported his findings that unrealistic demands of "perfection" in behavior and performance were made by 51 percent of the parents of children who stutter that he studied.

Although there is not extensive research in this area, there are many questions that must be asked about the attitudes of parents. However, Conture[38] has cautioned that parents come to us with feelings of guilt already. We should be careful not to increase that guilt. He also pointed out, and we agree, that although there is some research that identifies general characteristics of parents of children who stutter, we must remember that parents are individuals, too.

Recognizing the individuality of each parent and attempting to avoid increasing parental guilt must be done within the broader context of understanding that these parents are raising children in a highly technical, competitive society, and recognizing that some parents of stutterers do seem, as Neill[121] put it, to want to "speed up the pace." But this does not mean that all such parents are too demanding or time urgent or that even those parents who are somewhat demanding are necessarily demanding about every aspect of their child's behavior every hour of the day. Clinicians should work to understand the difference between normal parental concern and those concerns that frequently and consistently occur and that seem to inhibit the type of environment where a child's speech fluency can positively develop.

While we endorse the above cautionary observations, we also realize that living in today's society does include coping with a great deal of stress. Ramig[117] has highlighted some of these:

> Negative interpersonal interactions that cause a child to become angry, upset, frightened, or unsure of his/her family's ability to stay together are likely to aggravate his/her dysfluency. Such interactions may include, for example, a) loud arguments or yelling, b) parental threats to abandon the family, c) abuse directed at the dysfluent child or other family members, d) serious illness within the family, and e) belittlement of the dysfluent child, etc.

These same fears and family patterns of behavior affect the fluency of adults who stutter.

After working with many families of people who stutter, it has become clear to us that family dynamics that may appear to be unimportant can actually be an essential part of our therapy. In order to recognize this, and still heed the above caution urged by Conture, clinicians need to have a basic understanding of family therapy. Shapira[122] underscores the importance of working with family members, and highlights that anything happening to one person affects and is affected by other members of the family system. He says:

> For this reason alone, it is foolhardy to direct our clinical efforts to the person who stutters without consideration of the others with whom this person communicates regularly. The needs of all involved must be taken into account for the treatment to be effective and generalizable. (p. 145)

We will define the basic concepts here; applications to therapy will be expanded in Chapter 8. In order to fully grasp an understanding of family therapy, one must first understand the principles of counseling. We will, therefore, briefly introduce this concept here and devote Chapter 9 to expanding counseling issues that affect fluency.

Counseling

"Counseling" has become a catchall term, one that has evolved over the years but the meaning of which is still not universally agreed upon. Brammer[123] noted that there are two opposing views regarding counseling. One view emphasizes helping as a specialized enterprise based on a firm foundation in the behavioral and medical sciences. The other view sees helping as a broad human function using the skills possessed by most people.

Certainly, we know that we are not trained, professional counselors nor do we attempt to assume that role. However, as professionals who work with both children and adults who stutter, we know that we are in a position that requires us to counsel clients, parents, and families. Kennedy[124] has discussed this role as that of the "nonprofessional counselor." We have called this the role of the clinician/counselor[83] and believe it allows us to maintain our primary identity as speech-language pathologists and audiologists and yet adopt pertinent techniques of the counseling profession that can assist us in working with our clients. A synergistic approach to fluency necessitates our growth in awareness of the importance of this role.

The counseling process is characteristically supportive, insightful, reeducative, and usually short term. It is used to help individuals make practical changes in their lives without modifying established personality patterns. The essential task of the counselor is to help individuals work toward an understanding of themselves in order to learn new ways of coping with and adjusting to life situations.

This definition and most definitions of counseling point out that counseling includes an emphasis on relationships, self-understanding, and self-improvement. However, in our field we have traditionally used the term *counseling* to refer to giving information and advice. We hope to encourage professionals to expand this view in their own practice and to recognize that as clinician/counselors it is important for us to not only teach "targets of fluency" but to interact with the whole person. As clinician/counselors we should allow a relationship to be formed between ourselves and the client, parent, and family. As clinician/counselors, we help clients change not only their dysfluency but also their views of themselves and their environment. We hope that we can encourage our clients to identify their strengths and deficits, to develop assertiveness, and to change undesirable feelings and behaviors that have resulted because of their stuttering. As clinician/counselors, we strive to empower our clients to develop unused potential, to manage problem situations, and to achieve valued outcomes. We believe that clients will not achieve their therapeutic potential unless such a holistic approach is adopted. The major roles of the clinician/counselor will be expanded when we consider communication skills application in Chapter 8.

It is important to note here that success in any helping relationship is influenced heavily by not only the technical skills of the helper but also by his or her personal characteristics and traits. Many clinicians claim that the professional's own personality is the most significant resource that a clinician has. These attributes will be more fully discussed in Chapter 9; however, here we can at least say that "humanness" is the most important of all of these characteristics and that becoming more fully human is our constant goal because it is the basic characteristic of the effective clinician. It is this quality that will most assist us in engaging the family in a family-based therapy approach.

Family Therapy

As clinicians/counselors, we interact with and use our counseling skills with individual clients and with members of their families. We know that it is within the family that character is formed, self-esteem is developed, a sense of belonging is initiated, roles are established, and interpersonal skills are learned. As stated earlier, we believe that if we are to learn more about our dysfluent clients and to effect change in them, it is imperative that we include families in our assessment and rehabilitative process. Coming to understand interaction patterns with family members will assist us in determining some of the synergistic goals related to problem solving, self-esteem, assertiveness, coping, locus of control, and communication needs. Indeed, it seems impossible to know our clients outside of this context.

Rollin[125] noted that, as a profession of speech-language pathologists and audiologists, we have formally acknowledged the importance of treating the whole person but that in practice this seldom has been the case. Andrews and Andrews[126] pointed out that family members traditionally have been included in our treatment program as aides to carry out the structured plans of the clinician or as part of an attempt to educate them regarding the nature of the communication disorder. We agree with them that in order to fully utilize and integrate families into our synergistic therapy procedures we must have a systemic rather than an individual perspective.

Systems Theory   Hepworth and Larson[107] stated: "In family groups, each member is influenced by every other member. This creates a system that has properties of its own and that is governed by a set of implicit 'rules,' specific roles, power structures, forms of communication and ways of negotiating and solving problems." Because each family is a unique system, we believe that it is important for the clinician/counselor to develop a systems framework that will help to evaluate all clients in relation to their family groups.

Andrews and Andrews[126] have presented a rationale for the use of their family treatment model that is based on four systemic principles:

1. One part of the family cannot be understood in isolation from the rest of the family.
2. The parts of the family are interrelated; change in one part influences change in other parts of the system.
3. Transactional patterns of the family shape the behavior of family members.
4. A family's structure, organization, and developmental stage are important factors in determining the behavior of the family members.

If one believes in the validity of these principles, and we do, then it seems important to us to include as many family members as possible in both our assessment and rehabilitative processes in fluency therapy. This inclusion must be more than a token meeting. The clinician/counselor has to listen to all members of the family, observe interactional patterns, learn the family rules, and prepare the family for changes that will come about because of treatment. However, we are in no way implying that the clinician/counselor will become a family therapist. Lengthy assessments of family functioning and family interactions are not recommended. Clinician/counselors do not analyze pathologic functioning of the family. They concern themselves with "normal" reactions to a difficult situation. Nevertheless, it is important for us to realize that we might be the first "outsider" to be allowed into a closed, dysfunctional family system. Thus, we should be aware of possible referral services for these families. The effect of fluency disorders on a family system has not been researched adequately, and it is possible that family therapy may be an important recommendation for many families of people with fluency disorders.[127] It is also possible that there are certain patterns of family functioning that develop around a person who has a dysfluency problem.

As clinicians become more skilled in integrating counseling skills and family-based interactions into their assessment and treatment processes, we will be better able to assess this area. Family-based assessment and therapy techniques will be further explored in Chapter 8.

Summary   We have seen that understanding the communication patterns and attitudes of the family members of people who stutter is important. In addition, we believe that it is essential to expand the traditional view of environmental manipulation and to incorporate skills of counseling and family-based therapy techniques into our synergistic fluency programs.

It is important to have an understanding of family systems because intervention in any part of a system will effect change throughout the entire system. This interactive process of multiple factors is the essence of a synergistic approach to fluency therapy.

Multicultural Influences

General Considerations

Within the field of communication disorders, there is a growing awareness of our need to be sensitive to ethnic and cultural issues. Battle[128] has written:

> In 1968 at the annual convention of the American Speech-Language Hearing Association, the actions of a small group of individuals caused John Irwin, the president of ASHA, to forgo his usual presidential address to allow two members of ASHA to debate the question, "What is the role of a professional association in a conflict society?" This event marked the beginning of the recognition of the need for serious study of communication disorders in multicultural populations. The impact of that event was felt throughout the profession as the economic, social, and political events of the 1970s, 1980s, and 1990s changed the face and complexion of the nation.

Battle continues to highlight the importance for members of our profession to be aware of the increase in the number of racial and ethnic minorities that both already have come to our country in the recent past and who will come to our country in the next decade. Table 2.1 presents pertinent data from the 1990 census.[129]

Certainly one can see that the minority population has become a significant presence in our culture and we know that the predictions are that by the end of the twentieth century these numbers will have increased even more. This data calls us to recognize that very soon the minority will become the majority and the majority will become the minority.[130] It is imperative, therefore, that as speech-language pathologists and audiologists we become aware of the complexity of the issues involved in working with the communication disorders found among those in multicultural populations, and to then incorporate our knowledge into our practice.

This is not an area that has been heavily researched in our field. In general, we have just begun to recognize that not only speech and linguistic issues are im-

Table 2.1   1990 United States Population Statistics

Group	Population Count	Percentage
American Indian	1,959,234	0.75
Aleut	23,797	
Eskimo	57,152	
Asian/Pacific Islander	7,273,662	2.78
Black	29,986,060	11.48
Hispanic	22,354,059	8.56
Cuban	1,043,932	
Mexican	13,495,938	
Puerto Rican	2,727,754	
Other	5,086,435	
White	199,686,070	76.43
Total	261,259,085	100.00

Source: Data from Statistical Abstract of the United States: 1990. 110th ed. Washington, DC: U.S. Department of Commerce, 1990, p. xvi.

portant for us to examine and include in therapeutic approaches but that cultural values, learning styles, and the diversity found among the different peoples are also important. Our increased awareness has led us to recognize more clearly the interplay between culture and communication behavior and urged us to draw from the field of communication ethnography for increased understanding. Ethnography has been defined as a fully developed sense of the meaning of culture and the complicated manner in which one comes to understand the intricacies of the culture. An ethnographic understanding of a culture implies a full appreciation of the complex web of meanings, perceptions, actions, symbols, and adaptations that make a people who they are. Ethnography is the lens through which individuals view the world as they maneuver through life.[130]

The field of communication ethnography considers communication behavior to be one of the subsystems of culture. A person's requisite knowledge for communication includes not only rules for communication and shared rules for interaction but also the cultural rules and knowledge that are the basis for the context and the content of communicative events and the interactive process.[131] Ethnographic assessment considers linguistic abilities, sociocultural and cognitive knowledge, as well as pragmatics and other speech-language components. Micro-ethnographic methods focus on the quality of interaction as well as on the quantity of events.[132]

Through ethnographic study, we recognize that cultures tend to be characterized by modes of conduct that are different from our own in many areas. Saville-Troike[131] listed the following as culturally specific:

Family structure
Important events in life cycle
Roles of individual members
Rules of interpersonal interaction
Communication and linguistic rules
Rules for decorum and discipline
Standards for health and hygiene
Food preferences
Dress and personal appearance
History and traditions
Holidays and celebrations
Values and methods
Education
Perceptions of work and play
Perceptions of time and space
Explanation of natural phenomena
Attitudes toward pets and animals
Artistic and musical values and tastes
Life expectations and aspirations

Understanding these cultural differences should be part of the diagnostic and therapeutic process in communication disorders in general as well as of a synergistic approach to fluency disorders. Achieving such an understanding is a daunting task that many professions, including ours, have found necessary to attempt. Corey and Corey[133] have noted some of the recent developments that are the outgrowths of this attempt:

1. There is a trend toward cross-cultural courses and other means of acquiring knowledge about working with minority clients.
2. There is concern for adapting techniques and interventions in ways that are relevant to culturally diverse populations.
3. There is increasing recognition of the need for helpers to know themselves if they hope to understand clients from different cultures.
4. There are implications for practice in the value orientations and differing basic assumptions underlying eastern and western therapeutic systems.

We will consider some general diagnostic and therapeutic techniques that are culturally sensitive in Chapter 8 and we encourage clinicians to continue to avail themselves of the ever growing body of information that helps us to develop our profession.

Cultural Research in Fluency Disorders

Certainly the disorder of fluency has long been recognized as a culturally dependent behavior. Van Riper[3] believed that the universality of stuttering could be demonstrated by its present occurrence in a wide range of varying cultures. He compiled a list of words in various languages that refer to stuttering behavior:

Words Referring to Stuttering

Europe
Finnish: ankyttaa
German: stottern
French: begaiement
Portuguese: gagueira
Norwegian: stamning
Italian: balbuzie
Spanish: tartamundear
Yugoslav (Slovene): jeclijati
Latvian: stostisanas
Estonian: tolpkeel
Hungarian: dadogo
Czech: koktani
Russian: zaikatsia; zaikanie
Esperanto: babuti

American Indian, etc.
Salish: sutsuts
Nanaimo: skeykulskwels
Tlahoose: ha'ak'ok
Haida: kilekwigu'ung
Chocktaw: isunash illi
Asage: the'-ce u-ba-ci-ge
Cherokee: a-da-nv-te-hi-lo-squi
Sioux: eye-hda-sna-sna;
    iyi-tag-tag
Eskimo: iptogetok

Pacific
Fiji: kaka
Hawaiian: uu uus

Asian
Tagalog: patalutal
Chinese (Cantonese): hau hick;
    kong'-tak-lak-kak
Japanese: domori; kitsuon
Vietnamese: su noi lap

Eastern
Persian: lacknatezaban
Hebrew: gingeim
Arabic: fa faa; rattat
Hindi: khaha
Hindustani: larbaraha
Turkish: kekeke mek

African
Egyptian: tataha; tuhuhtuhuh
Ga: haamuala
Xhosa: ukuthititha
Luganda: okukunanagira
Ghana (Twi): howdodo
Nigeria (Ibo): nsu
Shangaan: manghanghamela
Somali: wuu haghaglayya

Van Riper[3] also pointed out that stuttering appeared to be fairly prevalent in Japan. He reported that one of their most famous doll plays, the *Domo Mata*, tells of an artist named Doma Matahei who stuttered severely:

"I am sorry for you, Matahei, but you must give up your cherished desires. You have two hands with ten fingers, but it is unfortunate that you stutter." She tells Matahei that the only thing he can do to gain fame is to commit suicide, but to paint his greatest masterpiece on a stone fountain before he dies. She brings him his brushes and prepares the ink, and Matahei draws his own portrait on the stone. The shogun who owns the fountain is enraged and cleaves the stone with his sword only to find that miraculously the portrait is also visible in the cleft, that it has penetrated the stone. And just as miraculously Matahei regains his speech. There is a touching scene in which he recites the vowels of the Japanese syllabary to convince himself that he no longer stutters. Then great rejoicings and honors and all ends well. The *Domo Mata* play was first performed in Osaka in 1752. Another more recent real life drama occurred in 1950 when, to the horror of all art loving and patriotic Japanese, a stutterer burned down the ancient temple of the Golden Pavilion.[3]

One can clearly recognize the cultural identifications that are present in this story. It is research like Van Riper's that has prompted us to recognize the importance of the social environment of people who stutter. This recognition was also promoted and expanded by the work of Johnson,[134,135] who was convinced that the difference between parents' child rearing practices brought about stuttering. His Diagnosogenic Theory of stuttering prompted Johnson to encourage one of his students to research stuttering on the Indian reservation where she had taken a job. She found that among the Bannock and Shoshone languages there was no word that described stuttering. Another of Johnson's students, Snidecor,[136] pursued this finding and reported that he could not find one pure-blooded Indian who stuttered. The Indians he interviewed were under no pressure to speak; they simply answered "yes" and "no." In addition, it was found that the parents of Indian children demanded less of their children while growing up. This research supported the ever growing acceptance of the Diagnosogenic Theory and the belief that stuttering did not exist among the Indians. It also highlighted the awareness of the importance of culture in determining stuttering. However, there was little data to support further understanding of the differences noted.

Cooper and Cooper[137] cited Lemert[138] as having found numerous Indians who stuttered among the Salish, Kwakiutl, and Nootka tribes of British Columbia and Vancouver Island. They also cited Liljeblad[139] and Zimmerman et al.[140] as presenting data that demonstrate that stuttering did and does exist among the Bannock and Shoshone tribes and that there is language to describe this behavior. Zimmerman et al.[140] helped to clarify the conflicting research by suggesting that the differences are directly related to our increasing sophistication in intercultural research, with the objectivity of the researcher being a key factor. We agree with this conclusion and recognize that this controversy is important background information for our pursuit of understanding cultural influences in fluency disorders.

The data, however, from multicultural research about fluency is not extensive. In our opinion, the Coopers[137] have provided the most up-to-date review of this area and they, too, noted that relatively few data exist concerning variations in fluency among cultures. In addition, they say, much of the data available are of dubious value in identifying significant cultural variations in stuttering primarily because of the lack of universally accepted definitions for terms such as *fluency, dysfluency, stuttering, cluttering,* and *stammering.* Shames[141] and Conrad[142] have agreed with them.

Summary   Based on previous research in the area of multicultural issues, ethnography, and fluency itself, we realize that there are many areas to be explored and understood before we succeed in integrating multicultural concerns into our synergistic approach to fluency. However, as a profession we have made great strides in promoting the awareness of cultural issues as they affect all disorders.[143] In the attempt to avoid cultural tunnel vision, we are prompted to integrate our new appreciation of cultural influences into both our assessment and remediation processes. Again, we encourage clinicians to join us as we continue to expand our own awareness and research in this area.

Multicultural Aspects of Fluency Disorders

As we explore the aspects of family life considered previously, we are aware that a central component of family life is its ethnicity. Ethnicity remains a major form of group identification:

> Every family's background is multicultural. All marriages are to a degree cultural marriages. No two families share exactly the same cultural roots. Understanding the various strands of a family's cultural heritage is essential to understanding its members' lives and the development of the particular individual as well.

Paulo Friere[145] has reinforced this view:

> No one goes anywhere alone, least of all into exile—not even those who arrive physically alone, unaccompanied by family, spouse, children, parents, or siblings. No one leaves his or her world without having been transfixed by its roots, or with a vacuum for a soul. We carry with us the memory of many fabrics, a self soaked in our history, our culture; a memory, sometimes scattered, sometimes sharp and clear, of the streets of our childhood.

In developing a synergistic approach to fluency disorders, it is clear that the physiologic, attitudinal, and environmental aspects of fluency that we have already considered must each be understood within the client's cultural context. A knowledge of that cultural milieu is necessary for both the assessment and the remediation of the individual with a fluency disorder. We will therefore briefly review the aspects of multiculturalism we have found to be important in our work with fluency clients.

Cultural Factors   "Culture" refers to something that most of us intuitively understand. It includes all aspects of a person's individual environment; perceptions; expectations; values; affective, behavioral and cognitive experiences; and social and psychological view points. Culture is like the air we breathe. We often accept our own culture as the "norm" and only recognize its influence when we are either deprived of our own culture or interacting with someone whose culture is different. Knowledge of the norms related to a client's culture is essential. The cognitive, attitudinal, behavioral, and interpersonal aspects of a person's life vary according to the culture. Hepworth and Larsen[107] noted that cultures differ in their prescribed patterns of child care, child rearing, adolescent roles, mate selection, marital roles, patterns of communication, and care of the aged. Views toward problem solving, autonomy and dependency needs, health and illness, and the acceptance of external help also depend upon one's ethnic background. Dava Waltzman[135] has provided some basic definitions related to multicultural issues:

> *Culture:* The total accumulation of an identifiable group's beliefs, norms, activities, institutions, and communication patterns.
>
> *Cultural Group:* People with common origins, customs, and styles of living. The group has a sense of identity and a shared language. The group's values, goals, expectations, beliefs, perceptions, and behaviors from birth until death are shaped by their shared history and experiences. This definition includes both ethnic and religious minorities.
>
> *Ethnocentrism:* The tendency to view one's own cultural group as the center of everything; the standard against which all others are judged. This view assumes that one's own cultural patterns are the correct and best way of acting. Judging culturally different clients in terms of values and behaviors of the dominant culture has led to racism and discrimination. In order to render culturally sensitive and appropriate care, it is necessary to identify how one's own cultural background impacts on ways of seeing and behaving.
>
> *Cultural Relativity:* The idea that any behavior must be judged first in relation to the context of the culture in which it occurs. To effectively intervene, one must first relate to the client's interpretations of experiences from his/her own background and cultural belief system.
>
> *Cultural Universals:* Structures or functions found in every extended culture: a family unit, marriage, parental roles, education, health care, forms of work, and forms of self expression. They include issues related to family structure, roles and relations, health beliefs related to illness and disability, and sexual attitudes and practices.

Different cultural perspectives can lead to verbal and nonverbal forms of miscommunication between cultural groups, as Cole[130] has pointed out. Wyatt[147] also compiled examples of how cultural perspectives can differ (see Table 2.2).

It is recommended that fluency clinicians develop cross-cultural sensitivity, awareness and competence with different cultural groups. Wyatt[147] defined cross-cultural sensitivity as "ways of thinking and behaving that enable members to work effectively with members of another group." In order to do this, she states that one must have an openness, appreciation, and respect for cultural differences:

Table 2.2 Cultural Perspectives

Western System Perspectives	*Other Cultural Perspectives*
Family: Biological parents and children	Family: Extended family and community
Relationships determine responsibilities	Family or community determines
Education is highly respected	Age and life experience more respected
Health related to body parts	Health combines physical, mental, and spiritual
Treatment: Specific to specific part	Treatment to "whole" person and family
Written agreements and signatures	Personal verbal agreements binding
Questions, eye contact show interest	Questions, eye contact are disrespectful
Silence during conversation is uncomfortable	Silence is appropriate: time for thought
Time is short. Seize the moment	Time is plentiful

Source: Reprinted with permission from Wyatt T. Multicultural Issues in Communication Disorders. Fullerton, CA: University of California, 1997 (unpublished manuscript).

Have a respect for differences (acknowledge integrity and value of all cultures); don't view differences as negative or threatening.

- Be eager to learn
- Be willing to accept the fact that there are different ways of viewing the world
- Be aware of one's own cultural limitations
- View intercultural interactions as learning opportunities

It is important to remember that the focus on the cultural issues in the environment of our clients does not render the client passive or irresponsible. Rather, it is our role to study the interactions of the environment and the client. This person–environment relationship was first termed an "ecological perspective" by Germain[148–150] and involves a consideration of the "fit" of human beings within their environment. Germain[148] wrote:

> The ecology of people is their "life space"; that is, all elements of the social and physical environments that impinge upon them. People are not viewed as passive reactors to their environments but rather are involved in dynamic and reciprocal interactions with them. The ecological perspective thus does not represent a swing of the pendulum from primary focus on the person to the other extreme of primary focus on the environment. Rather, problem-solving efforts may be focused on assisting people to adapt to their environments (e.g., training them in interpersonal skills), altering en-

vironments to meet the needs of the client more adequately, or a combination of the two.

Thus, the fluency clinician should adopt such an ecological approach when considering important cultural differences in assessment and remediation of persons who stutter.

Communication Disorders and Culturally Diverse Populations

Taylor[151] pointed out that, prior to 1968, there was little interest in addressing the needs of the culturally and linguistically diverse populations among the members of the professions of speech-language pathology and audiology. However, at the 1968 national convention of ASHA, a scheduled debate took place on "The Role of a Professional Association in a Conflict Society." Out of this debate came the following goals:

- To urge ASHA to require coursework in sociolinguistics and black history for clinical instruction.
- To urge ASHA to organize a committee to generate new ideas on training and research in sociolinguistics, especially as related to black language.

Taylor et al.[152] tracked the response of ASHA following the 1968 meeting:

1. ASHA opened an Office of Urban and Ethnic Affairs in 1969. This office was changed to the Office of Minority Concerns in 1979.
2. ASHA established Committees on Communication Behaviors and Problems in Urban Populations in 1969 (now the Committee on Cultural and Linguistic Differences and Disorders of Communication) and on the Status of Racial Minorities in 1973.
3. Several symposia, colloquia, and continuing education activities have been presented throughout the United States on normal and clinical issues pertaining to culturally and linquistically diverse populations. ASHA's 1985 National Colloquium on Underserved Populations is a good example of this type of activity.
4. Several universities have inaugurated special training projects to address the specific clinical needs of culturally or linguistically diverse populations.
5. Presentations in professional meetings and publications in professional journals have increased dramatically since 1969 on a myriad of topics pertaining to cultural and linguistic diversity.

Awareness of this issue relating to culturally diverse populations continued to grow within our professions and in 1990 the Executive Board of ASHA charged the Committee on the Status of Racial Minorities with the responsibility of developing a plan to promote parity among racial/ethnic minorities within the

Association. The result was the Multicultural Action Agenda 2000,[153] which consists of objectives and corresponding action steps in six areas: (1) membership, (2) leadership, (3) national office structure and staffing, (4) policies and programs affecting service, education, and research, (5) governmental and legislative issues, and (6) public image. The following objective and action steps are the ones that directly affect the service, education, and research areas in communication disorders:

> *Objective:* To institutionalize a commitment to sociocultural diversity throughout the Association and the professions, particularly in the areas of clinical practice, professional education, and research.
>
> *Action:* Establish an award program to honor distinguished achievements and contributions in the areas of multicultural professional education, multicultural research, and clinical service to multicultural populations, to be presented periodically.
>
> *Action:* Disseminate information on a regular basis to members on communication disorders, clinical materials and procedures, emerging research, model programs, new technologies, and legislation that have implications for service to culturally diverse populations through ASHA journals, other publications, special projects and educational programs.
>
> *Action:* Actively encourage federal agencies that fund research in the area of communication sciences and disorders, university programs in communication sciences and disorders, and the Council of Editors for the ASHA/NSSLHA scholarly publications to regard multicultural topics as high priority areas within their research agenda and to promote ethnographic paradigms in multicultural research design.

Clearly, our profession has set in place plans that will help us respond to the complexity of the multicultural issues that confront our changing society. In addition, the Executive Board and Legislative Council approved Resolution LC 50-85,[154] which states:

> RESOLVED: That the American Speech-Language-Hearing Association (ASHA) encourage undergraduate, graduate and continuing education programs to include specific information, course content, and/or clinical practicum which address communication needs of individuals within socially, culturally, economically, and linguistically diverse populations.

With such support and leadership to guide us, we eagerly look forward to expanding the research, further explored in Chapter 8, that increases our awareness of and response to the multicultural needs of fluency clients.

REFERENCES

1. Wall MJ, Myers F. *Clinical Management of Childhood Stuttering*. Baltimore: University Park Press, 1984.
2. Guitar B, Peters TJ. *Stuttering: An Integrated Approach to Its Nature and Treatment*. Baltimore: Williams and Wilkins, 1991.
3. Van Riper C. *The Nature of Stuttering* (2nd ed). Englewood Cliffs, NJ: Prentice Hall, 1982.
4. Kidd KK. A genetic perspective on stuttering. *J Fluency Disord* 1977;2:259–269.
5. Kidd KK. Genetic models of stuttering. *J Fluency Disord* 1980;5:187–202.
6. Kidd KK. Recent progress on the genetics of stuttering. In C Ludlow, J Cooper (eds), *Genetic Aspects of Speech and Language*. New York: Academic Press, 1983.
7. Kidd KK. Stuttering as a genetic disorder. In R Curlee, W Perkins (eds), *Nature and Treatment of Stuttering*. San Diego: College Hill Press, 1984.
8. Howie PM. Concordance for stuttering monozygotic and dizygotic twin pairs. *J Speech Lang Hear Res* 1981;24:317–321.
9. Howie PM. Intrapair similarity in frequency of disfluency in monozygotic and dizygotic twin pairs containing stuttering. *Behav Genet* 1981;1:227–238.
10. Hamm RE. *Therapy for Stuttering*. Englewood Cliffs, NJ: Prentice Hall, 1990.
11. Yairi E, Ambrose N, Cox N. Genetics of stuttering: A critical review. *J Speech Lang Hear Res* 1996;39:771–784.
12. Travis LE. *Speech Pathology*. New York: Prentice Hall, 1931.
13. Travis LE. The cerebral dominance theory of stuttering, 1931–1978. *J Speech Hear Disord* 1978;11:71–89.
14. Moore Jr.WH, Lorendo LC. Hemispheric alpha asymmetries of stuttering males and females for words of high and low imagery. *J Fluency Disord* 1980;5:11–26.
15. Moore Jr.WH, Lorendo LC. Hemispheric alpha asymmetries of stutterers and non-stutterers for the recall and recognition of words and connected reading passages: Some relationships to severity of stuttering. *J Fluency Disord* 1986;11:71–89.
16. Moore Jr.WH, Lorendo LC. Central nervous system characteristics of stutterers. In RJ Curlee, WH Perkins (eds), *Nature and Treatment of Stuttering*. San Diego: College-Hill Press, 1984.
17. Geschwind N, Galaburda AM. Cerebral lateralization: Biological mechanisms, associations, and pathology. A hypothesis and a program for research. *Archives of Neurology* 1985;42:429–459.
18. Fox PJ, Ingham R, Ingham J. A PET study of the neural system of stuttering. *Nature* 1996;382:158–162.
19. Hardin CE, Pindgola RH, Haynes NO. Hemispheric processing in children. *J Fluency Disord* 1992;17:265–281.
20. Kent RD. Stuttering as a temporal programming disorder. In RJ Curlee, WH Perkins (eds), *Nature and Treatment of Stuttering*. San Diego: College-Hill Press, 1984.
21. Guitar B. *Stuttering: An Integrated Approach to Its Nature and Treatment*. Baltimore: William and Wilkins, 1998.
22. St. Louis KO. Linguistic and motor aspects of stuttering. In NJ Lass (ed), *Speech and Language: Advances in Basic Research and Practice*. New York: Academic Press, 1979.
23. Hill HE. Stuttering II: A review and integration of physiological data. *J Speech Hear Disord* 1944;9:209–324.

24. Adams MR, Freeman FJ, Conture EG. Laryngeal dynamics of stutterers. In RJ Curlee, WH Perkins (eds), *Nature and Treatment of Stuttering*. San Diego: College-Hill Press, 1984.
25. Bloodstein O. *A Handbook on Stuttering* (3rd ed).Chicago: National Easter Seal Society, 1981.
26. Freeman FJ. Phonation in stuttering: A review of current research. *J Fluency Disord* 1979;4:78–79.
27. Starkweather CW. Stuttering and laryngeal behavior: A review. *American Speech and Hearing Association Monographs* 1982:21.
28. Adams MR. Stuttering theory, research and therapy: A five year retrospective and look ahead. *J Fluency Disord* 1984;9:103–113.
29. Zimmerman G. Articulatory dynamics of fluent utterances of stutterers and non-stutterers. *J Speech Lang Hear Res* 1980;23:95–107.
30. Zimmerman G. Articulatory behaviors associated with stuttering: A cine-fluorohrphic analysis. *J Speech Lang Hear Res* 1980;23:108–121.
31. Zimmerman G. Stuttering: A disorder of movement. *J Speech Lang Hear Res* 1980;23:108–121.
32. Zimmerman G. Articulatory dynamics of stutterers. In R Curlee, WH Perkins (eds), *Nature and Treatment of Stuttering*. San Diego: College-Hill Press, 1984.
33. Starkweather C, Myers M. Duration of subsegments within the intervocalic interval in stutterers and non-stutterers. *J Fluency Disord* 1979;4:205–214.
34. Van Riper C. *The Treatment of Stuttering*. Englewood Cliffs, NJ: Prentice Hall, 1971.
35. Perkins W, Rudas J, Johnson L, Bell J. Stuttering: Discoordination of phonation, articulation and respiration. *J Speech Hear Disord* 1980;55:370–382.
36. Perkins WH. What is stuttering? *J Speech Hear Disord* 1980;55:370–382.
37. Caruso A, Conture E, Colton R. Selected temporal parameters of coordination associated with stuttering in children. *J Fluency Disord* 1988;12:57–82.
38. Conture EG. *Stuttering* (2nd ed). Englewood Cliffs, NJ: Prentice Hall, 1990.
39. Brown SF. The influence of grammatical function on the incidence of stuttering. *J Speech Hear Disord* 1937;24:390–397.
40. Brown SF. A further study of stuttering in relation to various speech sounds. *Q J Speech* 1938;24:390–397.
41. Brown SF. The loci of stuttering in the speech sequence. *J Speech Hear Disord* 1945;10:181–192.
42. Wingate ME. A standard definition of stuttering. *J Speech Hear Disord* 1964;29:484–489.
43. Wingate ME. *Stuttering Theory and Treatment*. New York: Irvington Publishers, 1976.
44. Wingate ME. *The Structure of Stuttering: A Psycholingusitic Approach*. New York: Springer-Verlag, 1988.
45. Bloom C. Articulation assessment. In M Daniloff (ed), *Stuttering Therapy*. San Diego: College-Hill Press, 1985.
46. Crystal D. Towards a "bucket" theory of language disability: Taking account of interaction between linguistic levels. *Clin Linguistic Phonetics* 1987;1:7–22.
47. Bloodstein O. *Stuttering: The Search for a Cause and a Cure*. Needham Heights, MA: Allyn and Bacon, 1993.
48. Logan K, Conture E. Length, grammatical complexity and rate differences in stuttered and fluent conversational utterances of children who stutter. *J Fluency Disord* 1995;20:35–61.

49. Brundage S, Bernstein Rotner N. The measurement of stuttering frequency in children's speech. *J Fluency Disord* 1989; 14:351–358.
50. Bernstein Rotner N. Stuttering: A Psycholinguistic perspective. In RJ Curlee, G Siegel (eds), *Nature and Treatment of Stuttering: New Directions* (2nd ed). Boston: Allyn and Bacon, 1997.
51. Starkweather CW. *Fluency and Stuttering*. Englewood Cliffs, NJ: Prentice Hall, 1987.
52. Johnson W. A study of the onset and development of stuttering. In W Johnson (ed), *Stuttering in Children and Adults*. Minneapolis: University of Minnesota Press, 1955.
53. Bloodstein O. *Stuttering: The Search for a New Cause and Cure*. Boston: Allyn and Baron, 1993.
54. Bloodstein O. *Speech Pathology: An Introduction*. Boston: Houghton Mifflin, 1979.
55. Bloodstein O. *A Handbook on Stuttering* (4th ed). Chicago: National Easter Seal Society, 1987.
56. Sheehan JG. Conflict theory and avoidance-reduction therapy. In J Eisenson (ed), *Stuttering: A Second Symposium*. New York: Harper and Row, 1975.
57. Skinner BF. *Verbal Behavior*. New York: Appleton-Century-Crofts, 1957.
58. Goldiamond I. Effects of delayed feedback upon the temporal development of fluent and blocked speech communication. Bedford, MA: Air Force Cambridge Research Center, 1960.
59. Goldiamond I. Stuttering and fluency as a manipulable operant response class. In L Krisner, L Ulmann (eds), *Research in Behavior Modification*. New York: Holt, Rinehart and Winston, 1965.
60. Martin RR, Siegel GM. The effects of simultaneously punishing stuttering and rewarding fluency. *J Speech Lang Hear Res* 1966;9:466–475.
61. Azrin NH. Effects of punishment intensity during variable-interval reinforcement. *J Exp Anal Behav* 1960;3:123–142.
62. Shames GH, Egolf DB. *Operant Conditioning and the Management of Stuttering: A Book for Clinicians*. Englewood Cliffs, NJ: Prentice Hall, 1976.
63. Shames GH, Rubin H. Concluding Remarks. In GH Shames, H Rubin (eds), *Stuttering: Then and Now*. Columbus, OH: Charles E. Merrill, 1986.
64. Brutten GJ, Shoemaker DJ. Tow-factor behavior theory and therapy. In GH Shames, H Rubin (eds), *Stuttering: Then and Now*. Columbus, OH: Charles E. Merrill, 1986.
65. Costello J. Operant conditioning and treatment of stuttering. *Semin Speech Lang* 1980;1:311–325.
66. Costello J. Current behavioral treatment for children. In D Prins, R Ingham (eds), *Treatment of Stuttering in Early Childhood : Methods and Issues*. San Diego: College-Hill Press, 1984.
67. Ingham R. *Stuttering and Behavior Therapy*. San Diego: College-Hill Press, 1984.
68. Brutten GJ, Shoemaker DJ. *The Modification of Stuttering*. Englewood Cliffs, NJ: Prentice Hall, 1967.
69. Guitar BE, Peters TJ. *Stuttering—An Integration of Contemporary Theories*. Memphis Speech Foundation, 1980.
70. Branden N. *How to Raise Your Self-Esteem*. New York: Bantam Books, 1987.
71. Curlee R. Counseling with adults who stutter. In WM Perkins (ed), *Stuttering Disorders*. New York: Thieme-Stratton, 1984.
72. Sanford LT, Donovan ME. *Women and Self Esteem*. New York: Penguin Books, 1984.

73. Steinem G. *Revolution from Within*. Boston: Little, Brown, 1993.
74. Rosenberg M. *Conceiving the Self*. New York: Basic Books, 1979.
75. Sheehan J. Theory and treatment of stuttering as an approach-avoidance conflict. In Shames GH, Rudin H (eds), *Stuttering: Then and Now*. Columbus: Charles E. Merrill, 1986.
76. Rotter JB. Generalized expectancies for internal versus external control of reinforcement. *Psychol Monographs* 1966;80:1–28.
77. Hale WD. Locus of control and psychological distress among the aged. *Int J Aging Hum Dev* 1986;21:1–8.
78. Lefcourt H. *Locus of Control: Current Trends in Theory and Research*. New York: John Wiley, 1976.
79. Lefcourt H. *Research with the Locus of Control Construct*. Vols. 1–3. New York: Academic Press, 1981–1984.
80. Rohsinon D, O'Leary M. Locus of control research on alcoholic populations. *Int J Addictions* 1987:13:2:213–226.
81. Craig AR, Franklin JA, Andrews G. A scale to measure locus of control behavior. *Brit J Med Psychol* 1984:57:173–180.
82. McDonough A, Quesal R. Locus of control orientation of stutterers and non stutterers. *J Fluency Disord* 1988:13:97–106.
83. Bloom C, Cooperman D. *The Clinical Interview: A Guide for Speech-Language Pathologists and Audiologists* (2nd ed). Rockville, MD: National Student Speech Language Hearing Association, 1992.
84. Seeman M, Seeman L. Health behavior and personal autonomy. *J Health Soc Behav* 1983:24:14–160.
85. Stephens MW, Delys P. Internal control expectations among disadvantaged children at pre-school age. *Child Dev* 1973:44:670–674.
86. Wischner S, Nowicki S. Independence training practices and locus of control orientation in children and adolescence. *Dev Psychol* 1976;12:77–80.
87. Gordon DA, Jones RH, Nowicki S. An objective measure of parental punitiveness. *J Pers Assess* 1979;43:485–496.
88. Seifart K, Hoffnung J. *Child and Adolescent Development*. Boston: Houghton Mifflin, 1986.
89. Leigh G, Peterson G. *Adolescents in Family*. Cincinnati: South Western Publishing, 1987.
90. Crandell U, Crandell B. Maternal and childhood behaviors as antecedents of internal-external control perceptions in young adulthood. In Lefcourt H (ed), *Research with the Locus of Control Construct*. Vol. 2. New York: Academic Press, 1983.
91. Zastrow C, Kirst-Ashman B. *Understanding Human Behavior and the Social Environment*. Chicago: Neson-Hall Publishers, 1987.
92. Hayes D, Rose C. Concern with appearance, health beliefs, and eating habits. *J Health Soc Behav* 1987;28:120–130.
93. Paulhus D, Christie R. Spheres of control: An interactivist approach to assessment of perceived control. In Lefcourt H (ed), *Research with the Locus of Control Construct*. Vol. 1. New York: Academic Press, 1981.
94. Germain RB. Beyond the internal–external continuum: The development of formal operational reasoning about control of reinforcements. *Adolescence* 1985;20(80): 939–947.
95. Craig Ar, Howie P. Locus of control and maintenance of behavioral therapy skills. *Br J Clin Psychol* 1982;21:67–68.
96. Rotter JB. Some problems and misconceptions related to the construct of internal versus external control of reinforcement. *Psychol Monographs* 1975;43:56–67.

97. Ingham R. Modification of maintenance during stuttering treatment. *J Speech Lang Hear Res* 1990;23:732–741.
98. Conture E, Wolk L. Stuttering. *Semin Speech Lang* 1990;11(3):200–211.
99. Jakubowski-Spector P. Assertion training. *Counseling Psychologist* 1972;4:76–85.
100. Butler PE. *Self-Assertion for Women.* New York: HarperCollins, 1992.
101. Rieber RW, Wollock J. The historical roots of the theory and therapy of stuttering. *J Commun Disord* 1977;10:3–24.
102. Shames G, Egolf D. *Operant Conditioning and the Management of Stuttering.* Englewood Cliffs, NJ: Prentice Hall, 1976.
103. Gregory HH. Environmental manipulation and family counseling. In G Shames, H Rubin (eds), *Stuttering: Then and Now.* Columbus, OH: Charles Merrill, 1986.
104. Starkweather CW, Gottwald CR, Halfond MM, et al. *Stuttering Prevention: A Clinical Method.* Englewood Cliffs, NJ: Prentice Hall, 1979.
105. ASHA Division 4 Newsletter, Nov, 1992.
106. Bolton R. *People Skills.* Englewood Cliffs, NJ: Prentice Hall, 1979.
107. Hepworth D, Larsen J. *Direct Social Work Practice.* Chicago: Dorsey Press, 1986.
108. Egan G. *The Skilled Helper* (3rd ed). Monterey, CA: Brooks/Cole, 1986.
109. Carkhuff RR. *Helping Human Relations.* Vol 2. Amherst, MA: Human Resource Development Press, 1984.
110. Mallard AR. Using families to help the school-age stutterer: A case study. In L Rustin (ed), *Parents, Families and the Stuttering Child.* San Diego, CA: Singular Publishing Group, 1991.
111. Myers SC, Freeman FJ. Interuptions as a variable in stuttering and disfluency. *J Speech Lang Hear Res* 1985:428–435.
112. Myers SC, Freeman FJ. Mother and child speech roles as a variable in stuttering and disfluency. *J Speech Lang Hear Res* 1985;28:436–444.
113. Myers SC, Freeman FJ. Are mothers of stutterers different? An investigation of so-cial-communicative interaction. *J Fluency Disord* 1985;10:193–209.
114. Riley GD, Riley J. Evalauation as a basis for intervention. In D Prins, RJ Ingham (eds), *Treatment of Stuttering in Early Childhood: Methods and Issues.* San Diego: College-Hill Press, 1983.
115. Conture EH, Caruso AJ. Assessment and diagnosis of childhood disfluency. In L Rustin, H Purser, D Rowley (eds), *Progress in the Treatment of Fluency Disorders.* London: Whurr, 1987.
116. Fairbanks, G. *Voice and Articulation Drillbook* (2nd ed). New York: Harper and Row, 1960.
117. Ramig P. Parent-clinician-child partnership in the therapeutic process of the pre-school and elementary aged child who stutters. *Semin Speech Lang* 1993;XIV 3:226–236.
118. Gregory HH, Hill D. Stuttering therapy for children. *Semin Speech Lang* 1980; 1(4):351–363.
119. Moore M, Nystul N. Parent-child attitudes and communication processes in fami-lies with stutterers and non-stutterers. *Br J Disordord Commun* 1979;14:173–180.
120. Riley GD. *Stuttering Prediction Instruments.* Tigard, OR: C.C. Publications, 1981.
121. Neill A. *Summerhill: A Radical Approach to Child Rearing.* New York: Hart Asso-ciates, 1960.
122. Shapiro DA. *Stuttering Intervention.* Austin, TX: Pro-Ed, 1999.
123. Brammer LM. Who can be a helper? *Personnel Guidance J* 1977;55:303–308.
124. Kennedy E. *On Becoming a Counselor.* New York: Continuum, 1980.
125. Rollin WJ. *The Psychology of Communication Disdordorders in Individuals and Their Families.* Englewood Cliffs, NJ: Prentice Hall, 1987.

126. Andrews JR, Andrews MA. *Family Based Treatment in Communication Disorders: A Systematic Approach.* Sandwich, IL: Jonelle Publications, 1980.
127. Bloom C, La Salla M. Family Therapy and Those Who Are Communicatively Impaired. Unpublished manuscript.
128. Battle DE. *Communication Disorders in Multicultural Populations.* Stoneham, MA: Butterworth-Heinemann, 1993.
129. *Statistical Abstract of the United States* (110th ed). Washington DC: US Department of Commerce, 1990.
130. Cole LE. *Pluribus unum: Multicultural imperatives for the 90's and beyond.* ASHA 1989;31(9):65–70.
131. Saville-Troike M. Anthropological considerations in the study of communication. In O Taylor (ed), *Nature of Communication Disorders in Culturally and Linguistically Diverse Populations.* San Diego: College-Hill Press, 1986.
132. Cheng L. Asian-american cultures. In B Battle (ed), *Communication Disorders in Multicultural Populations.* Stoneham, MA: Butterworth-Heinmann, 1993.
133. Corey M, Corey G. *Becoming a Helper.* Monterey, CA: Brooks Cole, 1989.
134. Johnson W. The Indians have no word for it: Stuttering in children. *Q J Speech* 1944;30:330–337.
135. Johnson W, et al. A study of the onset and development of stuttering. *Q J Speech.* 1953;18:168–174.
136. Snidecor J. Why the Indian does not stutter. *Q J Speech* 1947;33:493–495.
137. Cooper EB, Cooper CS. Fluency disorders. In D Battle (ed), *Communication Disorders in Multicultural Populations.* Stoneham, MA: Butterworth-Heinemann, 1993.
138. Lemert EM. Some Indians who stutter. *J Speech Lang Hear Res* 1953;18:168–174.
139. Liljeblad S. The Indians Have a Word for It. Presented to the Nevada State Speech Association, May 6, 1967.
140. Zimmerman GN, Liljeblad S, Frank A, Cleveland C. The Indians have many terms for it: Stuttering amoung the Bannock-Shoshoni. *J Speech Lang Hear Res* 1983;26:315–318.
141. Shames GH. Stuttering. An RFP for a cultural perspective. *J Fluency Disord* 1989;14:66–67.
142. Conrad C. Fluency in multicultural populations. In L Cole, V Deal (eds), *Communication Disorders in Multicultural Populations.* Rockville, MD: American Speech and Language Association, 1996.
143. Multicultural Action Agenda 2000. *ASHA* 1991;33:39–41.
144. McGoldrick M, Giordano J, Pierce J (eds), *Ethnicity in Family Therapy.* New York: Guilford Press, 1996;6.
145. Friere, P. *The Pedagogy of Hope.* New York: Continuum, 1994, p. 32.
146. Waltzman D. Multicultural Issues in the Counseling Process. Presented to the New York State Speech Language Hearing Association, May, 1993.
147. Wyatt T. *Multicultural Issues in Communication Disorders.* Fullerton, CA: University of California, 1997. Unpublished manuscript.
148. Germain C. An ecological perspective in casework practice. *Soc Casework* 1973;54:323–330.
149. Germain C. Ecology and social work. In C Germain (ed), *Social Work Practice: People and Environment.* New York: Columbia University Press, 1979;1–2.
150. Germain C. The ecological approach to people: Environmental transactions. *Soc Casework* 1981;62:323–331.
151. Taylor O. Historical perspectives and conceptual framework. In O Taylor (ed), *Treatment of Communication Disorders in Culturally and Linguistically Diverse Populations.* Austin, TX: Pro-Ed, 1986.

152. Taylor O, Stroud R, Hurst G, Moore E, Williams R. Philosophies and goals of the ASHA Black Caucus. *ASHA* 1969;11:221–225.
153. Wyatt T. Multicultural Issues in Communication Disorders, 1993. Unpublished manuscript.
154. Committee on the Status of Racial Minorities. *Multicultural Professional Education in Communication Disorders: Curriculum Approaches.* Rockville, MD: ASHA Publications, 1987:2.

3

Principles of Assessment

THEORETICAL AND CLINICAL CONSIDERATIONS

In Chapter 1 we proposed that evaluation of the dysfluent client must include the examination of physical, psychological (emotional), linguistic, and psychosocial patterns. In keeping with our synergistic philosophy, our goal is to isolate the social, cognitive, and biologic factors that are operational in the lives of our clients and to understand how these interact and affect the stuttering.

Because our view is synergistic, we think of assessment less as an attempt to determine the underlying causes of the disorder and more as an attempt to evaluate the areas of normal speech production in which breakdown has occurred. We subscribe to the multicausality explanation of stuttering: some individuals may stutter as a result of learning, immature development, language delay, and/or emotional factors, while others may stutter as a result of a neurologic disorder or a physiologic predisposition. Regardless of the etiologic considerations, we aim to carefully assess the respiratory, articulatory, and phonatory aspects of the speech disorder and the impact that the stuttering has upon the individual and the significant people in his or her life. In addition, we assess, both formally and informally, the client's language and phonologic skills, attitudes, and the environment in which they function. We assess each component of the synergistic model.

Evaluation is a process that is unique to each person. Each client comes to us with a different mosaic of behaviors and experiences to be analyzed and understood. The assessment plan must therefore be developed over time, based upon the expanding knowledge and awareness of each particular client's needs. It follows, then, that we understand evaluation to be an ongoing process. Our evaluation begins with the initial telephone contact and continues throughout the entire treatment process. Since, in our view, the major purpose of evaluation is to determine the nature and direction of treatment, as behaviors are modified the thrust of treatment necessarily must be reviewed and modified.

OVERVIEW OF THE COMPONENTS OF THE FLUENCY EVALUATION

Our evaluation begins with obtaining a complete case history (Table 3.1). Whenever possible, we send this questionnaire home in advance of the first interview so that the client or parents may have sufficient time to consider the answers to our questions. With a completed questionnaire available during the interview, we are able to probe more deeply the areas that seem most significant for that client. In addition to the standard information sought by speech-language pathologists for all other communication disorders, our case history for the individual who stutters includes questions about the reasons why evaluation is being sought at this time, family history of stuttering, the client's/parents' ideas about onset of the stuttering, changes since onset, previous treatment, fluency with various significant others in the client's environment, and tensions related to employment, family, or other social interactions. We will discuss the various elements of the case history in greater detail throughout this chapter.

Table 3.1   Stuttering Case History Interview by C. Bloom and D. Cooperman

---

CLIENT: PARENT:

ADDRESS: REFERRED BY:

TELEPHONE: DATE OF BIRTH:

DATE OF EVALUATION:

1. Please describe the speech pattern about which you are concerned.

_____

_____

2. Please explain why you are seeking evaluation and treatment at this time.

_____

_____

3. What were the circumstances surrounding the onset of the stuttering?

_____

_____

4. Has the stuttering pattern changed since onset? If so, please describe the changes.

_____

_____

5. Please describe any previous history of evaluation or treatment for stuttering or any other communication problem.

_____

_____

6. Please note any remarkable developmental history (i.e., motor, speech, or language development).

_____

_____

7. Please note any early or continuing medical concerns.

_____

_____

8. Please comment on educational issues or concerns.

_____

_____

9. Please describe the social skills of the client.

_____

_____

10. Does the fluency change with different family members? Please describe.

_____

_____

11. Is there a family history of stuttering or other speech disorders? Please describe:

_____

_____

12. Please describe any tension related to employment, family, or social interactions.

_____

_____

The questions that follow relate to children.

13. Please describe how family members respond to the child's dysfluency.

_____

_____

14. Please describe the child's social interactions at home and away from home.

_____

_____

15. Please describe the child's academic performance. Have there been recent changes?

_____

_____

16. Please describe the child's awareness and level of concern about stuttering.

_____

_____

_____

Using the case history form as our starting point, we spend time conducting personal interviews with the client and with as many significant others in the client's life as possible. In the case of a child, we might interview not only the parents and siblings but members of the extended family, the teacher, or other school personnel as well. It is through these interviews that we begin to gain some insight into the client's attitudes and feelings, as well as his or her environmental support system.

The formal and informal evaluation segments cover the speech and language components, of course, but they also include a close examination of the client's attitudes and feelings (with emphasis upon self-esteem, locus of control, and assertiveness) and the client's environment (with emphasis upon family support, interpersonal communication, and the influence of cultural factors). The initial interview with the client, during the first face-to-face meeting, is a time for both gathering information from as well giving information to the client and family. In an earlier publication, we more fully set forth our philosophy of the clinical interview and the procedure we follow in conducting it.[1]

SYNERGISTIC EVALUATION: CHILDREN AND ADULTS

The basic evaluation plan that we use with our adult clients is modified for children in various ways, depending upon the age of the child being treated. Using the synergistic model as our guideline, we divide our individualized assessment plan into three major areas: (1) Speech and Language, (2) Attitudes and Feelings, and (3) the Environment. As depicted in our diagram of the synergistic model (see Figure 1.1), the Speech and Language dimension includes physiologic, psycholinguistic, and learned factors; the Attitudes and Feelings dimension includes self-esteem, locus of control, and assertiveness factors; and the Environment dimension includes communication, family, and cultural factors. A description of each of these separately assessed areas follows.

ASSESSMENT OF SPEECH AND LANGUAGE

Physiologic Factors

As we earlier saw in Chapter 1, the physiologic factors subsumed under the Speech and Language dimension of a synergistic approach to fluency are those related to the elements of normal speech production: respiration, articulation/co-articulation, and phonation. We assess these dimensions by obtaining (and recording with both audio and videotape) a speech sample including reading, monologue, and conversation with a variety of partners.

Respiration

We observe respiratory patterns during structured and nonstructured speaking tasks to determine the adequacy of breath stream management. We are interested in learning whether the client's breathing pattern is deep or shallow, clavicular or abdominal, quiet or noisy. Does he hold his breath during speech attempts? Is there wastage of air? Is the airstream stopped at any point during the moment of stuttering? These are selected respiratory variables to be observed and noted in all spontaneous speech attempts during the interview and subsequent evaluation.

Phonation, Articulation, and Co-Articulation

The sample, as we mentioned above, is recorded (videotape is preferable to audiotape), and, as is the case with assessment of respiration, elements of articulation, co-articulation, and phonation are subjected to careful analysis. We may also administer formal articulation tests to both children and adults. In the case of a child, we might use the Goldman-Fristoe Test of Articulation[2] along with the Khan-Lewis Phonological Analysis,[3] since these are quickly administered and easily interpreted. For adults we might choose the sentence subtest of any frequently used tool including the Photo Articulation Test,[4] the Templin Darley Test of Articulation,[5] or the Arizona Articulation Proficiency Scale.[6]

Voice

We consider the voice evaluation to be a significant assessment area, since we have frequently seen individuals with fluency disorders who present with hoarseness, breathiness, and extreme vocal tension as a function of the vocal abuse that accompanies their stuttering patterns. Although we do not evaluate phonation instrumentally, in the event that a client's voice quality is judged to be perceptually abnormal, we refer him to a laryngologist for a medical opinion about vocal cord pathology.

Hearing

All clients routinely receive a hearing screening and an examination of the oral peripheral speech mechanism. These are the last of the physiological factors to be assessed.

Psycholinguistic Factors

The second level of analysis within the Speech and Language dimension is the psycholinguistic domain. We understand psycholinguistic factors to have a significant impact upon fluency skills. This area includes such elements as basic language competence (syntax, semantics, phonology), discourse skills, and pragmatic behaviors. We are interested in determining if the client demonstrates acceptable syntactic and semantic skills and age appropriate phonologic patterns, and whether she can maintain conversational rules and use language as a comfortable social tool. We often begin our analysis by reviewing client responses to the case history interview.

In the sections that follow, we will describe the psycholinguistic evaluation first of children and then of adults.

Special Considerations for Evaluating the Language of Dysfluent Children

Syntax and Semantics   When evaluating young dysfluent children who are nonreaders, we structure the evaluation session as we would for a language-delayed child in that we obtain a free speech language sample through structured play. We invite the parent or parents to participate in this play session so differences in fluency with familiar and unfamiliar conversational partners can be observed. A 100-utterance portion of the sample is transcribed, which is then subjected to a syntactic and semantic analysis based upon the conventions described by Miller.[7] The results of this analysis help us to determine whether the child needs language goals added to the fluency treatment plan, since this is a systematic way to assess such variables as acquisition of grammatical morphemes, use of age appropriate sentence structures (e.g., noun and verb phrase elaborations, questions, negatives), or knowledge and use of a wide variety of word meanings.

We use Riley's Stuttering Severity Instrument (SSI)[8] to obtain an objective measure of the client's stuttering severity based upon evaluation of the frequency of stuttering, the duration of stuttering blocks, and the physical concomitants of the stuttering pattern (Table 3.2). In addition, this tool gives us another opportunity to observe the linguistic complexity of the child's speech pattern. The synergistic model allows us to use the information obtained from this analysis of the SSI to plan treatment that emphasizes not only the remediation of the areas of normal speech production most clearly affected by the client's stuttering behavior, but the language-based issues related to the child's dysfluency as well. We will discuss our language-based approach to stuttering treatment in Chapters 4 and 5.

In addition to the SSI, we use the Ryan Interview[9] to help us understand the client's stuttering frequency in a hierarchy of speaking situations (Figure 3.1). Ryan's protocol divides specific speaking tasks into reading, monologue, and conversation, a division that further reinforces our individualized assessment philosophy, permits us to corroborate the severity rating of our subjective assessment, allows us to compare the severity rating with that obtained from the SSI, and enhances our ability to view our client's stuttering pattern in a variety of linguistic contexts.

We further measure frequency of stuttering by recording a speech sample and counting the number of stuttered words per minute, which can be converted into a score of percent of dysfluency.

Discourse   Discourse is one of the pragmatic areas of language. Bernstein and Tiegerman[10] stated that discourse relates to a child's ability to manage a communicative interaction with precision and clarity. Frequently, we see dysfluent children who have particular difficulty demonstrating the ability to initiate and/or maintain a conversation. Breakdowns may occur as a result of the absence of some fundamental skill such as eye gaze or a more linguistically so-

Table 3.2 Stuttering Severity Instrument by G. Riley

Name:_____ Sex:_____ Age:_____

Examiner:_____ Date:_____

Frequency (Use A or B, not Both)

A. For readers: Use 1 and 2   B. Nonreaders: Use Picture Task

1. Job Task		2. Reading Task		Picture Task	
% Score	Task Score	% Score	Task Score	% Score	Task Score
1	2	1	2	1	4
2–3	3	2–3	2	2–3	6
4	4	4–5	5	4	8
5–6	5	6–9	6	5–6	10
7–9	6	10–16	7	7–9	12
10–14	7	17–26	8	10–14	14
15–28	8	27+	9	15–28	16
29+	9			29+	18

TOTAL FREQUENCY SCORE A 1 & 2_____ or B:_____

DURATION: Estimated Length of Three Longest Blocks

Task Score	
Fleeting	1
One half second	2
One full second	3
2–9 seconds	4
10–30 seconds (by second hand)	5
30–60 seconds	6
More than 60 seconds	7

Total Duration Score:_____

PHYSICAL CONCOMITANTS

Evaluating Scale: 0=none; 1=not noticeable unless looking for it; 2=barely noticeable to the casual observer; 3=distracting; 4=very distracting; 5=severe and painful looking

1. Distracting Sounds. Noisy breathing, whistling, sniffing, blowing, clicking sounds..1 2 3 4 5

2. Facial Grimaces. Jaw jerking, tongue protruding, lip pressing, jaw muscles tense...1 2 3 4 5

3. Head movement. Back, forward, turning away, poor eye contact, constant looking around..1 2 3 4 5

4. Extremities movement. Arm and hand movement, hands about face, torso movement, leg movements, foot tapping or swinging.................1 2 3 4 5

Total Physical Concomitant Score:_____

TOTAL OVERALL SCORE:_____

Reprinted with permission from Riley GD. A stuttering severity instrument for children and adults. *J Speech Hear Disord* 1972;37:321. Reprinted by permission of the American Speech-Language-Hearing Association.

STUTTERING INTERVIEW
Procedure and Recording Form

Date:_____

Name:_____Birthdate:_____Age:_____

Speech Pathologist:_____

Time Sec.	Number of Stuttered Words	
		A. Automatic: 1. Count from 1-20 (less for younger children). 2. Say the alphabet or days of week or month. 3. Say a poem" or nursery rhyme.
		B. Echoic:. 4. cat man ice goodbye paper table stuttering cooperation yesterday competition over it near there on the table He can go. They won't do it. The cat jumped up. Mother and he will go to the store. Yesterday it rained for hours.
		C. Read: (Select material at or below reading level.) 5. "Read aloud." (1 minute)
		D. Pictures: (Any magazine or set of pictures) 6. Name 10 pictures 7. Tell a story about 2 pictures
		E. Speak with Puppet: (optional) 8. Have two puppets talk to each other (1 minute)
		F. Monologue: 9. Talk about recent movie, trip or TV show. (1 minute)
		G. Talk and Gesture: (optional) 10. Tell and show me how you would get a drink of water or put on clothes or hit a ball.
		H. Talk and Draw: (optional) 11. Draw something and tell about it. I will close my eyes and try to guess what it is from your talking.
		I. Questions: 12. "What is your name? Where do you work or attend school? What do you do there? Do you have brothers or sisters? Tell me about them. 13. "Ask me five questions."
		J. Conversation: 14. Engage in conversation. (2 minutes)
		K. Telephone: 15. Place three calls. (Total time 1 minute). Call airlines, bus, friend, relative. Answer a classified ad.

Figure 3.1 Stuttering Interview by B. Ryan. (Reprinted with permission from Ryan B. *Programmed Therapy for Stuttering Children and Adults.* Springfield, IL: Charles C. Thomas, 1974, p. 47.)

phisticated skill such as topic maintenance. Some of these children have particular difficulty engaging in narrative discourse.

Depending upon the age of the younger client, we may select a variety of formal language tests to aid in the determination of linguistic competence. We find that a valuable tool in the language assessment of the younger child (usually

STUTTERING INTERVIEW (SI)
FORM B
(Bruce Ryan)

Elementary/Junior High/Senior High/Adult

Name:_____   Age:_____Sex:_____

Tester:_____   Total: SW/M_____ Severity: 0 1 2 3 4

Data:_____   Reliability:_____%

Time Sec.	Number of Stuttered Words	
		A. Automatic: 1. "Count to 20" 2. "Say alphabet" or "days of week or "months of year" 3. "Say a poem" or "The Pledge of Allegiance" 4. "Sing a song"
		B. Echocic: (say after tester one at a time) 5. car Ann man goodbye paper interest stuttering amphibians cooperation specialization organizational representational constitutional some-day the-house into-the-car I can't find her. It's a good idea. Yesterday it rained for hours.
		C. Read: ("Amplifier" Passage with 300 words or comparable passage) 6. "Read aloud"
		D. Pictures: (any magazine) 7. Name 10 pictures
		E. Speak alone: (tester leaves room) 8. "Talk about anything" (1 minute)
		F. Monologue: 9. "Tell me about recent TV program or movie you saw" (1 minute)
		G. Questions: 10. "What is your name? Where do you work or attend school? What exactly do you do there? What does your father/husband do? What does your mother/wife do? How many are in your family? Tell me about them." 11. "Ask me five questions."
		H. Conversation: (tester may take case history) 12. Tester engages in conversation with person about his speech; history of the problem, previous therapy, therapy goals, difficult speaking situations, other problems (3 minutes).
		I. Telephone: 13. Place three calls. Call airlines or bus lines. "What time does the __ from __ arrive?" Call a friend or relative and chat. Answer a classified ad or call a store about a desired item. (Total time 1 minute).
		J. Observation in a natural setting: 14. Observe the person in conversation with someone other than the tester in a setting other than the test room. (3 minutes) Location_____ Other Person_____
		TOTAL: Total SW = _____ _____SW/M Total Time in Minutes

NOTES:

Figure 3.1   (continued)

age 8 and younger) is the Preschool Language Assessment Instrument (PLAI).[11] Although this is not a standardized instrument, it allows us to evaluate the child's fluency skills at four different levels of abstraction (see Chapter 5). The test probes both receptive and expressive language and calls upon higher levels of reasoning than many of the available standardized tools. Children are asked to match their perception, to selectively analyze their perception, to reorder their

Item, Mode, and Rate:

Readings: Total SW__WR__
Time____ =SW/M__WR/M__

Monologue: Total SW__WS__
Time____ =SW/M__WS/M__

Conversation: Total SW__WS__
Time____ =SW/M__WS/M__

Types:

W/W whole word
P/W part word
P Prolongation
S Struggle (secondaries)
O Other

\# one type
\# total types x 100 = %Types

Other (describe)_____

Severity	0	1	2	3
SW/M	0-.5	.6-5	6-10	11+
WS/M or	100+	90-99	70-89	69-
Type	W/W	P/W	P or O	S

TOTAL SCORE = _____
3

	SCALE	SEVERITY
0-.4	Normal	0
.5-1	Mild	1
1.1-2	Moderate	2
2.1-3	Severe	3

Figure 3.1 (continued)

perception, and to reason about their perception of various language-based tasks. We particularly like this tool because it allows us to observe varying levels of fluency while the child engages in verbal problem solving. It presents the child with tasks that tap the language of school discourse demands and gives us a sense of how well they will perform linguistically in a classroom setting.

We also use the Stocker Probe[12] as an evaluation tool for the young child because, like the PLAI, this instrument allows us to hear and assess the child's stuttering pattern at different levels of communicative demand (i.e., either-or and yes/no questions, simple wh-questions, more abstract wh-questions, listing of attributes, and story narrative tasks). Stocker hypothesized that as the level of communicative demand increases, the likelihood that there will be a breakdown in fluency also increases. Rather than relying solely upon parent report, using the Stocker Probe actually facilitates a breakdown in fluency in children who might otherwise remain fluent during a standard stuttering evaluation, thereby allowing the clinician to hear a sample of the child's dysfluent speech pattern.

The scoring conventions of the Stocker Probe require only the counting of dysfluencies. Stocker suggests that 1–10 dysfluencies equate to a normal to mild stutter; 11–20 dysfluencies equate to a moderate stutter; 21–30 dysfluencies equate to a severe stutter; and 31 or more dysfluencies equate to a very severe stutter. In addition to the suggested scoring protocols, when examining a child's response to the probes, we note the nature and type of dysfluencies that occur at each level of communicative demand. This gives us insight into the relationship between severity characteristics and the level at which breakdowns in fluency occur. In many of the children we have evaluated, the higher the level of communicative demand, the more severe the stuttering pattern, so that Level I questions may be answered with easy initial-sound repetitions, while Level V questions often are answered with blocks or prolongations accompanied by rising inflection.

Pragmatics　The pragmatic dimension of language relates to the individual's ability to engage in communicative interaction in a socially acceptable manner. Normally developing children learn very early to manage the communication context with such strategies as humor, requests, complaints, and demands. The child's pragmatic skills may be assessed formally, using a tool such as Shulman's Test of Pragmatic Skills,[13] or more informally, using Prutting's[14] or Roth and Spekman's[15] protocols for pragmatic assessment. With any of these tools, the goal is to learn something of the child's understanding of such conversational rules as turn taking, topic maintenance, and understanding speaker and listener roles. In addition, we want to assess the communicative functions language serves for the child and how he expresses communicative intentions.

Of course, observational skills used during the clinician's interaction with the younger client are still fundamental, since the pragmatic aspect of language is most clearly noted in the child's typical social interactions. It has been our experience that many children with fluency problems have difficulty, as well, in the use of language as a social tool. We think it important to define the nature of the pragmatic disorder, if it is present, so that we may include specific pragmatic tasks in our treatment program.

Special Considerations for Evaluating the Language of Adults

In evaluating the speech and language skills of an adult, our objective is to obtain a speech sample that will yield an adequate analysis of the verbal and nonverbal stuttering symptom pattern. We believe that it is important to engage the client in conversation, usually while obtaining history information. An additional sample can be obtained through various structured activities including reading, monologue, questions, automatic speech tasks, and conversation while using Ryan's Interview format.

In the event that there is a question about the adequacy of the adult client's linguistic competence, we might administer a formal language assessment tool appropriate for the evaluation of more sophisticated levels of impairment. We have used such instruments as the Test of Language Competence,[16] the Detroit Tests of Learning Aptitude (DTLA-2),[17] or the Test of Adult and Adolescent Word Finding.[18] These standardized tests provide a broad picture of the full range of language skills and help determine if the adult client's stuttering is influenced by word finding problems, an inability to organize and engage in abstract thinking, or difficulty focusing on linguistic tasks. In some cases, the fluency disorder may be secondary to a neurologic insult or deterioration. We have seen adult clients who, after improving their fluency, demonstrate difficulty engaging in logical, sequential, organized, and concise conversation. We suspect that this language deficit is more a result of lack of practice in conversational interaction—a deficit more in linguistic performance rather than in linguistic competence.

Learned Factors

The third and final assessment area to be considered under the dimension of speech and language is that of learned factors. Here, the attempt is to identify the behaviors of struggle, avoidance, and expectancy that the client may have learned in his efforts to abort or prevent stuttering. To this end, we use Woolf's Perceptions of Stuttering Inventory (PSI),[19] reproduced in Table 3.3, a tool that helps us understand how the client views his own stuttering behavior while allowing us to match his perceptions of that stuttering with our own. The PSI also yields a measurement of severity that can be compared with the severity levels of our informal assessment, the Riley SSI,[8] and the Ryan Interview[9] described previously.

Of course we continue to use our observational skills, as well, in the attempt to identify behaviors that might be characterized as struggle (overt physical behaviors that include tension, breathing irregularities, facial grimaces, etc.), avoidance (attempting to stay out of conversations, or to avoid talking in certain situations, etc.), and expectancy (feeling that stuttering is going to "happen" to them regardless of how hard they try to prevent it).

Since many of the components of stuttering are learned, we believe they can be changed. Whatever the etiology of their stuttering, people learn habits to compensate for or cope with their difficulty in speaking fluently. These habits should be identified and the frequency of their appearance recorded. A listing of the physical concomitants of stuttering should be completed once careful observation has been combined with the results of the Riley Instrument and Ryan Interview. This listing completes our assessment picture of the learned behaviors that accompany our client's stuttering.

ASSESSMENT OF ATTITUDES AND FEELINGS

Because stuttering is a multidimensional, synergistic disorder, we must include in our assessment the dimension of attitudes and feelings, which is the second spiral in our depiction of the synergistic approach to fluency therapy (see

Table 3.3 Perceptions of Stuttering Inventory by G. Woolf

The symbols S, A, and E after each item denote struggle (S), avoidance (A), and expectancy (E). In practice, these symbols are not included in the Inventory, but are listed on a separate scoring key.

Name:_____Age:_____#_____

Examiner:_____Date:_____%:_____

Directions:

Here are 60 statements about stuttering. Some of these may be characteristic of your stuttering. Read each item carefully and respond as in the examples below.

Characteristic of me:

_____Repeating sounds

Put a check mark under characteristic of me if "repeating sounds" is part of your stuttering; if it is not characteristic, leave the space blank. "Characteristic of me" refers only to what you do now, not to what was true of your stuttering in the past and which you no longer do, and not what you think you should or should not be doing. Even if the behavior described occurs only occasionally or only in some speaking situations, if you regard it as characteristic of your stuttering, check the space under characteristic of me.

THE ASSESSMENT OF STUTTERING

Characteristic of me:

_____ 1. Avoiding talking to people in authority (e.g., a teacher, employer, or clergyman). (A).

_____ 2. Feeling that interruptions in your speech (e.g., pauses, hesitations, or repetitions) will lead to stuttering. (E).

_____ 3. Making the pitch of your voice higher or lower when you expect to get "stuck" on words. (E).

_____ 4. Having extra and unnecessary facial movements (e.g., flaring your nostrils during speech attempts). (S).

_____ 5. Using gestures as a substitute for speaking (e.g., nodding your head instead of saying "yes" or smiling to acknowledge a greeting). (A).

_____ 6. Avoiding asking for information (e.g., asking for directions or inquiring about a train schedule). (A).

_____ 7. Whispering words to yourself before saying them or practicing what you are planning to say long before you speak. (E).

_____ 8. Choosing a job or a hobby because little speaking would be required. (A).

_____ 9. Adding an extra and unnecessary sound, word, or phrase to your speech (e.g., "uh," "well," or "let me see") to help yourself get started. (E).

_____ 10. Replying briefly using the fewest words possible. (A).

_____ 11. Making sudden, jerky, or forceful movements with your head, arms, or body during speech attempts (e.g., clenching your fist, jerking your head to one side). (S).

_____ 12. Repeating a sound or word with effort. (S).

Table 3.3 Perceptions of Stuttering Inventory by G. Woolf (continued)

_____ 13. Acting in a manner intended to keep you out of a conversation or discussion (e.g., being a good listener, pretending not to hear what was said, acting bored, or pretending to be in deep thought). (A).

_____ 14. Avoiding making a purchase (e.g., going into a store or buying stamps in the post office). (A).

_____ 15. Breathing noisily or with great effort while trying to speak. (S).

_____ 16. Making your voice louder or softer when stuttering is expected. (E).

_____ 17. Prolonging a sound or word (e.g., m-m-m-my) while trying to push it out. (S).

_____ 18. Helping yourself to get started talking by laughing, coughing, clearing your throat, gesturing, or some other body activity or movement. (E).

_____ 19. Having general body tension during speech attempts (e.g., shaking, trembling, or feeling "knotted up" inside). (S).

_____ 20. Paying particular attention to what you are going to say (e.g., the length of a word, or the position of a word in a sentence). (E).

_____ 21. Feeling your face getting warm and red (as if you are blushing) as you are struggling to speak. (S).

_____ 22. Saying words or phrases with force or effort. (S).

_____ 23. Repeating a word or phrase preceding the word on which stuttering is expected. (E).

_____ 24. Speaking so that no word or sound stands out (e.g., speaking in a singsong voice or in a monotone). (E).

_____ 25. Avoiding making new acquaintances (e.g., not visiting with friends, not dating, or not joining social, civic, or church groups). (A).

_____ 26. Making unusual noises with your teeth during speech attempts (e.g., grinding or clicking your teeth). (S).

_____ 27. Avoiding introducing yourself, giving your name, or making introductions. (A).

_____ 28. Expecting that certain sounds, letters, or words are going to be particularly "hard" to say (e.g., words beginning with the letter "s"). (E).

_____ 29. Giving excuses to avoid talking (e.g., pretending to be tired or pretending lack of interest in a topic). (A).

_____ 30. "Running out of breath" while speaking. (S).

_____ 31. Forcing out sounds. (S).

_____ 32. Feeling that your fluent periods are unusual, that they cannot last, and that sooner or later you will stutter. (E).

_____ 33. Concentrating on relaxing or not being tense before speaking. (E).

_____ 34. Substituting a different word or phrase for the one you had intended to say. (A).

_____ 35. Prolonging or emphasizing the sound preceding the one on which stuttering is expected. (E).

_____ 36. Avoiding speaking before an audience. (A).

_____ 37. Straining to talk without being able to make a sound. (S).

Table 3.3 Perceptions of Stuttering Inventory by G. Woolf (continued)

_____ 38. Coordinating or timing your speech with a rhythmic movement (e.g., tapping your foot or swinging your arm). (E).

_____ 39. Rearranging what you had planned to say to avoid a "hard" sound or word. (A).

_____ 40. "Putting on an act" when speaking (e.g., adopting an attitude of confidence or pretending to be angry). (E).

_____ 41. Avoiding the use of the telephone. (A).

_____ 42. Making forceful and strained movements with your lips, tongue, jaw, or throat (e.g., moving your jaw in an uncoordinated manner). (S).

_____ 43. Omitting a word, part of a word, or a phrase that you had planned to say (e.g., words with certain sounds or letters). (A).

_____ 44. Making "uncontrollable" sounds while struggling to say a word. (S).

_____ 45. Adopting a foreign accent, assuming a regional dialect, or imitating another person's speech. (E).

_____ 46. Perspiring much more than usual while speaking (e.g., feeling the palms of your hands getting clammy). (S).

_____47. Postponing speaking for a short time until certain you can be fluent (e.g., pausing before "hard" words). (E).

_____ 48. Having extra and unnecessary eye movements while speaking (e.g., blinking your eyes or shutting your eyes tightly). (S).

_____ 49. Breathing forcefully while struggling to speak. (S).

_____ 50. Avoiding talking to others of your own age group (your own or the opposite sex). (A).

_____ 51. Giving up the speech attempt completely after getting "stuck" or if stuttering is anticipated. (A).

_____ 52. Straining the muscles of your chest or abdomen during speech attempts. (S).

_____ 53. Wondering whether you will stutter or how you will speak if you do stutter. (E).

_____ 54. Holding your lips, tongue, or jaw in a rigid position before speaking or when getting "stuck" on a word. (S).

_____ 55. Avoiding talking to one or both of your parents. (A).

_____ 56. Having another person speak for you in a difficult situation (e.g., having someone make a telephone call for you or order for you in a restaurant). (A).

_____ 57. Holding your breath before speaking. (S).

_____ 58. Saying words slowly or rapidly preceding the word on which stuttering is expected (E).

_____ 59. Concentrating on how you are going to speak (e.g., thinking about where to put your tongue or how to breathe). (E).

_____ 60. Using your stuttering as the reason to avoid a speaking activity. (A)

Reprinted with permission of Woolf G. Assessment of stuttering as struggle, avoidance and expectancy. *Br J Disord Commun* 1967;2:168–171.

Figure 1.1). A treatment program that ignores the role of attitudes and feelings and refuses or fails to address them is doomed to failure. Although we think it possible to establish fluency skills without addressing the issues of attitudes and feelings, we do not think it possible for the client to stabilize and maintain those fluency skills over time unless this important area is systematically addressed. We use the Modified Erickson Scale of Communication Attitudes S-24,[20] reproduced in Table 3.4, as a tool to assess the general communication attitudes of adults in our program. Brutten's Children's Attitude Test[21] or Andre and Guitar's[22] A-19 Scale for Children Who Stutter serve a similar purpose in the assessment of our younger clients.

As we discussed in Chapter 2, positive attitudes and feelings are understood as part of the synergistic approach to promote or enhance one's self-esteem, help to internalize one's locus of control, and facilitate the development of assertiveness. At the same time, high self-esteem, internal locus of control, and a healthy level of assertiveness are likely to result in positive attitudes and feelings, as well as promote fluency. As we examine each of these factors separately below, it is important to remember their synergistic interaction.

Self-Esteem

Self-esteem begins to develop early in childhood. When the child is successful, she comes to believe she can be successful; when she is unsuccessful, she comes to believe that success is not within reach. The young child who struggles with fluency may soon learn that speaking is difficult and that she is not capable of speaking smoothly. Communication situations may become increasingly difficult for these children, whose self-esteem suffers as a result of these negative experiences.

We evaluate our clients' self-esteem through ongoing counseling and various paper and pencil tasks where appropriate. We may use such tools as the S-24 scale[20] (see Table 3.4), Rosenberg's Self-Esteem Scale[23] (see Table 3.5), or Woolf's Perceptions of Stuttering Inventory[19] to aid in our understanding of this crucial dimension of self-esteem.

Locus of Control

According to Craig, Franklin, and Andrews,[24] internal locus of control of one's personal behavior is an essential component of the ability to maintain behavior change. If an individual sees himself as capable of and responsible for control of his problem behaviors, there is a greater likelihood of long-term control of those behaviors. The Locus of Control of Behaviour Scale (LCB)[24] is a tool that is sensitive to issues of internality or externality of control of one's personal behaviors (Table 3.6). We use this scale to evaluate our clients' locus of control at the start of treatment, and then reassess this dimension periodically to determine if specific tasks should continue to be incorporated into the treatment program targeted at internalization of locus of control. Stuttering behavior revolves around

Table 3.4 Scale of Communication Attitudes S24 by G. Andrews and J. Cutler

1.	I usually feel I am making a favorable impression when I talk.	True	False
2.	I find it easy to talk with almost anyone.	True	False
3.	I find it very easy to look at my audience while speaking.	True	False
4.	A person who is my teacher or my boss is hard to talk to.	True	False
5.	Even the idea of giving a talk in public makes me afraid.	True	False
6.	Some words are harder than others for me to say.	True	False
7.	I forget all about myself shortly after I begin to give a speech.	True	False
8.	I am a good mixer.	True	False
9.	People sometimes seem uncomfortable when I am talking to them.	True	False
10.	I dislike introducing one person to another.	True	False
11.	I often ask questions in a group discussion.	True	False
12.	I find it easy to keep control of my voice when speaking.	True	False
13.	I do not mind speaking before a group.	True	False
14.	I do not talk well enough to do the kind of work I'd really like to do.	True	False
15.	My speaking voice is rather pleasant and easy to listen to.	True	False
16.	I am sometimes embarrassed by the way I talk.	True	False
17.	I face most speaking situations with complete confidence.	True	False
18.	There are few people I can talk with easily.	True	False
19.	I talk better than I write.	True	False
20.	I often feel nervous while talking.	True	False
21.	I find it very hard to make talk when I meet new people.	True	False
22.	I feel pretty confident about my speaking ability.	True	False
23.	I wish that I could say things as clearly as others do.	True	False
24.	Even though I know the right answer, I have often failed to give it because I was afraid to speak out.	True	False

SCORE_____

Reprinted with permission from Andrews G, Cutler J. Stuttering therapy: the relation between changes in symptom level and attitudes. *J Speech Hear Disord* 1974;39:318–319. Reprinted by permission of the American Speech-Language-Hearing Association.

issues of control, which therefore must be considered in the planning and implementation of a treatment program. We recommend a balance of internal and external responses as optimum for a positive outcome in stuttering treatment over the long term.

Paulhus and Christie[25] have introduced the concept of spheres of control, which we find to have a clear application to the control issues facing individuals

Table 3.5 Rosenberg Self-Esteem Scale

The Rosenberg Self-Esteem Scale (RSE) is a ten-item Guttman Scale with a Coefficient of Reproducibility of 92 percent and a Coefficient of Scalability of 72 percent. Respondents are asked to strongly agree (SA), agree (A), disagree (D), or strongly disagree (SD) with the following items (asterisks represent low self-esteem responses):

(1) On the whole, I am satisfied with myself.	SA	A	D*	SD*
(2) At times I think I am no good at all.	SA*	A*	D	SD
(3) I feel that I have a number of good qualities.	SA	A	D*	SD*
(4) I am able to do things as well as other people.	SA	A	D*	SD*
(5) I feel I do not have much to be proud of.	SA*	A*	D	SD
(6) I certainly feel useless at times.	SA*	A*	D	SD
(7) I feel that I'm a person of worth, at least on an equal plane with others.	SA	A	D*	SD*
(8) I wish I could have more respect for myself.	SA*	A*	D	SD
(9) All in all, I am inclined to feel that I'm a failure.	SA*	A*	D	SD
(10) I take a positive attitude toward myself.	SA	A	D*	SD*

Scoring conversions: This scale is based on contrived items and yields a seven-point scale.

Scale Item I is contrived from the combined responses to items 3, 7, and 9. If the respondent answers 2 out of 3 or 3 out of 3 positively, he receives a positive (that is, low self-esteem) score for Scale Item I. Scale Item II is contrived from the combined responses to items 4 and 5. One out of 2 or 2 out of 2 positive responses are considered positive for Scale Item II. Scale Items III, IV, and V are scored simply as positive or negative based on responses to items 1, 8, and 10. Scale Item VI is contrived from the combined responses to items 2 and 6. One out of 2 or 2 out of 2 positive responses are considered positive.

who stutter. They suggested the possibility that people have varying expectations for their ability to exercise control over their problem behaviors that are dependent upon the social situation. They further suggested that there are three major spheres in which an individual may express control: (1) the nonsocial, achievement domain in which a person gains control over various nonshared challenges or personal achievement goals; (2) the interpersonal domain in which one gains control over situations involving communicative interaction with others in a social setting; and (3) the sociopolitical domain in which the individual gains control over communicative interactions in the larger arena, usually when one takes a public position against some aspect of the status quo or in the face of conventional thinking.

In our synergistic view, we suspect that individuals who stutter may have particular difficulty exercising control primarily in the interpersonal domain, although the sociopolitical domain may surface as an area of difficulty as fluency

Table 3.6 Locus of Control Behavior Scale by A. Craig, J. Franklin, and G. Andrews

Directions: Below are a number of statements about how various topics affect your personal beliefs. There are not right or wrong answers. For every item there are a large number of people who agree and disagree. Could you please put in the appropriate bracket the choice you believe to be true. Answer all the questions.

0	1	2	3	4	5
Strongly Disagree	Generally disagree	Somewhat disagree	Somewhat agree	Generally agree	Strongly agree

1. I can anticipate difficulties and take action to avoid them. ( )
2. A great deal of what happens to me is probably just a matter of chance. ( )
3. Everyone knows that luck or chance determines one's future. ( )
4. I can control my problem(s) only if I have outside support. ( )
5. When I make plans, I am almost certain that I can make them work. ( )
6. My problem(s) will dominate me all my life. ( )
7. My mistakes and problems are my responsibility to deal with. ( )
8. Becoming a success is a matter of hard work; luck has little or nothing to do with it. ( )
9. My life is controlled by outside actions and events. ( )
10. People are victims of circumstances beyond their control. ( )
11. To continually manage my problems I need professional help. ( )
10. When I am under stress, the tightness in my muscles is due to things outside my control. ( )
13. I believe a person can really be the master of his fate. ( )
14. It is impossible to control my irregular and fast breathing when I am having difficulties. ( )
15. I understand why my problem(s) varies so much from one occasion to the next. ( )
16. I am confident of being able to deal successfully with future problems. ( )
17. In my case maintaining control over my problems is due mostly to luck. ( )

Score = _____ + _____   Sum Score = _____

Scoring: The 17-item test is scored in the same direction as the Rotter I-E scale, that is, high scores indicate externality. The ten items that relate to externality are tallied from the left-hand column of response boxes and the scores for the seven items related to internality (items 1, 5, 7, 8, 13, 15, and 16) are transposed so that 5 is scored as 0 (strongly disagree), 4 (generally agree) becomes 1 (generally disagree), etc. in the right-hand column of response boxes. After transposing the seven items the test is scored by summing the scores for all 17 items.

Reprinted with permission from Craig AR, Franklin JA, Andrews G. A scale to measure locus of control of behavior. *Br J Med Psychol* 1984;57:175.

develops, since the client may venture into more public and controversial situations as he gains confidence in his ability to control the stuttering. This area of research in locus of control and spheres of control offers promise in terms of increasing our understanding of how best to assess and then address issues of control in our stuttering treatment programs.

Assertiveness

An assertive speaker is one who is confident that her message will be of interest to or well received by the conversational partner(s). We understand assertiveness to be an essential component in successful communication experiences. It is assessed informally throughout treatment as a part of the ongoing counseling component of our program. We attempt to heighten our clients' awareness of assertiveness issues by engaging in what Butler[26] has called the "assertive analysis." As shown in Table 3.7, Butler predicted that when clients are encouraged to identify situations in which they are least apt to assert themselves, four areas of difficulty would likely be chosen by nonassertive individuals: expressing positive

Table 3.7   Assertiveness Scale by P. Butler

Checklist for Assertiveness with Different People

Category	Positive Feelings	Negative Feelings	Setting Limits	Self-Initiations
1. Strangers	_____	_____	_____	_____
2. People in authority	_____	_____	_____	_____
3. Members of opposite sex	_____	_____	_____	_____
4. Older people	_____	_____	_____	_____
5. People I want to like me	_____	_____	_____	_____
6. People close to me	_____	_____	_____	_____
7. People I supervise	_____	_____	_____	_____
8. My partner (spouse)	_____	_____	_____	_____
9. My father	_____	_____	_____	_____
10. My mother	_____	_____	_____	_____
11. Teenagers	_____	_____	_____	_____
12. My children	_____	_____	_____	_____
13. Others	_____	_____	_____	_____
Difficulty factor	_____	_____	_____	_____

Reprinted with permission from Butler PE. *Self-Assertion for Women.* San Francisco: Harper, 1982:22.

feelings, expressing negative or protective feelings, engaging in the setting of limits, and acting as the initiator in a communicative interaction. Our clients examine their assertiveness in relation to these four areas with various people with whom they are bound to interact. They are encouraged to ask themselves how assertive they are in expressing positive and negative feelings, setting limits, and initiating conversations or interactions with people. Each of these areas is then ranked from least difficult (1) to most difficult (4) by the client for each of the 13 categories of people with whom they interact. Once this has been completed, the total scores for each area are added and the areas of greatest difficulty and least difficulty can be clearly defined. This process facilitates a heightened awareness of assertiveness for the client.

Through this analysis procedure, clients become sensitized to those areas in which they have particular difficulty expressing themselves. The resulting information may then serve as a topic in the counseling portion of the treatment process, as well as assisting the therapist in planning role plays or other treatment activities.

ASSESSMENT OF THE ENVIRONMENT

The final area of assessment in the synergistic approach to fluency therapy is the environment in which the client functions. This environment is defined by the client's interpersonal communication skills, family composition and support, and cultural background. It is the clinician's responsibility to identify and understand the nature and interaction of these variables and to determine the role each one plays in an individual's stuttering history.

Interpersonal Communication Skills

Interpersonal communication is anchored in the pragmatic dimension of language and relates to the ways in which the client uses both verbal and nonverbal behaviors to manage social situations. We have found that many of the individuals whom we treat have increasingly more difficulty as the environmental demands or the number of communicative partners in any given interaction increases. The assertive analysis described in the previous section helps to shed light upon areas of communicative difficulty within the environment of the client. In addition, we apply Butler's[25] Influence Analysis procedure, one which facilitates the clients' ability to identify the significant people in their lives—that is, those who exert the greatest influence—and to examine how they deal with these influential people. Once these "influencers" have been identified, we suggest that the clients consider what kind of influence each of these people exerts, whether it is positive or negative. Next, clients are asked to examine how they respond to the "influencers," and finally they are asked to note any patterns of their behavior with these significant people. By working through this sort of analysis, our clients may learn to change their behavior.

Family-Related Issues

The variable of the family is a significant one in our understanding of the synergy of stuttering in our clients. We seek to understand not only the impact of family members on the individual's stuttering pattern but also the family history as it relates to stuttering incidence. The Influence Analysis[26] described above is one tool that may be helpful in uncovering family dynamics, since many of the "influencers" may be members of the client's immediate or extended family.

In order to obtain additional information in this assessment of issues related to the family, we must obtain a careful case history as described above. This provides a picture of the family interactions as well as the larger context of the environment in which our client functions.

First we question our clients as to why an evaluation is sought at that particular time and the level of family support for the client's decision to seek treatment. We are frequently surprised by the variety of answers we receive to the first question. Some clients seek treatment for work-related reasons (e.g., job advancement, job selection, career change) while others tell us that they no longer want to give up personal control and have come for stuttering treatment because it's time they took their lives into their own hands. Often we are able to predict outcomes based upon the perceived level of motivation at the outset of treatment and the level of commitment demonstrated not only by the client but by the significant others in his life.

Questions related to onset of stuttering behavior help us to understand the client's or family's perceptions about possible etiology. We are interested not only in whether onset was related to environmental change or stress but also whether there have been changes in the stuttering pattern since onset. It has been interesting to note the various theories that clients or their families have about the reasons for the development of stuttering. One parent suggested that her 13-year-old son stuttered because he "worshipped" his grandfather whose speech was very dysfluent, and the boy imitated his grandfather to keep his memory alive after the older man died. Another parent thought her son stuttered because he rode in the "way-back" of a station wagon on a long and bumpy trip from New York to Michigan when he was three years old. Questions about onset help us to understand which issues may be suitable topics for counseling of the client or family members.

Medical, developmental, educational, and social histories are obtained including the changing patterns of fluency with various family members and others. The family history of fluency disorders or other speech and language disorders is explored, as is the presence of tension related to employment, family, or current social interactions. Again, the information obtained from these kinds of questions helps in planning the topics for counseling throughout therapy. In the case of a child, we are interested in learning about the family members' responses to stuttering, the level of social interaction at home and away from home, the child's academic performance, especially changes in long-term performance, and the child's level of awareness and concern relative to the frequency and severity of the stuttering.

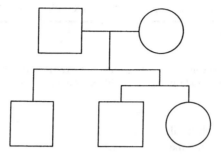

Figure 3.2 Genogram from C. Bloom and D. Cooperman. Directions: A marriage is indicated by drawing a line from a square (man) to a circle (woman); the marital date is added to the line. Children are added according to age, beginning with the oldest on the left. A divorce generally is portrayed by a dotted line and date. A death is indicated by drawing an "X" through the figure and dating it. (Reprinted with permission from Bloom CM, Cooperman DK. *The Clinical Interview: A Guide for Speech-Language Pathologists and Audiologists.* Rockville, NY: NYSSLHA, 1992, p. 82.)

It is sometimes helpful to draw a genogram, as shown in Figure 3.2, as a more formal tool to assist understanding complex family relationships and how they impact upon our client's fluency.[1] Some of the information that can be diagrammed with the genogram includes naming patterns, birth order, major family losses, relationships, educational backgrounds, family functioning, and other critical events.

Cultural Factors

The area of ethnographic study discussed in Chapter 2 is in its infancy in its clinical application in speech-language pathology. Nevertheless, we believe that an understanding of the cultural background of one's clients is often imperative in assessing the prognosis for learning and maintaining a stuttering control. Each culture, each community, has its communication "values." Until we know these values, we may be expecting behaviors and attitudes that are in direct conflict with the clients' cultural traditions and taboos. While some cultures may accept the presence of stuttering with little concern or notice, others may interpret it as a punishment of the family or one of its members. Clearly, the way in which one's family culture views this communication disorder will have a significant impact upon the ultimate outcomes of treatment. It is through the process of gathering a case history that we are most likely to identify the pertinent cultural factors.

Once the case history has been obtained either through interview alone or the combination of interview and parent/client questionnaire, we will have a clearer idea of the client's interpersonal communication skills, family composi-

Table 3.8   Fluency Evaluation Summary Sheet by C. Bloom and D. Cooperman

---

I. Speech and Language

    A. Physiologic Variables

    1. Observations of Respiration: please note abbreviations that apply: wnl = within normal limits; sh = shallow; aud = audible. Comment where appropriate.

      a. Reading

      b. Monologue

      c. Conversation with familiar partners

      d. Conversation with unfamiliar partners

    2. Observations of Articulation: please note abbreviations that apply: wnl = within normal limits; pra = phonological rules apply; ad = articulation disorder noted. Describe your observations.

      a. Reading

      b. Monologue

      c. Conversation with familiar partners

      d. Conversations with unfamiliar partners

    3. Observations of Phonation: please note abbreviations that apply: wnl = within normal limits; q = voice quality draws attention to itself; hp = pitch too high; lp = pitch too low. Describe your observations.

      a. Reading

      b. Monologue

      c. Conversation with familiar partners

      d. Conversation with unfamiliar partners

    4. Stuttering Severity Scale

      a. List formal measures and indicate ratings

      b. Therapist's observations

    5. Hearing Screening Results (check appropriate item)

      _____Passed

      _____Failed

    6. Oral Peripheral Examination Results (check appropriate items)

      _____Wnl

      _____Movements slow (describe)

      _____Movements imprecise (describe)

      _____ Drooling noted

    B. Psycholinguistic Variables

    1. Syntactic skills. List formal measures and include scores:
Informal observations:

    2. Semantic skills. List formal measures and include scores:
Informal observations:

    3. Pragmatic skills. List formal measures and include scores:
Informal observations:

Table 3.8 Fluency Evaluation Summary Sheet (continued)

    C. Learned Factors. List formal measures and includes scores:
    1. Struggle behaviors (describe briefly)
    2. Avoidance behaviors (describe briefly)
    3. Expectancy behaviors (describe briefly)

II. Attitudes and Feelings
    A. Self-esteem. List formal measures and include scores:
        Informal observations:
    B. Locus of control. List formal measures and include scores:
        Informal observations:
    C. Assertiveness. List formal measures and include scores:
        Informal observations:

III. Environment
    A. Interpersonal skills (describe):
    B. Observations of family composition and support (describe):
    C. Cultural considerations (list and describe cultural influences noted by the
        examiner):

---

tion, and cultural background and values. Once our evaluation has been completed, the results are entered on the fluency evaluation summary sheet (Table 3.8), where they can be summarized in an organized and systematic manner. It is from this summary that specific elements of treatment can be identified and targeted. Those domains that are most deviant from the normal speech production model will be targeted most specifically, although each of the areas outlined in our synergistic approach will naturally be targeted to some degree.

SYNERGISTIC EVALUATION

Some Additional Concerns and Issues Specific to Children

As we have described, the assessment of the dysfluent child includes the same elements as that of the adult—namely, a speech and language evaluation, an attitudinal evaluation, and an environmental evaluation. The assessment process assists the clinician in making a number of important decisions. In the case of the young child, it is the assessment that allows the clinician to judge whether the communication pattern should be considered stuttering or normal nonfluency. We use the criteria described by Adams[27] and Pindzola and White[28] as the primary tools for making this determination.

There is a consistency between the areas described and the criteria formulated by Adams and Pindzola and White, the major difference being that Pindzola's work has been organized for the clinician as a convenient assessment checklist. Pindzola's

PROTOCOL FOR DIFFERENTIATING THE
INCIPIENT STUTTERER

Rebekah H. Pindzola, Ph. D.
Auburn University, Alabama

Date of birth___

Age___ Sex___
Name_____ Date of Test
Clinician

Address_____

I. AUDITORY BEHAVIORS

TYPE OF DISFLUENCY (mark the most typical)

Interjections	Hesitations/Gaps- Repetitions	Prolongations- Coexisting Struggle
Probably Normal	Questionable	Probably Abnormal

SIZE OF SPEECH UNIT AFFECTED (mark the typical level at which dysfluencies occur)

Sentence/phrase	Word/Sound	Syllable
Probably Normal	Questionable	Probably Abnormal

Figure 3.3 Protocol for differentiating the incipient stutterer by R. Pindzola. (Reprinted with permission from Pindzola R. White D. Protocol for differentiating the incipient stutterer. *Lang Speech Hear Services in Schools* 1986;17:12–15.)

protocol includes assessment of such auditory behaviors as the type and frequency of dysfluency; the size of the speech unit; the frequency of prolongations and dysfluencies in general; the duration of dysfluencies including number of reiterations; the audible effort present including glottal attacks, disrupted airflow, vocal tension, and pitch variations; the rhythm of speech; schwa intrusion; and the use of substitutions, circumlocutions, and avoidances. She has further evaluated the visual evidence of stuttering commonly referred to as "concomitant" or "associated" behaviors, as well as the historical and psychosocial symptoms including such areas as

DURATION OF DISFLUENCIES

Typical Number of Reiterations of the Repetition=

Less than 2	2 to 5	More than 5
Probably Normal	Questionable	Probably Abnormal

Average Duration of Prolongations=_____

Less than 1 sec.	One or more seconds
Probably Normal	Probably Abnormal

AUDIBLE EFFORT (mark those that apply)

Lack of the following:	Presence of the following:
Probably Normal	Probably Abnormal

_____hard glottal attacks
_____disrupted airflow
_____vocal tension
_____pitch rise
_____others:

Figure 3.3 (continued)

family history, awareness and concern of the client and/or significant family members, and client fears and avoidances (Figure 3.3).

We do not agree with the position taken by some clinicians that the speech-language pathologist can only evaluate a nonfluent child if he is actually stuttering during the assessment. We understand that nonfluency in young children varies with many factors, and that a child may be an incipient stutterer and still present fluent speech during the diagnostic evaluation session. We make every effort to place the child in a variety of speaking situations during the assessment, planning a hierarchy of speaking tasks that might be likely to facilitate stuttering behavior, and including such formal evaluation tools as the Stocker Probe[12] and the

FREQUENCY OF DISFLUENCIES (compute from speech sample and mark values on continua)

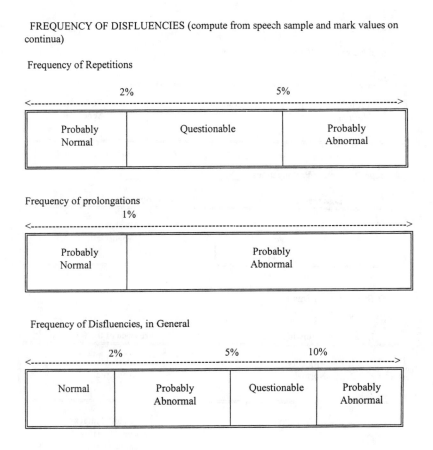

Frequency of Repetitions

Frequency of prolongations

Frequency of Disfluencies, in General

Figure 3.3 (continued)

Preschool Language Assessment Instrument[11] mentioned earlier (and later discussed in Chapter 5), which expose the client to increasingly higher levels of communicative and linguistic demand. However, in the event that we hear no dysfluent speech, we initially accept the parent's assessment of the communication disorder. We attempt to objectify parent information by using, for example, Riley's Stuttering Prediction Instrument,[29] a parent questionnaire protocol that serves much the same function as the Pindzola and White inventory.

We are influenced in our approach by the work of Starkweather and his associates[30] in taking the position that all parental concerns about dysfluency must be treated seriously. It is better to treat a normally dysfluent child and family, a child who might ordinarily "outgrow" the tendency to nonfluent speech, than to take the chance of denying treatment to an incipient stutterer. We also believe that early intervention is more efficient and cost effective than the "wait and see"

RHYTHM/TEMPO/SPEED OF DISFLUENCIES

Slow/normal; evenly paced	Fast, perhaps, irregular
Probably Normal	Probably Abnormal

INTRUSION OF SCHWA VOWEL DURING REPETITIONS

Schwa not heard	Presence of Schwa
Probably Normal	Probably Abnormal

AUDIBLE LEARNED BEHAVIORS (mark those that apply)

Lack of the following:	Presence of the following:
Probably Normal	Probably Abnormal

_____ word/ phrase substitutions
_____ circumlocutions
_____ Avoidance tactics (starters, postponers, and the like)

Figure 3.3   (continued)

approach, because it has been our experience that early treatment is generally short term with an excellent prognosis.

SUMMARY

In this chapter, we have described a comprehensive evaluation procedure that includes assessment of the Speech and Language, the Attitudes and Feelings, and the Environment of the individual who stutters. Each of these three areas was viewed as a separate but related dimension with its own components that, when integrated, would yield a more complete and synergistic analysis of the factors affecting a client's fluency. Our model underscores the notion that each client is an individual with his or her own issues, and that in order to be effective, treatment must be tailored to these individual factors.

II. VISUAL EVIDENCE (list behaviors observed)

FACIAL GRIMACES/ ARTICULATORY POSTURING:

HEAD MOVEMENTS:

BODY INVOLVEMENT:

III. HISTORICAL/ PSYCHOLOGICAL INDICATORS (comment on the following based on client and/ or parent interviews, observations, and supplemental test or questionnaires, if any.)

AWARENESS AND CONCERN (of child; of parents):

LENGTH OF TIME FLUENCY PROBLEM HAS EXISTED:

CONSISTENT VERSUS EPISODIC NATURE OF PROBLEM:

REACTION TO STRESS:

PHONEME/WORD/SITUATION FEARS AND AVOIDANCES:

FAMILIAL HISTORY:

OTHER COVERT FACTORS:

IV. SUMMARY OF CLINICAL EVIDENCE AND IMPRESSION

Figure 3.3   (continued)

REFERENCES

1. Bloom CM, Cooperman DK. *The Clinical Interview: A Guide for Speech-Language Pathologists and Audiologists.* Rockville, NY: NYSSLHA, 1992.
2. Goldman R, Fristoe M. *Test of Articulation.* Circle Pines, MN: American Guidance Service,1986.
3. Khan L, Lewis N. *Phonological Analysis.* Circle Pines, MN: American Guidance Service, 1986.
4. Pendergast K, Dickey S, Selmar J, Soder A. *Photo Articulation Test.* Danville, IL: Interstate, 1969.
5. Templin MC, Darley FL. *The Templin Darley Tests of Articulation.* Iowa City, IA: Bureau of Educational Research and Service, University of Iowa, 1969.
6. Fudala J. *Arizona Articulation Proficiency Scale.* Los Angeles: Western Psychological Services, 1974.
7. Miller J. *Assessing Language Production in Children: Experimental Procedures.* Baltimore, MD: University Park Press, 1981.
8. Riley GD. A stuttering severity instrument for children and adults. *J Speech Hear Disord* 1972;37:314–322.

9. Ryan B. *Programmed Therapy for Stuttering Children and Adults*. Springfield, IL: Charles C. Thomas, 1974.
10. Bernstein D, Tiegerman EM. *Language and Communication Disorders in Children*. Columbus, OH: Merrill, 1985.
11. Blank M, Rose S, Berlin L. *Preschool Language Assessment Instrument*. New York: Grune and Stratton, 1978.
12. Stocker B. *The Stocker Probe Technique: For Diagnosis and Treatment of Stuttering in Young Children*. Tulsa, OK: Modern Education Corp., 1980.
13. Shulman B. *Test of Pragmatic Skills*. Tucson, AZ: Communication Skill Builders, 1987.
14. Prutting C. Pragmatic assessment tool. *J Speech Hear Disord* 1987;52:105–119.
15. Roth F, Spekman N. Assessing the pragmatic abilities of children: Part 2. Guidelines, considerations and specific evaluation procedures. *J Speech Hear Disord* 1984;49:12–17.
16. Wiig EH, Secord W. *Test of Language Competence: The Psychological Corp*. San Antonio, TX: Harcourt Brace, Jovanovich, Inc., 1988, 1987.
17. Baker HJ, Leland B. *Detroit Tests of Learning Aptitude (DTLA-2)*. Indianapolis, IN: Bobbs-Merrill, 1967.
18. German DJ. *Test of Adult and Adolescent Word Finding*. Austin, TX: Pro Ed, 1990.
19. Woolf G. Assessment of stuttering as struggle, avoidance and expectancy. *Br J Disord Commun* 1967;2:158–171.
20. Andrews G, Cutler J. Stuttering therapy: the relation between changes in symptom level and attitudes. *J Speech Hear Disord* 1974;39:312–319.
21. Brutten G, Dunham S. The communication attitude test: A normative study of grade school children. *J Fluency Disord* 1989;14:371–377.
22. Andre S, Guitar B. A-19 scale for children who stutter. In B. Guitar (ed), *Stuttering: An Integrated Approach to Its Nature and Treatment*. Baltimore, MD: William and Wilkins, 1998.
23. Rosenberg, *Self-Esteem Scale: From Conceiving the Self*. New York: Basic Books, Inc., 1979.
24. Craig AR, Franklin JA, Andrews G. A scale to measure locus of control of behavior. *Br J Med Psychol* 1984;57:173–180.
25. Paulhus D, Christie R. Spheres of control: An interactionist approach to assessment of perceived control. In H. Lefcourt (ed), *Research with the Locus of Control Construct*. Vol. 1. New York: Academic Press, 1981.
26. Butler PE. *Self-Assertion for Women*. San Francisco: Harper, 1982:22.
27. Adams M. The differential assessment and direct treatment of stuttering. In J Costello, A Holland (eds), *Handbook of Speech and Language Disorders*. San Diego, CA: College Hill Press, 1986;261–290.
28. Pindzola R, White D. Protocol for differentiating the incipient stutterer. *Lang Speech Hear Services in Schools* 1986;17:2–15.
29. Riley GD, Riley J. A component model for diagnosing and treating children who stutter: Part 1. Organization and assessment parameters. *J Fluency Disord* 1979;4:279–294.
30. Starkweather CW, Gottwald CR, Halfond MM. *Stuttering Prevention: A Clinical Method*. Englewood Cliffs, NJ: Prentice Hall, 1991.

4

Overview of Treatment

By its very nature, synergy implies change, growth, and movement. Our view of treatment is grounded in the belief that good clinical practice requires frequent assessment and revision of the plan based upon client performance and client progress. We do not offer a single or didactic scripted program; such an approach is not best suited to meeting the needs of people who stutter. Instead we offer a philosophy of treatment that requires a strong theoretical foundation in the communication process as it relates to the disorder of stuttering. This philosophy combines elements of both fluency shaping and symptom modification approaches to stuttering treatment (see Table 4.1). As we introduce and develop our approach, we hope that readers will consider adopting our treatment process rather adhering to some rigid, step-by-step protocol for the delivery of stuttering treatment. This brief chapter is a general overview of treatment and serves only to introduce various concepts. The chapters that follow will describe our treatment process in greater detail.

A PHILOSOPHICAL FOUNDATION FOR TREATMENT

We view stuttering treatment as a long-term, in fact a life-long, process. Our active treatment stage lasts from four to five years, and our maintenance stage continues for an indefinite period, depending upon the requirements of the individual. We understand the clinician to be a partner in the treatment process rather than a mere instrument for the delivery of fluency. Clients are involved from the start in goal setting and lesson planning. Treatment is individualized for each client based upon the results of the assessment described in Chapter 3 and upon the needs and concerns brought by these clients as they enter the program. Goals are revised frequently, as clients or therapists identify new concerns. Each phase of treatment brings changes in all the treatment domains (speech and language, attitudes and feelings, environmental management). As these changes occur, client or therapist priorities may change with them.

Table 4.1 Integration of Treatment Approaches[1]

(Compares the synergistic approach to treatment with fluency shaping and stuttering modification approaches in order to highlight the way in which we integrate the two with a more holistic philosophy.)

Fluency Shaping	Stuttering Modification	Synergistic
Little or no attention to attitudes, fears, or avoidances	Major interest and focus on attitudes, fears, and avoidances	Major interest and focus on attitudes, fears, and avoidances
Little or no attention to client analysis of stuttering behaviors	Major interest and focus on client analysis of stuttering behaviors	Major interest and focus on client analysis of stuttering behaviors
Does not deal with modification of stuttering spasms	Primary goal is to modify stuttering spasms	Major goal is to modify stuttering spasms
Primary goal is to establish fluency	Does not deal with establishment of fluency	Major goal is practice of specific fluency targets
Self-monitoring may or may not be emphasized	Self-monitoring is emphasized	Self-monitoring is emphasized
Baselines are described in quantitative terms	Baselines are described in qualitative terms	Baselines are described in quantitative terms
Progress is measured in quantitative terms	Progress is measured in qualitative terms	Progress is measured in both quantitative and qualitative terms
Treatment emphasizes conditioning or programming	Treatment emphasizes rapport, motivation, teaching, and counseling	Treatment combines conditioning with such cognitive strategies as rapport, motivation, teaching, and counseling
Treatment is the same for all clients; may be scripted	Treatment is based on individual client needs	Treatment is individualized for each client, but the structure is preplanned
Little attention to pragmatic language	Little attention to pragmatic language	Major goal is improved pragmatic language
Transfer activities occur early and are generally planned	Transfer activities are generally planned and occur after establishment of modification techniques	Transfer activities occur early and are carefully planned
Maintenance is generally planned and gains are evaluated for varying follow-up periods	Maintenance may be planned but is often unsystematic and dependent on client interest	Maintenance is carefully planned and monitored for a five-year period

Adapted from Ham R. *Therapy of Stuttering*. Englewood Cliffs, NJ: Prentice Hall, 1990, p. 119.

THE PROGRAM

The first year of treatment emphasizes the learning and transfer of new speaking skills and the exploration of affective (assertiveness, self-esteem, locus of control), and environmental (family, communicative stress, cultural) issues. The next three years of treatment are devoted to maintaining these newly learned skills while taking an ever-increasing leadership role in the support group structure. The last year of formal treatment encourages more independent maintenance with access to a professional at the request of the client.

As is the case with all forms of communication intervention, the treatment cycle may be divided into four separate components: establishment, stabilization, transfer, and maintenance. Although these frequently overlap, it is convenient to examine them separately.

Components of the Establishment Phase

In the establishment phase, the fluency skills are taught and practiced in a highly structured and preferably intensive treatment environment. In our setting we offer an intensive Weekend Workshop each year to introduce newcomers to our treatment program. During this workshop, a theme is presented that serves as the vehicle for the weekend's activities. The "theme concept" has become a strong motivational device that energizes the participants and fosters a powerful group dynamic. Clients are taught target fluency facilitating behaviors that are compatible with normal speech production. In addition, they are exposed to strategies for enhancing self-esteem, internalizing locus of control, increasing assertiveness, and exercising control over the various environments in which they function. After the completion of the workshop, participants are invited to attend weekly sessions at what we refer to as the "Council for Fluency," a combined individual and group therapy program that serves both treatment and support group purposes. The Council meets throughout the year one night each week. The first hour of each Council meeting functions as a support group; it is planned and led by Council members with professionals and graduate students monitoring the group and serving as consultants to Council members. The second hour of each Council meeting is dedicated to individual treatment sessions.

Individuals who are unable to participate in the Weekend Workshop may enter our program through the campus clinic. We attempt to maintain the intensive nature of the experience during this establishment phase by recommending four 30-minute sessions per week for the first four weeks of treatment. Subsequently, we recommend two full hour sessions per week for the next month and, finally, one hourly session per week for an additional two months. Once clients complete the first month of treatment (the establishment phase), they are invited to join the Council for Fluency as a supplement to their clinic visits. After the first four weeks of treatment, they generally have a sufficient familiarity with the target behaviors to allow them to practice these skills in the less-structured environment of the Council.

In this first phase of treatment in the clinic (the first four weeks), emphasis is on teaching techniques that enhance natural respiration, phonation, and articulation. Although attitudes are examined and environmental issues are explored, these areas are not emphasized while the new speech behaviors are being established. This phase, then, is taken up with teaching behaviors that are compatible with fluency and that approximate the patterns of normal speech production.

Components of the Stabilization Phase

It is during the stabilization phase of treatment that the newly learned fluency skills are habituated. This is a period of intensive drill and practice that will ultimately allow the individual to "own" the new behaviors. Activities include practicing fluency skills in reading, monologue, and conversation in contexts that are carefully structured and controlled by the clinician. Although this is described as the stabilization phase of treatment, transfer activities actually begin at this time. We are committed to encouraging the early transfer of skills to minimize reliance on the therapist and the therapy room as secure havens for the individual who stutters. The client therefore begins to use these fluency skills in the context of the support group meetings as an early transfer activity. Treatment is carefully coordinated between the clinic and the Council, with ongoing communication between the therapists in each setting.

Components of the Transfer Phase

This eight-week phase entails one hourly session per week in the clinic setting. A variety of interactive activities are introduced in which our clients practice fluency skills outside of the therapy room, first on campus and then in settings off campus in the surrounding community.

Shopping trips, conversations with strangers, asking for directions, and offering assistance are some of the frequently used activities. Keeping a journal has proved to be a successful technique for assisting our clients to heighten their awareness of the factors that affect their fluency. It is at this juncture of the treatment process that we begin to introduce activities that deal with the upper levels of the client's fear hierarchy and to initiate direct intervention targeting avoidance behaviors. We also direct our attention and to further increasing assertiveness and continued focus on the process of internalizing the locus of control of behavior. There is an increase in the number of home based-assignments during this critical phase of treatment.

COMPONENTS OF THE MAINTENANCE PHASE

This final phase of treatment is actually composed of two subphases: guided maintenance (six months) and maintenance (three years). During the first six months of maintenance (guided maintenance) clients attend weekly Council meetings during which they receive one hour of group support and one hour of individual treatment. Our goal during this phase is to prepare clients for more independent monitoring of their speech and to build the skills necessary for functioning in their own environments without the need for constant therapist support. The skills introduced during the first six months of treatment are practiced and reinforced, as many more out-of-clinic treatment assignments are added. Clients choose various people, times, and situations in their daily lives as targets for transfer practice. They then accept responsibility for reporting outcomes of these activities to their clinicians. These reports serve as the content for individual therapy sessions during this six-month phase.

This part of treatment combines issues of the client's actual speech behaviors with affective and environmental factors. Therapy sessions might, for example, be devoted to a range of issues from managing negative environmental elements or modifying the environment in general to the concept of control (who has it?, how to get it?, when to take control?), or assertiveness (how it can help reduce communicative stress), or self-esteem (how to realistically evaluate one's communicative competence). The work done in any one session will depend upon the client's report of weekly experiences. Some sessions may be devoted primarily to practicing fluency control techniques, if this is indicated by the client as a need.

During the final phase of maintenance (three years), the client assumes more responsibility each year for managing, monitoring, and evaluating fluency. Clients are encouraged to take on leadership roles in the Council. They become officers of the Council, address community and parent groups, participate in interviews with the media, and act as mentors for new members entering the Council of Fluency. It is during this last phase that clients generally begin to talk about readiness to leave the Council and, knowing that they may return at any time, move on to other life concerns.

SUMMARY

The four phases of treatment—establishment, stabilization, transfer, and maintenance—when viewed together form a synergistic matrix. They combine the acquisition of fluency skills based upon a model of normal speech production (the fluency shaping component of the program) with the systematic attention to feelings, attitudes, and management of the communicative environment (the symptom modification component of the program). Treatment takes place over a period of five years beginning with an intensive Weekend Workshop or with frequent clinical sessions (four meetings per week) during the first four weeks. Once fluency skills have been introduced, the affective, cognitive, and environmental elements of treatment are presented.

REFERENCE

1. Ham R. *Therapy of Stuttering*. Englewood Cliffs, NJ: Prentice Hall, 1990.

5

Early Intervention

HISTORICAL PERSPECTIVE

The popularity of the notion of early intervention for children with fluency disorders is relatively new. Although indirect therapy for young children who stutter has been provided since the early days of our profession (particularly following the popularity of the theories of Wendell Johnson), we have only recently begun to think in terms of providing direct service to these children.

According to Bloodstein,[1] in the 1980s we began to treat young children more directly with a combination of parent counseling, increasing the child's feelings of success as a speaker through simple exercises that guaranteed success (e.g., reciting nursery rhymes, choral speaking), and simple behavior modification techniques (e.g., easy, slow speech, controlling length and complexity of utterances). The decade of the 1990s has seen an increase in research related to stuttering treatment for children. Yairi and his colleagues[2-4] have investigated a variety of variables related to stuttering in young children, including speech and voice characteristics and the genetic basis of recovery. The works of Starkweather,[5] Starkweather and Givens-Ackerman,[6] Starkweather, Gottwald, and Halfond,[7] and Perkins[8] have emphasized that stuttering can be prevented when treated early enough, and Starkweather has further suggested it be treated directly if necessary.

Whether we believe that this disorder can be prevented or just successfully treated at a very early age, for us the course of action remains the same. We are committed to the concept of early intervention and endorse the combination of direct and indirect treatment procedures for young, sometimes very young, children. We agree with many of our colleagues—Adams,[9] Costello,[10] Peters and Guitar,[11] Ryan,[12] Shine,[13] Starkweather and Gottwald,[14] Starkweather and Givens-Ackerman,[6] and Starkweather, Gottwald, and Halfond[7]—who have suggested that with early intervention there is a far more positive prognosis than when treatment is delayed. Starkweather has written that "most young children who successfully completed early intervention or prevention programs have natural sounding speech, no need to be vigilant, and only a remote possibility of relapse."[5]

TREATMENT TECHNIQUES FOR EARLY INTERVENTION

A number of programs are available as options for direct treatment of young children who stutter. These early intervention programs have a common thread in that they all introduce the child to one or more known fluency facilitation techniques. Wall and Myers[15] identified the reduction of rate of speaking and reduction of linguistic complexity as activities that can facilitate fluency. Most of the approaches combine one or both of these direct treatment strategies with elements of parent and family counseling. In this section we will review some of the systematic programs that are available to the clinician, and then add a description of our own approach.

As early as 1971, Ryan[16] treated children who stutter with behavioral techniques designed to diminish and eventually eliminate the stuttering. Ryan and his associates[17] have used a combination of gradual increase in length and complexity of utterances (GILCU) and carefully scheduled social and token reinforcement through the establishment, transfer, and maintenance stages of treatment. They continue to report high levels of fluency in children who have been treated with this program.

Like the Ryans, Shine[13] controls the length and complexity of utterances and uses token reinforcement to establish and maintain fluent speech in stuttering children between the ages of three and nine. Shine believes that children's dysfluent speech reflects overly forceful use of the muscles of respiration, articulation, and phonation. His program targets the diminishing of this excessive force, encouraging the child to use an easy voice or prolonged speech in order to establish initial fluency. He introduces a hierarchy of structured speaking activities beginning with picture identification, a task that carries a low level of linguistic demand, and concluding with spontaneous language elicited by a "surprise box" activity (requiring a much higher level of linguistic demand).

Stocker[18] devised yet another behaviorally based program that employs a hierarchy of linguistic demands to assess and treat young stuttering children. The Stocker Probe is based upon the notion that young children (preschool and early elementary school age) become more dysfluent as the linguistic demands of their communicative interactions increase. Stocker presents questions at five different levels of linguistic demand, practicing each of these levels with the child until fluency is achieved, before moving to the next level. Although the original version of this instrument is no longer commercially available, it continues to be used by clinicians in a variety of treatment settings. Recently (1995) a revised version of the Probe has been introduced by Stocker and Goldfarb.[19]

Starkweather[5] and his associates[6,7,14] have described a model of treatment based upon the idea that a child's fluency is at risk when that child's capacity for fluency does not equal the cognitive, motoric, emotional, and environmental demands for fluency that may be placed upon him. They maintain that children have a certain capacity for fluency that is related to their speech motor control abilities, language formulation abilities, social-emotional maturity, and cognitive skills. This varies from child to child and from one age to another. They further note that there are certain demands placed upon the child for fluency that may be internal (i.e., child driven) or environmental. The more mature the child, the greater the expectation or demand for fluency. Demands may take the form of time pressure, uncertainty born of changes in the security base of the child (e.g., moving, marital problems, family illness, new baby), or the family's reaction (or lack of reaction) to the child's difficulty with speech. When demands exceed the child's capacity for fluency, stuttering occurs.

This Demands and Capacities Model combines direct intervention with a strong parent counseling component. Starkweather has suggested that after careful assessment, the focus of therapy becomes increasing the child's capacities for fluency (cognitive, motor, linguistic and emotional) while decreasing the parallel demands. He has recommended that parent counseling include education about stuttering as well as answering parents' questions and helping them to bring stuttering out in the open with their child. Starkweather has also focused on exploring, identifying, and confronting parents' attitudes in a supportive way. Finally, through a process of self-discovery with family members, he has addressed the issue of changing the way parents and other family members behave in relation to their participation in the communicative environment.

In working with the child, Starkweather targets the removal of struggle, reducing speech rate and controlling the linguistic level during speaking events. When necessary, he has recommended the introduction of such fluency shaping activities as gentle onsets, light articulatory contacts, and improved resonance. This may be accomplished by modeling desired behaviors, including easy whole word and phrase repetitions, and by highlighting slowed conversation and "polite" turn-taking behavior.

Richardson and Oyler[20] endorse the Demands and Capacities Model and have used it as a foundation for their therapy program for children that they call "Interactive Fluency Treatment." They use a modified form of traditional speech therapy as well as principles derived from cognitive psychology and counseling in order to modify the beliefs and perceptions of people who stutter. The primary vehicle for service delivery is play, with some structured activities and ongoing counseling sessions. They examine the internal capacities of the child with regard to linguistic skills, speech intelligibility, behavior, and personality in order to compare these to the external demands placed upon the child. As is the case with Schneider's treatment philosophy,[21] this program relies upon a collaboration with the parents in making decisions about possible environmental modifications. According to Richardson and Oyler[20]:

> Therapy sessions with the young child are interactive and involve several different levels of play. Discussions or scenarios played out with small dolls often focus on strengthening the child's linguistic skills and emotional capacities. Specific skills may be taught, reactions modeled, and feedback provided to strengthen the child's sense of personal empowerment.

Parents are taught to engage in "theme centered play" in which the child is the leader and the parent uses slow speech, increased pauses, and good listening while modeling calm, positive, assertive behaviors during play. Toys are selected that allow for functional, symbolic, and dramatic play scenarios.

Meyers and Woodford[22] also developed a program that combines parent counseling techniques with decreasing the child's speaking rate, using smooth and easy speech, and practicing appropriate pragmatic skills (e.g., turn-taking behavior). Their approach relies heavily upon a systematic analysis of the interaction between stuttering children and their conversational partners. The direct intervention is described as a behavior modification approach in which children are taught to contrast fast and slow speech, use smooth and relaxed speech rather than bumpy speech, and understand and practice certain pragmatic strategies (turn taking, sequencing, acknowledging disagreement, and retrieving thoughts). The parent training/counseling component is quite similar to the Starkweather approach described above. Portions of this treatment program have been adapted by and widely used by many clinicians, especially the device known as "talking like a turtle" as opposed to "talking like a racehorse," or using "turtle speech" as opposed to "racehorse speech."

More recently, the work of Walton and Wallace[23] was reported at the Second World Congress of the International Fluency Association. This interesting approach, one which endorses both fluency shaping (without the use of punishment and negative reinforcement) and stuttering modification principles, is the most direct of the treatment strategies suggested for young children. They endorse moving from a direct focus on techniques that facilitate fluency (e.g., easy speech, stretchy talk, bouncy speech) to a direct focus on the differences between fluent and dysfluent speech (e.g., "speech villains" like hard speech and pushing).

This therapy approach incorporates Ryan's GILCU strategy as well as what they call "desensitization and empowerment" therapy.[24] The desensitization principles include voluntary stuttering that they call "bouncy talk" or "Tigger talk" and games in which the child is asked to catch the therapist who is not using easy speech. Later the child is taught to speak fluently in the presence of speech fluency disrupters. The empowerment program helps the child to identify "speech villains" that can be captured by drawing pictures of them and then engaging in such activities as tying them up, locking them up, and/or sending them away.

The parent training component includes education and training with the use of available written materials from the Stuttering Foundation of America and the National Stuttering Project, as well as a thorough explanation of Walton and Wallace's philosophy of treatment. Parents are then assisted in developing conversational and listening strategies that will facilitate fluency. Parent participation is enlisted in practicing carryover activities at home. Parents are taught the therapy techniques and asked to practice them for specified periods each day.

Onslow and his associates[25-28] have reported the results of the Lidcombe Program, a parent-administered early intervention stuttering program that has been utilized in Australia during the past several years. In this program, parents are trained to identify stuttering in their children and to respond to their children's stuttered speech by requesting that they repeat stuttered utterances fluently (i.e., without "bumpy words"); they are taught, as well, to respond to fluent speech with praise and tokens or other desired rewards. This occurs during a number of daily ten-minute sessions and is demonstrated by the parent in weekly sessions in the clinic setting so that the supervising therapist may monitor and provide feedback. Parents are taught to chart their children's stutter-free and stuttered speech and to provide "on-line" feedback in nontreatment situations both in the home and outside. This "on-line" feedback consists of intermittent praise when speech is fluent and intermittent requests for correction when speech is stuttered. Results have been reported to be highly favorable for the four subjects in the first study[25] and the 12 subjects in the second study.[27]

Schneider[29] described a program that he calls Self-Adjusting Fluency Therapy (SAFT), an approach that he has found to be successful with preschool and school age children who are overtly dysfluent but who do not tend to avoid speaking situations. This treatment paradigm involves teaching "children [to] integrate fluency enhancing speech adjustments by repeatedly experiencing the effects of volitional increases and decreases in loudness and pausing."[29] The clinician first models variations in loudness and rate (e.g., pausing) to demonstrate that "choice" is possible. These choices are presented as different options for speaking as the therapist uses self-talk to demonstrate which speaking style he or she chooses to use at any given time. The child is then encouraged to choose how he wants the therapist to speak. This can be presented in a game format in which the child has the therapist shift from one speech style to another (e.g., fast rate to pauses between words; loud voice to gentle or quiet voice). Once the child understands the concept of self-adjustment, he is encouraged to try this technique himself, shifting at will from one speech style to another and being positively reinforced for making the choices. Ultimately the child is asked to make these adjustments before beginning to speak and during what Schneider calls "periods of fluency interruption."

Parents are involved in this treatment program from the outset. In fact, parent counseling begins with the initial telephone contact, during which Schneider attempts to enlist the parent's partnership in the treatment process by engaging immediately in shared decision making about the need for face-to-face consultation. Before a child is scheduled for therapy, the parents are invited for a consultation. An environment is created in which the parents feel comfortable enough to discuss their fears, concerns, perceptions of the child's communication effectiveness, and notions about why their child is dysfluent.

Schneider attends particularly to the family's communication dynamics, its process for setting limits, and the parent's pattern of asserting the role of being the "person-in-charge." He also pays particular attention to the child's desire to communicate and the response of family members.

During the child's treatment period, parent counseling takes the form of shared problem solving about ways in which fluency can be facilitated and ways in which family members may respond to periods of fluency and dysfluency. Parents are cautioned not to expect the child to be able to use self-adjustments to control dysfluency consistently. They are taught the process of self-adjustment, and learn that successful use of this technique takes time and patience. The therapist's observations of family communication patterns and parental concerns and issues form the basis for ongoing counseling sessions. Parents are encouraged to work with the therapist to devise less demanding communication experiences at home.

Tepperman,[30] who has been influenced in her clinical work by our synergistic philosophy of treatment, also combines direct fluency shaping techniques with a strong parent counseling component and environmental modification. She uses language-based stuttering treatment techniques that include GILCU as well as reinforcement of the child's well-planned and clearly sent messages (see next section under treatment of speech and language). Like Schneider,[29] Tepperman incorporates fluency facilitation techniques that may include slowing the speech rate and softening the intensity of the child's utterances. She talks about "smooth and easy speech," contrasting it with "hard speech" that consists of "big bumps" (i.e., whole-word repetitions), "little bumps" (i.e., part-word repetitions), "getting stuck" (i.e., blocks), and "skidding" (i.e., prolongations).

Parent counseling and environmental modification are major components in Tepperman's treatment program. She emphasizes the importance of listening both in her direct therapy and in her work with families. In order to achieve positive changes in the environment, "Family Speech Rules" are presented and discussed with parents and are then introduced into the home via "refrigerator pictures," one rule at a time. These "rules" are suggestions for becoming a good conversational partner and benefit all members of the household since they are relevant for all speakers. They include such suggestions as refraining from interrupting others when they are speaking, taking turns when speaking, looking at each other when speaking and listening, allowing for silent time, and being a good listener.

As is the case with most other children's treatment programs, Tepperman's counseling program includes educating parents regarding therapy techniques and including them in the treatment process; reviewing progress on a regular basis; viewing informational videotapes as well as video and audiotapes of their child's therapy sessions; explaining communication alternatives to be used at home; and identifying time pressure, emotional, motoric and linguistic demands, complex language, feelings regarding stuttering, and attitudes about communication.

SYNERGISTIC APPROACH TO EARLY INTERVENTION

The treatment program that we recommend for young children combines features of many of the programs described above. The synergistic approach to early intervention in stuttering is compatible with our adult synergistic approach in that it, too, considers the dimensions of normal speech production as well as the child's attitudes and feelings and the home and communicative environment. We endorse the combined fluency shaping and stuttering modification philosophies seen in so many of the child-oriented treatment programs available today.[22,31,32]

We begin with a careful assessment of the child, as we do with our adult clients, but pay special attention to the client's linguistic maturity. It has been our experience that young children who stutter often have difficulty with the organizational (categorization and sequencing) and pragmatic (conversational rules) aspects of language, as well as difficulty with such higher level language functions as expressing abstract concepts, verbal problem solving, verbal reasoning, and expressing relationships among words and ideas.

This linguistic fragility of some young children who stutter has been noted by various investigators.[11,15,33,34–36] Although there remains much controversy regarding the language abilities of young stuttering children,[37–39] the role of language should not be overlooked in the treatment of this age group, since the period of greatest language development (2.5 to 5 years) frequently coincides with the period of greatest risk for the development of stuttering.

Our assessment entails the administration of a variety of formal tests including the Preschool Language Assessment Instrument (PLAI).[40] We chose this tool, despite the fact that it has not been standardized, because it reveals the child's ability to handle four different levels of abstraction: (1) matching perception, (2) selective analysis of perception, (3) reordering perception, and (4) reasoning about perception. If fluency breaks down at a particular level, we have an increased understanding of the role of linguistic complexity on the child's fluency. For example, if stuttering occurs or increases markedly when the child is asked to predict, explain, or find a logical solution to a problem (level 4), then we may predict that this child would benefit from treatment that targets higher level language tasks and that the lower levels of abstraction (identifying or labeling, describing, defining by concept) do not present a problem to the child.

Treatment of Speech and Language

In treating the young stuttering child, we believe that a language-based approach is most efficient and effective. We therefore begin with a focus on communication, teaching the child, as Yovetich[36] has recommended, that communication is the sending of good messages. We explain that a "good message" means that the other person understands what we said. We spend several sessions establishing the concept of good messages, exploring various ways of deciding if the conversational partner understands our messages (facial expressions, nods, sounds like "ah-ha"), and practicing sending messages to each other and to mom and dad, brother and sister, and friends. Once the idea of a good message has been established, we introduce the idea of smooth or easy messages as opposed to rough, bumpy, or hard messages. Whenever possible we use the child's language to describe the stuttering. If the child does not have a word for his stuttering we may suggest the terms *rough, bumpy,* or *hard.* Then good messages that are hard or bumpy can be made easy or smooth. We continue to reinforce good messages and encourage the child to problem solve how to make a hard message easy. Children are remarkably skillful at figuring out their own ways of converting stuttered utterances into fluent ones. The words *easy speech, smooth talk,* and *turtle speech* are frequently introduced to facilitate fluency.

Many clinical investigators have suggested that simplifying the linguistic demands will increase the child's fluency.[10,12,13,22] We often begin our treatment by requiring only single word responses and gradually increasing the length and complexity of required responses while practicing the fluency facilitation techniques described above. We also introduce Tepperman's "Family Speech Rules" considered above, which can be pictured in rebus form to convey waiting until it's your turn to talk, listening to what the other person is saying, and talking about the same thing that the other person is talking about. Again, even very young children respond positively to these pragmatic language requirements, quickly learning the conversational rules and, in so doing, giving themselves more time to organize their language responses to conversational demands.

When the results of language testing suggest that there are more significant language concerns, our treatment plan includes goals and objectives that address those concerns. Language goals are easily incorporated into fluency practice. After all, language is the context in which we present all of our teaching of fluency skills. What difference does it make whether we practice smooth and easy speech or turtle talk in picture naming tasks, verbal problem solving activities, or narrative construction? The important consideration is to engage in a careful task analysis before teaching a new language concept, so that the level of difficulty of the linguistic demand is compatible with the child's capacity for the use of the fluency facilitation techniques we have previously taught.

Like Starkweather and his associates,[7] we sometimes introduce easier ways to stutter, helping the child move back down through the stages of stuttering severity. We use easy voluntary stuttering ourselves, sometimes pointing it out to the child, sometimes not. We assure the children we treat that there are times it is hard for all of us to say things, but that we always listen because what they have to say is important to us.

Treatment of Feelings and Attitudes

Feelings and attitudes are as important to us in treating children as they are in treating adults. The negative impact of unsuccessful speech attempts and failed communicative interactions must be countered by strong positive reinforcement of successful communication. In keeping with the synergistic model, our focus is on building self-esteem and assertiveness and increasing an internal locus of control. Our young clients are taught to realistically evaluate the success of their communicative attempts on an ongoing basis. They are constantly assessing whether their messages are "good messages"—that is, understood by the other person. Unrealistic beliefs about what other people think are directly confronted as we teach our clients to read such nonverbal responses as body language, facial expression, and eye contact. They come to feel more successful because they are experiencing the total communication event rather than just the role of their fluency in their social and communicative interactions. We believe children are empowered by the knowledge that they are in charge of their messages, thereby helping to internalize their locus of control, even at the very youngest ages.

In addition, this sense of empowerment makes our young clients more confident and assertive. Success in therapy is transferred to success in real life situations over the course of treatment, and the children come to believe that they are as special as we, their parents, and others who know them think they are. Please note that success in therapy is not necessarily defined as "fluency"; rather it is defined as effective communication, making certain that the people we talk to understand the meaning of our messages. The goal is that children learn that others value what they have to say more than how they say it.

Treatment of Environmental Issues

All treatment programs for children who stutter must concern themselves with the social and communicative environments within which the children function. The Synergistic Model seeks to specifically address those issues identified during the comprehensive assessment in addition to the more typical parental concerns regarding stuttering children, which might include wondering whether the child will outgrow his stuttering or what to do if the child is teased by classmates or playmates. It is here that we address parental concerns, sibling issues, family and school or teacher questions, and cultural factors related to such ideas as shame, fear, pride, or custom.

Issues are addressed through parent/family counseling and systematic parent training. Both counseling and training are tailored to the individual needs of the families of our clients. For example, if discipline is a problem for parents, we might discuss various standard approaches to this issue during a counseling session and facilitate the exploration of the parents' comfort level with each approach. If a family's cultural background has negatively influenced the way in which family members view the child's stuttering, we seek to understand this and find ways to mitigate their acting on these negative attitudes. Some issues are more sensitive than others. Our job is to uncover issues, whether sensitive or not, and bring them to the open forum of family problem solving.

Counseling occurs in various ways. For children who are enrolled in our clinic-based program, counseling sessions are held during the child's regular therapy time or during additional sessions that are scheduled as necessary. While the child is seen by a graduate student, the family member or members who accompany the child to the clinic view the session with a clinical supervisor who specializes in the treatment of fluency disorders in children. The supervisor explains the techniques that are being used and encourages the family members to ask questions or comment on the child's participation. The supervisor models techniques and gives the family members an opportunity to practice using some of these techniques under her guidance. Later in the course of treatment, parents and other family members (siblings, grandparents, caregivers) are introduced into the actual treatment sessions and begin to interact with the child and therapist using the techniques that have been modeled for them.

Parents are given a variety of home-based observation tasks to complete, and these are discussed during this clinical period. These tasks include analyses of fluent periods with an emphasis on such variables as the conversational partners, topics of conversation, who initiated the interaction, what the environmental conditions were at the time, and how the fluency was reinforced by the conversational partner. These tasks highlight for the family those environmental variables that serve to facilitate fluency. Parents are asked to heighten their awareness of the role that specific events might play in their child's fluency successes and breakdowns.

As family-related issues surface that require more discussion time, parents are invited to return to the center without the child for in-depth exploration of these issues. Often parents are confused about how to handle well-meaning grandparents or other significant family members who offer advice that is counter to what they are learning in the clinic sessions; sometimes other siblings begin to "act out" in negative ways during the treatment period; in other cases parents need to talk about their own fears for the future. These and other topics can be addressed in these sessions without the child.

Another form of counseling takes place in a group with other parents of children who are, or were, at risk for stuttering. The group is facilitated by an experienced fluency therapist. We have found that families learn important strategies from each other that they might not be able to learn from us. There is a built-in credibility that exists when parents who have lived through an experience share it with those who have not. No amount of "telling" on the clinician's part can compare to the impact of the words of a parent who has "been there."

These counseling sessions take place at least one evening a month for as many weeks as the group members choose to participate. The format of the session generally includes brief introductions, an open forum for discussion of any issues raised by the group, and the presentation of a planned topic by the therapist. This last part should remain flexible enough that it can be canceled if group members wish to continue discussing the issues that surfaced during the open forum.

Adult members of the Council for Fluency Support Group are invited to attend some of these parent counseling sessions to answer questions and to demonstrate their effectiveness as communicators to parents who may feel that stuttering means their children will never be able to speak in public or make a favorable communicative impression. We have found this to be a most effective teaching tool for parents as well as a powerful transfer activity for the Council members who choose to participate.

SUMMARY

This chapter reviewed a number of popular stuttering treatment programs for young children and described how they have influenced our synergistic approach to treating preschoolers who stutter or are at risk for developing stuttering. We demonstrated how the synergistic philosophy of treating the speech and language domain, the attitudinal domain, and the environmental domain is reflected in our treatment of this population. We emphasized the importance of both direct and indirect treatment strategies for children, and included a brief description of both individual and group counseling approaches.

REFERENCES

1. Bloodstein O. *A Handbook on Stuttering*. Chicago: National Easter Seal Society, 1987.
2. Ambrose NG, Cox NJ, Yairi E. The genetic basis of persistence and recovery in stuttering. *J Speech Lang Hear Res* 1997;40:567–580.
3. Yairi E, Ambrose NG, Cox N. Genetics of stuttering: A critical review. *J Speech Lang Hear Res* 1996;39:771–784.
4. Yairi E, Ambrose N. Onset of stuttering in preschool children. *J Speech Lang Hear Res* 1992;35:782–788.
5. Starkweather CW. Therapy for younger children. In RF Curlee, GM Siegel (eds), *Nature and Treatment of Stuttering: New Directions* (2nd ed). Boston: Allyn and Bacon, 1997.
6. Starkweather CW, Givens-Ackerman CR. *Stuttering*. Austin, TX: Pro-Ed, 1997.
7. Starkweather CW, Gottwald SR, Halfond MM. *Stuttering Prevention: A Clinical Method*. Englewood Cliffs, NJ: Prentice Hall, 1990.
8. Perkins WH. *Stuttering Prevented*. San Diego, CA: Singular Publishing, 1992.
9. Adams M. The young stutterer: Diagnosis, treatment and assessment of progress. *Semin Speech Lang* 1980;1:289–298.
10. Costello JM. Treatment of the young chronic stutterer: Managing fluency. In RF Curlee, WH Perkins (eds), *Nature and Treatment of Stuttering: New Directions*. San Diego, CA: College Hill, 1984.
11. Peters TJ, Guitar B. *Stuttering: An Integrated Approach to Its Nature and Treatment*. Baltimore: Williams and Wilkins, 1991.
12. Ryan B. Stuttering therapy in a framework of operant conditioning and programmed learning. In HH Gregory (ed), *Controversies About Stuttering Therapy*. Baltimore: University Park Press, 1979:129–173.
13. Shine R. Direct management of the beginning stutterer. *Semin Speech Lang* 1980;1: 339–350.
14. Starkweather CW, Gottwald SR. The demands capacities model II: Clinical applications. *J Fluency Disord* 1990;15:143–157.
15. Wall MJ, Myers FL. *Clinical Management of Childhood Stuttering* (2nd ed). Austin, TX: Pro-Ed, 1995.
16. Ryan B. Operant procedures applied to stuttering in children. *Top Lang Disord* 1995;15:32–47.
17. Ryan B, Van Kirk B. *Monterey Fluency Program*. Palo Alto, CA: Monterey Learning Systems, 1978.
18. Stocker B. *Stocker Probe Technique: For Diagnosis and Treatment of Stuttering in Young Children*. Tulsa, OK: Modern Education Corp., 1980.

19. Stocker B, Goldfarb R. *The Stocker Probe for Fluency and Language.* Vero Beach, FL: The Speech Bin, 1995.
20. Richardson M, Oyler M. Stuttering vulnerability, demands, and capacity model and treatment. Mini-seminar presented at Second World Congress of the International Fluency Association, San Francisco, August 1997.
21. Schneider P. *Self-Adjusting Fluency Therapy.* Personal correspondence, 1998.
22. Meyers SC, Woodford LL. *The Fluency Development System for Young Children (Ages 2-9).* Buffalo, NY: United Educational Services, 1992.
23. Walton P, Wallace M. Stuttering in young children: Direct early intervention. Mini-seminar presented at the Second World Congress of the International Fluency Association, San Francisco, August 1997.
24. Wallace M. Personal correspondence, 1997.
25. Onslow M, Costa L, Rue S. Direct early intervention with stuttering: Some preliminary data. *J Speech Hear Disord* 1990;55:405–416.
26. Onslow M. Choosing a treatment procedure for early stuttering: Issues and future directions. *J Speech Lang Hear Res* 1992;35:983–993.
27. Onslow M, Andrews C, Lincoln M. A control/experimental trial of an operant treatment for early stuttering. *J Speech Lang Hear Res* 1994;37:1244–1259.
28. Onslow M, Packman A. Issues in treatment of early stuttering. Mini-seminar presented at the Second World Congress of the International Fluency Association, San Francisco, August 1997.
29. Schneider P. Personal correspondence, 1998.
30. Tepperman L. Personal correspondence, 1998.
31. Cooper E, Cooper C. *Cooper Personalized Fluency Control Therapy—Revised.* Allen, TX: DLM Teaching Resources, 1985.
32. Healy EC, Scott LA. Strategies for teaching elementary school-age children who stutter: An integrative approach. *Lang Speech Hear Servs Schools* 1994;26: 151–161.
33. Bloodstein O. *Stuttering: The Search for a Cause and Cure.* Boston: Allyn and Bacon, 1993.
34. Ratner NB. Language complexity and stuttering in children. *Top Lang Disord* 1995;15:32–47.
35. Wingate M. *The Structure of Stuttering: A Psycholinguistic Analysis.* New York: Springer-Verlag, 1988.
36. Yovetich WS. Message therapy: Language approach to stuttering therapy with children. *J Fluency Disord* 1984;9:11–20.
37. Bernstein Rotner NB, Sih C. Effects of gradual increases in sentence length and complexity on children's dysfluency. *J Speech Lang Hear Res* 1987;52:278–287.
38. Nippold M. Concomitant speech and language disorders in stuttering children: A critique of the literature. *J Speech Hear Disord* 1990;55:51–60.
39. Ryan B. Articulation, language, rate and fluency characteristics of stuttering and non-stuttering preschool children. *J Speech Lang Hear Res* 1992;35:333–342.
40. Blank M, Rose S, Berlin L. *Preschool Language Assessment Instrument.* New York: Grune and Stratton, 1978.

6

Synergistic Treatment of the Speech and Language Domain

The first spiral in our Synergistic Model (see Figure 1.1), the one comprising the Speech and Language domain, includes the physiologic, linguistic, and learned factors associated with stuttering. It is in this spiral that treatment most clearly combines elements of fluency shaping and stuttering modification. This chapter will describe our approach to the treatment of these elements of normal speech production in adults as we introduce the therapeutic phases of identification, modification or establishment, stabilization, and transfer and maintenance.

TREATMENT PRINCIPLES

The treatment principles of the synergistic approach are based on the same principles that relate to normal speech production. Normal speech consists of the smooth integration of the processes of respiration, phonation, and articulation. It is our belief that the person who stutters has, to some degree, learned habits that interfere with normal speech production. Therefore, we teach the targets of speech that will produce more fluent performance and practice these targets in structured and nonstructured situations, in keeping with a basic fluency shaping philosophy.

We first teach the mechanics of normal speech. Our clients learn about the general processes of respiration, phonation, and articulation through films and pictures of the larynx, explanation of the process of breathing, explanation of the process of articulation including the various sound classes (vowels, voiced and unvoiced sounds, fricatives, and plosives), and by increasing their awareness of the dynamic moving properties of speech (co-articulation).

We then engage the client in activities to heighten his awareness of the moment of stuttering, a common practice in most stuttering modification programs. At the moment of stuttering the client must feel what parts of the diaphragm, throat, face, tongue, and lips are being tensed. This is a crucial time in treatment because the client's commitment to change may break down at this point; he may feel that there is no time for this specific kind of analysis as the demands of the conversational flow urge him onward. He may complain of mental "blackout," of not knowing what is happening or what he is doing. This is the identification phase, the phase in which the client must be taught to recognize and feel the tension at the levels of the diaphragm, larynx, and articulators.

The client is next taught to release this tension whether it is felt in the diaphragm, larynx, articulators or any combination of these structures. The client must choose and practice the process of releasing tension. For a person who may have always pushed and forced during this stuttered moment, this may seem an impossible task. Initial attempts often meet with frustration. The therapist must demonstrate a "tighten and release" pattern in the physiologic structures so that the client may learn to contrast tension and relaxation and, ultimately, to tighten and release tension in the speech mechanism at will. This is the first step in modification of the stuttering behavior.

The next step requires teaching the respiratory, phonatory, and articulatory targets of normal speech production that are full breath (or passive airflow if necessary), gentle onset, and movement. The full breath target is important to us because we have noted that people who stutter tend to cut off the flow of air at the level of the larynx. The gentle onset target is important because sound is produced when the vocal folds come together gently, allowing the air to pass through, and people who stutter demonstrate the larynx as their prime area of tension. The importance of the movement target is that people who stutter frequently fail to move smoothly from one sound to another, from the initial consonant to the vowel or from the initial vowel to the rest of the word.

PHYSIOLOGIC FACTORS

Treatment Techniques in the Identification Phase

The physiologic factors with which we are concerned, therefore, are respiration, phonation, and articulation/co-articulation. It has been our experience that adults who stutter demonstrate unnatural patterns in one or more of these areas, and we have noted as well that tension is a major contributing factor to these unnatural patterns. For this reason, we begin our treatment with instruction in the mechanics of speech production and experience in tensing and easing the tension in the speech mechanism on command.

Clinicians are urged to use diagrams, films, and experiential exercises to educate the client with the processes of normal speech production. These diagrams are available in anatomy and physiology texts, Netter drawings, or in various sites on the Worldwide Web. Clients must learn to name and feel the systems of respiration, phonation, and articulation. They must also learn the interactive, synergistic properties of these systems in order to recognize their application to their own speech processes. Although this instruction takes place at the beginning of treatment, clinicians are urged to frequently refer to the description of the physical behaviors of speech production and to the client's control of these behaviors throughout the treatment process. Even in the identification phase of treatment, the introduction of control as a meaningful variable is explored.

In order to execute an utterance in a continuous, forward flowing, and sequentially ordered fashion, a speaker must be able to do the following: maintain airflow from the lungs; modify the airflow with appropriate opening and closing of the cords in the larynx to promote continuous phonation and the voiceless/voiced contrast as demanded by the composition of sounds in the utterance; sustain progressive articulatory movement; and coordinate breathing, voicing, and articulation as the movement from sound to sound occurs. This complex series of speech events is taught through the introduction of targets of normal speech production, described in the following section.

The experience of tensing and easing the tension of the diaphragm, larynx, and articulators on command is a very important step for the client in achieving control of the stuttering behavior. We engage the client in practice contrasting tension and relaxation in these structures at the syllable, word, and conversational levels. The client is encouraged to feel the tension, feel the release, and recognize the she is the person who controls the strength of the tension. Here, again, the notion of exercising control is introduced and explored. Clients are taught to monitor tension in the speech of others, in tape recordings of their own speech, and in their spontaneous speech. The clinician must be able to stop the client, analyze the tension, demonstrate the tension, and have the client do the same.

Treatment Techniques in the Modification and Establishment Phases

Armed with the knowledge of normal speech processing and the awareness of one's own ability to control the production of speech, the client is ready to learn more about the individual components of the speech mechanism. It is at this point that the three targets of normal speech production are taught and practiced. The respiratory or "breath" target, phonatory or "easy onset" target, and articulatory or "movement" target are explained, modeled by the therapist, and practiced by the client until they become automatic.

Respiration is a frequently noted point of difference between normal speakers and the stuttering clients we have treated. If our individualized assessment suggests that our client has an unnatural breathing pattern, we analyze that pattern to determine the appropriate respiratory target behavior. For the majority of clients we introduce a full breath target, since this is most like the respiratory pattern of normal speakers. For those who are unable to utilize the full breath target naturally, we may choose instead to teach a passive airflow target[1] that we consider less natural but that frequently is successful for individuals who tend to hold their breath before initiating phonation.

Full Breath Target

The full breath target consists of teaching the client to inhale (through the mouth) in a relaxed manner, with particular attention to relaxation of the throat and a smooth downward movement of the diaphragm. We carefully distinguish between a "full breath" and a "deep breath," since for many people the latter encourages expansion of the chest by raising the shoulders instead of lowering the diaphragm. Two different locations are monitored by the client: the throat and the diaphragm. The diaphragm must move smoothly during the inhalation, making room in the thoracic cavity for the expansion of the lungs; at the same time the vocal tract (including the articulators) must be relaxed. At the top of a comfortably full inhalation, the client is cautioned to refrain from hesitating or tightening the throat region. He is asked to simply begin the exhalation by relaxing the diaphragm. At the same time that the exhalation begins, he is instructed to commence speaking without any hesitation. The air and the voice must start at precisely the same time. Once the diaphragm is relaxed, returning to its high position in the abdominal cavity, speech ceases. The client is instructed never to speak on residual air. Once the voice stops, the diaphragm will be able to relax a bit more without speech. It is critical that the exhalation be completed by relaxing the diaphragm without speech before beginning a new inhalation.

The full breath target is taught first without phonation, achieving a silent relaxed full breath; the client should then be taught the full breath target with phonation as quickly as possible, first in vowels and one-syllable words, then in automatic speech (counting, days of the week, months of the year), phrases, short sentences, reading, monologue, and conversation. We attempt to elicit this target in all contexts in a three-minute period with 100 percent accuracy before moving on to the gentle onset target.

For some clients, extreme laryngeal tension prevents them from initiating phonation and exhalation at the same time. For these clients, we may choose to introduce a passive airflow target similar to the one described by Schwartz.[1] In this case the client is asked to take a natural, relaxed inhalation (again through the mouth), to let a little air out, and then to speak, slightly stretching the first vowel while keeping the exhaled flow moving gently forward. A length of vinyl tubing (5/8" in diameter) has been helpful in allowing the client to hear his own airflow. One end of the tube is placed next to the client's ear, while the other end is placed just below the lower lip. With the tube in this position it is possible for the client to hear the exhaled airstream and to monitor whether it is stopped just prior to phonation.

Gentle Onset Target

Gentle onset of voicing addresses the harsh, abrupt initiation of phonation that is common in many of those who stutter. Because initiation of the gentle onset of phonation requires a sufficient amount of air, the full breath target is taught first. Therapy begins by exaggerating the gentle onset with the client to demonstrate a very low amplitude vibration of the vocal cords, followed by a gradual increase in the loudness of phonation, and finally a decrease in loudness to the initial amplitude level. This process is practiced first with vowels. At this time, the client is encouraged to stretch or prolong his speech so that the details of movement can be felt, analyzed, and studied. This stretched speech is never used outside of the therapy room. It is merely a training tool to enhance the client's awareness of vocal cord vibration and articulatory movement patterns.

Once the client practices the gentle onset target in one- and two-syllable words beginning with vowels, he may move on to phrases, sentences, reading, monologue, and conversation. We encourage clinicians to introduce the full breath and gentle onset targets within the first two or three treatment sessions. Once these targets have been established, the final target may be introduced.

Movement Target

The movement target provides for the smooth transition from sound to sound and from word to word. The client is taught to recognize the different properties of the sounds of the language and to utilize the first two targets, full breath and gentle onset, to master the third.

Teaching the movement target requires that the client learn about the four classes of sounds: (1) vowels, (2) voiced consonants, (3) voiceless consonants, and (4) plosives. She is taught that the vowels are produced with the most open vocal tract and require little concern regarding movement variables. Vowels would have already been addressed in learning the full breath and gentle onset targets, and are merely reviewed at this point.

The second class of sounds, the voiced consonants, require a full breath, gentle onset, continuous voicing, and reduced articulatory pressure—that is, all contact points of the articulators (tongue, lips, teeth, palate) are reached with a minimal amount of pressure between the articulation points. These class II sounds are again practiced in one- and two-syllable words, phrases, sentences, reading, monologue, and conversation. The client is encouraged to note the class II sounds that were stuttered and to analyze them according to which targets were misapplied.

The third class of sounds, the voiceless consonants, require a reduced amount of airflow in conjunction with the full breath and gentle onset targets. Excessive airflow prevents correct initiation of voicing on the next phoneme, usually a vowel. If the next phoneme is a vowel, the client is advised to prolong that vowel slightly before moving on to the next sound. Gentle onset must be applied to the phoneme that follows the voiceless consonant; movement proceeds from unvoiced to voiced production.

The fourth class of sounds, the plosives (both voiced and voiceless), require the application of both reduced airflow and reduced articulatory pressure. For the voiceless plosives, the client must again learn to move from unvoiced to voiced phonemes with a gentle onset of the voiced sound. Class III and IV sounds are practiced, once again, in the previously described hierarchy from one-syllable words to conversation with an analysis of misapplied targets for all stuttered words.

These three targets, then, (full breath, gentle onset, and movement) comprise the first small segment in the Synergistic Model of treatment. Clients learn new ways to control those elements of speech that they may already have had to learn to manage differently from normal speakers. New behaviors are established slowly and precisely. Clients practice the patterns used by those of us who do not stutter, learning to make adjustments to their habitual, nonfluent patterns of communication.

Treatment Techniques in the Stabilization Phase

The stabilization phase of treatment requires a commitment to drill with total concentration on correct target behavior. It is during this stage of treatment that new behaviors are habituated. Stabilization requires hours of mass practice both within the clinical setting and at home. The targets are practiced in reading, monologue, and conversation in both individual and group sessions. The clinician monitors the client's accurate production and counts and charts the number of dysfluent words per minute at the beginning and end of every therapy session. Then the client is asked to chart and analyze his own stuttered words in group and individual sessions according to target breakdown and class of sounds. Treatment sessions are always tape recorded in order to facilitate these types of analyses.

Clients are encouraged to monitor and analyze each other's speech when they meet either during the weekly group sessions or during individual sessions in which two therapists combine their lessons to foster this monitoring and analysis. Clients are also encouraged to achieve 100 percent accuracy within the clinical situation, since this is considered the laboratory where total concentration on targets is essential. Although we assure clients that 100 percent fluency in conversation is an unrealistic goal and that fluency is a less important goal than effective communication, we do encourage strict self-monitoring and self-correction during all individual therapy sessions.

If target production breaks down in these structured settings, the client must learn how to self-correct. Instead of using Van Riper's[2] hierarchy of cancellations, then pullouts, and finally preparatory sets, we encourage the use of preparatory sets first; if these are unsuccessful, we then encourage the use of pullouts; finally, if these are unsuccessful, we recommend the use of cancellations. Self-corrections are monitored by the clinician and counted as fluent utterances. The client is required to engage in conscious target production during all self-corrections.

Homework assignments are an essential part of every client's work. Homework should include daily practice during which a high level of self-awareness is developed. Each client should have a small tape recorder to use for these daily practice sessions. Clients need to practice each of the targets in reading, monologue, and conversation for brief sessions several times each day. These practice sessions should be used for maintaining the "feel" of the targets. If the client is at the syllable, word, or phrase level of any target, that is the level to be practiced.

Treatment Techniques in the Transfer and Maintenance Phases

Once a client has moved to the sentence level or beyond, individual hierarchies must be identified and transfer activities, individualized for each client, should be practiced for homework. Transfer activities must be designed to correspond to the individual's hierarchy of feared or difficult situations and must comprise a sufficient number of activities each day to enable the client to have practice in different situations. These activities are presented through a process of systematic desensitization[3,4] so that the client's comfort level increases in difficult speaking situations over time. Transfer activities may include phone calls, role plays, and general communication activities with a variety of communication partners. Activities are planned to enhance felt fluency by building successful speaking experiences first at lower levels of communicative fear and demand, and then at increasingly higher levels. The nature of the actual activities is limited only by the level of creativity of the therapist.

PSYCHOLINGUISTIC FACTORS

It is during the identification phase of treatment that the person who stutters is assisted in examining her communication style and evaluating its effectiveness. Psycholinguistic factors that we have noted frequently to occur in treating people who stutter relate to the pragmatic dimension of language. It has been our experience that many adults, despite their ability to learn techniques that result in successful control of stuttering behavior, frequently have difficulty engaging in or maintaining satisfactory social conversational interactions. Perhaps this is due to an early history of withdrawing from social contact, feelings of inadequacy as a speaker, negative communicative experiences, or lack of experience or confidence in a social environment. Whatever the initial cause, these individuals continue to be confounded by the demands of social intercourse. They may shift topics frequently, fail to take the perspective of the conversational partner, interrupt other speakers to make a point, say things that seem irrelevant or immature—all while being unaware of their violation of the simple conversational rules taken for granted by other speakers.

Identification of these pragmatic language issues assists the individual in prioritizing appropriate personal communication goals in the Psycholinguistic domain. Client and therapist engage in joint identification and analysis of elements of effective communication. We then negotiate acceptable communicative behaviors and select strategies for their development. The concept of effective communication is emphasized during this part of the treatment process. The client is motivated to think of herself as a communication partner, and to consider the possible effect she has on the other member or members of the conversational unit. For some, this is a new realization. People who stutter may not think of themselves as "partners" in a communication event. Rather, they may dwell on their own inadequacies in speaking, losing sight of the interactive quality of social interaction and feeling isolated by their history of negative communicative experiences. It is for these reasons that the identification phase of treatment of the Psycholinguistic domain plays so significant a role in the client's ultimate success in the treatment process.

In the establishment and modification phases of treatment, the client is encouraged to experiment with a variety of strategies that address the pragmatic dimension of language. One might introduce activities related to initiating a conversation with a stranger at a party, trying a number of different conversation openers or developing those skills necessary to be a good conversational partner (e.g., active listening, practicing eye contact while another is speaking, responding in a reflective manner when another is describing an event or experience). In addition, other psycholinguistic factors are introduced that relate primarily to the practice of exercises and drills in a carefully constructed hierarchy of linguistic demand. Each new skill is taught first in the most simple linguistic context available to the therapist. This simplicity may be at the level of syntax, richness of vocabulary, or length of utterances.

Then, in the stabilization phase of treatment, clients are encouraged to select those strategies they found to be most comfortable and effective in assisting them to communicate more easily, and to habituate them. They are introduced to a wide variety of practice drills at the word, phrase, sentence, and connected speech levels in reading, monologue, and conversation. It is during this phase that the clinician introduces the strategy of "mass practice," which is the highly repetitive, intensive practice of drills and activities performed frequently each day at designated times.

Although we speak of transfer as a separate dimension of treatment, in reality transfer activities are built into every stage of the treatment process. Once a new skill is introduced, it is practiced in as many speaking situations as possible in order to encourage generalization. It is during these transfer activities that the client is encouraged to use his fluency facilitation skills with new conversational partners and during specific intervals throughout each day, adapting to the differing communicative requirements inherent in any social situation.

It is also during this later stage of treatment that "conversational risk" is introduced. This technique sends the client into the larger community outside of the secure therapeutic environment to further select and refine those strategies that he believes will enhance effective communication. A trip with a church group, a social mixer, a party, or other social event at which new conversational partners are likely to be present—all become opportunities to try, evaluate, incorporate, or discard possible strategies for effective communication. The "message" becomes just as important, if not more so, than how it is delivered.[5] Many clients choose to join Toastmasters at this point in treatment since the focus of Toastmasters' meetings is effective speaking.

LEARNED FACTORS

Learned factors relate to those ultimately unsuccessful behaviors that the client employs in order to prevent stuttering and that in time become characteristic of the stuttering. These include what the client does to avoid certain words, speaking situations, or conversational partners, what the client does that suggests the anticipation or expectation that stuttering will occur, and what the client does physically that suggests a struggle to produce an utterance. These learned factors interfere with effective communication, as they distract the attention of the communicative partner from the message to the manner of its presentation.

During the identification phase of treatment, the client may view video-tapes or listen to audiotapes of conversations between people who stutter and their nonstuttering conversational partners. At first the subjects might be un-known to the client. The analysis of behaviors is then more objective, since ano-nymity precludes the viewer from attributing motives, feelings, or attitudes based upon known personality traits. The client is encouraged to identify the obvious uses of avoidance, anticipation, and struggle in the taped samples.

Next, the client may analyze taped samples of his own conversation with familiar conversational partners. Again the emphasis is on learned behaviors and how they promote or interfere with effective communication. The client's reac-tions to his own use of these learned behaviors is explored. The client's sugges-tions for diminishing these behaviors is solicited. Therapist and client spend as much or as little time on this variable as they deem necessary, based upon the sig-nificance of client's reliance on these behaviors or the severity of the stuttering.

During the modification and establishment phases, the client tries various techniques to diminish those learned behaviors that have been identified earlier. The point that must be emphasized is that learned behaviors can be modified, they can be replaced with a new set of learned behaviors that more closely paral-lel nonstuttered speech. For many, the very act of preparing for more fluent speech by consciously using and monitoring their use of fluency facilitating tech-niques serves to eliminate the interfering struggle behaviors. In addition, both anticipation and avoidance are diminished as unsuccessful speaking experiences are replaced with more successful ones.

Of course, it is our belief that managing stuttering behaviors alone does not ensure long-term maintenance of fluency. Old fears must be confronted and re-placed with feelings of confidence and increased self-esteem. Environmental is-sues related to family, communication skills, and cultural influences must be con-sidered and often modified. Counseling is an important therapeutic tool in this regard and will be discussed in detail in Chapter 9.

During the stabilization phase, new behaviors are once again mass prac-ticed until they are habituated. Home practice is key to successful completion of this phase of treatment. Then, during the transfer and maintenance phases, these new behaviors are tried in the world, first in low-stress situations and later in more complex, stressful communication experiences. Each spiral of the Speech and Language domain is introduced within the framework just described, from identification of existing behaviors through modification of these behaviors, sta-bilization of the newly learned behaviors, transfer of these behaviors into nontherapeutic environments, and maintenance of the new behaviors over time with little or no input from the clinician. It is through this systematic process that successful communication may become a reality for people who stutter.

SUMMARY

In this chapter we have explored the first of the three spirals of the Synergistic Model, the Speech and Language spiral. We have described a philosophy of treatment related to the physiologic, psycholinguistic, and learned behaviors found in individuals who stutter. We have made suggestions for treatment of these variables in the identification, modification and establishment, stabilization, transfer and maintenance phases.

REFERENCES

1. Schwartz MF. *Stuttering Solved.* New York: Lippincott, 1976.
2. Van Riper C. *The Treatment of Stuttering.* Englewood Cliffs, NJ: Prentice Hall, 1973.
3. Wolpe J. *Psychotherapy by Reciprocal Inhibition.* Stanford, CA: Stanford University Press, 1958.
4. Brutten EJ, Shoemaker DJ. *The Modification of Stuttering.* Englewood Cliffs, NJ: Prentice Hall, 1967.
5. Yovetich WS. Message therapy: Language approach to stuttering therapy with children. *J Fluency Disord* 1984;9:11–20.

7

Attitudes and Feelings

As we have noted in the preceding chapters, attitudes have long been acknowledged as a component in the stuttering equation. While there is a general conclusion that there is not a typical "stuttering personality," and our research does not support a single emotional or anxiety-based cause of stuttering, we believe that there is significant support from the research and from people who stutter that attitudes and feelings are an integral part of the synergistic pattern of stuttering. We agree with Conture[1] when he stated, "In my opinion, to understand the psychosocial aspects of stuttering without understanding the physiological aspects (or vice versa) means that one doesn't really understand the problem at all."

Drever[2] defined an attitude as "a more or less stable set or disposition of opinion, interest or purpose, involving expectancy of a certain kind of experience and readiness with an appropriate response." It would seem that this definition highlights the underlying expectancy of the experience of stuttering that dominates the attitudes and feelings reported by people who stutter. Some of the attitudes attributed to people who stutter are chronic fear, frustration, and embarrassment[3] and self demands for perfection.[4] People who stutter have also been described as anxious, shy, insecure, and hostile.[5] Conture[1] observed the following common traits in people who stutter: self-critical behavior; perfectionistic attitudes toward performance; extreme resistance to change; low self-esteem and self-confidence; and denial of increased fluency.

These attitudes have been found in both adults and children. Bloodstein[6] wrote:

> From age nine to sixteen the verbal reactions reported are substantially the ones with which clinicians are familiar through clinical experience with older people who stutter. Subjects admit more frequently that they are embarrassed or concerned about their stuttering, that they rehearse speech situations mentally beforehand, that they find it difficult to talk to other people about their stuttering, and that they are hurt or angered by the reactions of some of their listeners.

REVIEW OF THE LITERATURE: ATTITUDE ASSESSMENT

Adults

The relationship between stuttering and attitude has been studied by researchers and clinicians for many years.[3,7-10] A review of this literature is often complicated by confusion in terminology and difference in focus for research. Although many clinicians, using stuttering modification, recognize this difficulty in measuring attitudes, they nevertheless support the need for including attitudinal components in an intervention program. These clinicians often use reported scales for measuring attitudes and attempt to include some aspects of attitude in their therapy. Clinicians using fluency shaping therapy do not include attitudinal focus in rehabilitation techniques, yet they sometimes use the available tests to support their belief that improved speech will bring a corresponding improvement in attitude. Since these tests of attitude are used in some fashion by most clinicians, we will briefly review them here.

One of the first attempts to measure attitudes toward stuttering was the Iowa Scale of Attitude Toward Stuttering.[11] In this scale, a person was asked to indicate agreement or disagreement with a series of questions about stuttering. The purpose of this test was to identify the cognitive expectancies that contributed to stuttering. Although used for many years, this test contained the weakness of many attitudinal inventories in that the approved or desirable choices were too obvious.[12]

In 1967, Lanyon devised the Stuttering Severity Scale,[13] which was a self-report inventory of 64 true-false questions that measured the severity of the reactions of people who stutter. This scale included behavioral reactions such as avoidance, effort, and breathing difficulty as well as attitudes of worry, sensitivity, and dissatisfaction. Later, Lanyon reported that the behavioral and attitudinal components of this test demonstrated two distinct phenomena.[14] A popular clinical tool for the measurement of attitudes was developed by Woolf in 1967, the Perceptions of Stuttering Inventory.[15] This test measures the struggle, avoidance, and expectancy aspects of stuttering. Clinicians are encouraged to develop therapy goals and to measure progress based on this inventory. We have found that for the purposes noted, this instrument has been especially helpful in our approach to therapy (see Chapter 3).

The Erickson Scale of Communication Attitudes[16] was developed in 1969. This "S Scale" measures attitudes of people who stutter toward communication. In 1976, Guitar[17] found this measure to be a valid predictor of long-term improvement after treatment. In 1976, Guitar and Bass[18] found that attitude change appeared to be an important factor in treatment outcome. Based on the work of Bandura,[19] Ornstein and Manning[20,21] developed a technique to measure the confidence of by a person who stutters. Termed the "self-efficacy" technique, it assesses whether a person who stutters can (1) enter into speaking situations typically found outside treatment and (2) achieve a predetermined level of fluency in the speaking situation. They maintained that people who stutter show less confidence in regard to speaking situations and maintaining fluency. The Stuttering Problem Profile (SPP) was developed by Silverman in 1980.[22] The purpose of this inventory is to provide the clinician assistance in determining goals for therapy. Attitudes of the person who stutters are thought to be contained in their determination of the sort of statements they would like to be able to make at the end of therapy.

Watson and associates[23–25] developed an inventory to assess affective, cognitive, and behavioral attitudes to stuttering. Thirty-nine different situations are rated according to whether the client enjoyed a speaking situation, that is, whether their speech skills were good in the situation. In 1993, Leith and colleagues[10] attempted to review and summarize the tests that measure attitudes and feelings toward stuttering. They devised five well-developed scales that tested orientation toward oral communication in general, perceived influences of stuttering on life adjustments, and attitudes toward stuttering. This comprehensive study demonstrated that negative attitudes and beliefs do exist among people who stutter and that these attitudes and beliefs influence the success of treatment. Consequently, the "treatment program should include specific procedures designed to modify those attitudes and beliefs that are counter-productive in the stuttering person's treatment, life-style, and social interactions."[10]

Children

There has been conflicting research regarding the attitudes of children who stutter. Janis Costello said in 1984 that "[t]here is essentially no literature that demonstrates that children who go through stuttering treatment have attitudinal problems."[26] In 1970, Silverman[27] concluded from his research with children who stutter that dysfluent children are not typically concerned about their speech. More recently, Culatta[28] repeated Silverman's study and confirmed the previous results that children were not concerned about their speech. Devore, Nandur, and Manning[29] found no difference between the speech attitudes of five stuttering children and five nonstuttering children. As in the research on adult attitudes, the conflicting parameters of the research in children often seem to cloud the issue. Despite these differences, researchers have continued to explore the possibility of a communication attitude test (CAT) for children. In 1985, Brutten and Dunham[30] reported no difference between males and females who stutter. Their findings suggest, however, that children who stutter responded to the CAT in a clearly different way than did children who do not stutter. De Nil and Brutten[31] used a Dutch version of the test (CAT-D) and their results led them to conclude that young children have already developed a relatively firm negative self-concept about their communicative abilities.

These findings were confirmed by Vanryckeghem and Brutten,[32] who reported that the CAT test is reliable over time and that it has considerable utility for clinicians who are concerned with the attitudes of children whose fluency is problematic. Vanryckeghem[33] investigated the extent that the parents' view of their school-aged child's attitude reflected that of their child's attitudes about stuttering. She found that neither parent is likely to be a useful source of information about their child's attitudes toward speech:

> The relative lack of parent-child agreement as to the grade-schoolers' attitude toward speech, be they stutterers or nonstutterers, is consistent with the findings of similar studies in the field of psychiatry. There, too, parent-child agreement has proven to be very limited, especially as it relates to beliefs, feelings, anxieties and worries.[33]

We support the use of the CAT test of attitudes for children and we urge clinicians to continue to integrate the reports of children's attitudes toward their stuttering behavior found by assessment techniques and observational reports.

Riley and Riley[34] listed the following attitudes found among stuttering children who place themselves under pressure to be "perfect":

1. Excessive self-blame
2. Excessive anxiety
3. Excessive withdrawal
4. Excessive dependency
5. Poor ego strength

Such children also resent disruptive communication conditions that influence their attitudinal response to speaking:

1. Child has difficulty getting the speaker's attention
2. Family members rush the child's speech
3. Listeners interrupt or "butt in" while the child is speaking
4. Child is teased about his speech problem by siblings, playmates, or others
5. People make negative comments about the child's speech

We believe that these descriptions give evidence of the interaction of attitudinal and environmental forces, especially the interaction among self-esteem, assertion, locus of control, communication skills, and family.

Conture[1] expanded upon the necessity for the close observation of children's attitudes when he wrote: "With children, who cannot as easily articulate their psychosocial concerns, one may have to look for behavioral indexes." A partial listing of additional behavioral indexes includes the following:

1. A child that other children routinely shun or avoid
2. A child that other adults report that they can't manage or won't allow in their home
3. A child who refuses to speak to the clinician, no matter what the topic or approach, after 30 to 90 minutes of trying, but who readily talks to the parent once the clinician leaves the room

4. A child who routinely acts out against other children
5. A child whose strong fear of fire, loud noises, the dark, and anything new or unusual is so routine and long-term as to disrupt home life
6. Any combination of 1–5 above

While we do not believe that negative attitudes, beliefs and psychosocial problems cause stuttering, we believe that the varied attitudes toward stuttering develop as a result of the general synergistic interaction of the child's self-esteem, locus of control and assertiveness. In turn, these aspects synergistically interact with the physiologic and environmental levels of dysfluency.

SYNERGISTICALLY INTEGRATED APPROACH TO ATTITUDES AND FEELINGS

As we have seen, the reported literature on attitudes has provided us with a variety of tools for assessment. Although each of these tests assesses attitude, few of them test the same thing. One tests the feelings and attitudes about stuttering.[16] Another one tests the stutterer's perception of the presence of struggle, avoidance, and expectancy of stuttering in communication.[15] Yet another assists the therapist in defining goals for therapy.[22] Each of these can play a valuable role in therapy, but we believe that it is important that clinicians understand what is being tested and how their own understanding of the role of attitudes in the development of stuttering plays a major role in both their assessments and development of therapeutic processes.

Although all people who stutter do not share the same attitudes about themselves or their stuttering, Silverman and Zimmer[35] demonstrated that speech attitudes can strongly affect the lives of people who stutter. They found that students who stuttered took little part in classroom activities and avoided speaking privately with teachers. As adults, they spoke of taking jobs they were overqualified for and from which they experienced little success because of their inappropriate attitudes toward communication. We agree with these findings, and although there is less research on the attitudes of people who stutter than on the other components of stuttering, we believe that a clearer focus on the attitudes of people who stutter will provide valuable data and a greater understanding of the roles attitudes play in the lives of those who stutter.

Culatta and Goldberg[36] have written:

If clinicians decide it is important to directly work on a client's attitude to facilitate successful accomplishment of the desired goals, then it is necessary to determine what goals should be selected. A review of the literature reveals there are essentially five types of attitudes, not all compatible, that clinicians attempt to develop in their clients: 1. acceptance of responsibility for behavioral change, 2. realistic understanding of both negative and positive effects of stuttering on the client's life, 3. acceptance of stuttering as a life-long condition, 4. acceptance of monitored fluency as a life-long condition, and 5. acceptance of nonmonitored normal fluency as a life-long condition.

We believe that clinicians can best pursue such goals by understanding the three areas of self-esteem, locus of control, and assertiveness. These were analyzed in Chapter 2, and we reintroduce them here as what we choose to call "Empowerment Attitudes." It is the synergistic interaction of these elements that we believe underlies the development of both negative and positive attitudes in those who stutter and that therefore must be addressed with our clients. In order to include these areas in their approach to therapy, it is important that clinicians reflect on their role as clinician-counselors as defined by Bloom and Cooperman[37] and develop the therapeutic skills that are considered in Chapters 8 and 9.

Self-Esteem

Everyone understands that each of us has a self-image. We are also aware that we act out whatever image we have of ourselves. However, we are not born with our self-concept. It is something that we learn from our environment. As noted in Chapter 2, self-esteem is the measure of how much we like and approve of our self-concept. It is our belief that people who stutter have incorporated the negative elements of stuttering into their self-concept. Our research currently in progress strongly supports this view.

Carol Prutting[38] has written:

It has been said that in America no less than 95 percent of us somehow manage to develop low self-esteem by the young age of 7. At our core is a vital, alive, perfect being equipped with all that is needed and is with us from our first breath to our last. Sadly though, most people do not reside in that being. By age 7 a second core has formed which has too much to do with the nagging question of what is incomplete or wrong with us. In conjunction with this second circle, a third one emerges. This one is depicted as involving what we do to try and hide and compensate for our believed set of impurities. Our behavior can take on many forms and we become vulnerable to others when finding out just how inadequate we are.

Certainly, we know that people who stutter have gone so far as to create a second identity to prevent others from knowing that they stutter. Prutting continued:

The challenge here is to believe in ourselves and to trust ourselves for everything external depends on trust within. What we are to the outer world is a mirror or reflection of our inner world. When we achieve high self-esteem and we are emotionally well-grounded and self-accepting, we are able to accept others unconditionally. The result is an enhancement of our relationships with others.

Our goal is to expand our client's world of communication and this necessarily implies that our clients will become more self-actualized and independent people. In 1962, Maslow[39] described the fully functioning person with a positively developed self-esteem as one who had the following characteristics:

1. Acceptance of the inner core of self
2. Expression of the inner core of self
3. Minimal presence of ill health, neurosis, psychic loss, or dimunition of basic human personal capacities; this inner core is good, but although biologically based is weak
4. Selfishness and unselfishness fused into higher superordinate unity
5. Conscious, preconsciousness, unconsciousness integrated
6. Cognitive, affective, and motor more synergistic
7. Aesthetic, perceiving, creating, and peak experiences are central aspects of life and of psychology and educational rather than peripheral

As speech-language pathologists and audiologists, we know that our clients have battled with their acceptance of self as a person who stutters and that their expression of that same self is generally limited. At the end of therapy, it is rewarding to be told by a client that their understanding of self is as a person who happens to stutter sometimes. They have come to value their inner core and to express the same with great enthusiasm. Combs[40] describes the person with high self-esteem as:

1. Seeing himself in positive ways
2. Having an identification with others
3. Being open to experience and acceptance
4. Having a rich and available perceptual field

These characteristics form what we call a "healthy self-concept" and result in a positive self-esteem. This is best understood as a process, not a fixed or rigid idea of self, and the goals listed above are ones toward which we all strive throughout our life. Consciousness of these goals is important for our development as clinician-counselors and for our work with those who stutter. Frey and Carlock[41] surveyed how leading psychologists of our day have understood the importance of self-esteem:

1. Carl Rogers: "If I were to search for the central core of difficulty in people as I havecome to know them, it is that in the great majority of cases they despise themselves, regarding themselves as worthless and unlovable."
2. Eric Fromm: "Love of others and love of ourselves are not alternatives. On the contrary, an attitude of love toward themselves will be found in all those who are capable of loving others."
3. Stanley Coopersmith: "Probably the most important requirement for effective behavior, central to the whole problem, is self-esteem."

4. Virginia Satir: "My dream is to make families a place where adults with high self-esteem can develop. I think we have reached a point where if we don't get busy on dreams of this sort, our end is in sight. We need a world that is as good for human beings as it is for technology."
5. Bruno Bettelheim: "With some qualifications I suggest that nothing is more characteristic of mental well being than a healthy self respect, a regard for one's body and its functions, and a reasonably optimistic outlook on life."
6. Abraham Maslow: "No psychological health is possible unless this essential care of the person is fundamentally accepted, loved and respected by others and by himself."

As our understanding of the importance of self-esteem deepens, we continue to research techniques for enhancing the self-concept of our clients who stutter. Stanley Coopersmith[42] conducted extensive research on self-esteem and concluded that there are four different fundamental experiences that lead to increased self-esteem: (1) feelings of significance, (2) feelings of competence, (3) feelings of power, and (4) feelings of virtue.

Feelings of Significance

According to Coopersmith, this experience lies in "the acceptance, attention and affection of others." The individual high in self-esteem feels important to, involved with, and valued by the other significant people in his life. No one is immune from this need, but it is of special importance to those who stutter. As a young child, a person who stutters derives feelings of importance, significance, involvement, and worth from their family. Many of our clients tell us that no one ever spoke about their stuttering to them. It was as if it wasn't there, which made them also feel as if this was a "bad" part of themselves and unacceptable to their families. In addition, as children move into adolescence, it is necessary for them to separate from their parents and find sources of validation outside their family. Most typically, feelings of significance and connectedness with adults are obtained through teachers and other school staff. Adults find significance from personal relationships, professional achievement, and interpersonal communication. When considering the important role of teachers and clinicians, as well as clients' families, it was disquieting to note that in a survey of 818 students attending a suburban high school in Portland , Oregon, only 27 percent of the students answered yes to the item: "I feel wanted and needed at this school." It is important that we incorporate techniques that will enable our clients to feel both significant and positively connected to others.

Feelings of Competence

Coopersmith[42] defined competence as "successful performance in meeting demands for achievement." The individual with high self-esteem generally feels capable, adequate, competent, and successful in one or more of the important aspects of her life. Many people who stutter have developed feelings of competence in other areas of their lives: music, sports, and even business. However, the lack of the ability to communicate freely may shadow their self-concepts. Their failure to speak as they perceive others do often has a detrimental impact on both their feelings of competence and their self-esteem. In order to grow in a feeling of competence, we must know and accept our individual strengths and our weaknesses. We learn to cope with failure by recalling past successes and triumphs. We can also learn to accept our weaknesses and strive to change what can be changed. It is an interesting fact that when one has been affirmed sufficiently for the strengths that one possesses, it is not difficult for that person to confront weaknesses. It is our job as clinicians to assist our clients in developing their self-esteem by reinforcing the strengths we see and leading them to both accept and change what can be changed. Carl Rogers[43] observed: "The curious paradox is that when I accept myself just as I am, then I can change."

It is important that we recognize that it is not sufficient to praise someone lavishly or unduly. Praise must be an honest response to what the person accomplished. It is through competence and mastery that we begin to change our negative self-concept and to feel good about ourselves. We must afford our clients many opportunities to feel successful and to recognize their success. In addition, we must be available for our clients when they experience failure. David Daly[44] wrote:

> We must be there for the client to support, to encourage, and to genuinely praise. We also must be there to catch them and help them back up when they fail. And they will fail at some point. Failure is common along the road to success. Remind clients of the fact that successful people fail more than unsuccessful people. Invite them to read histories of successful people. Show them samples of people who failed and then succeeded because they kept on trying. To be more successful they must be willing to fail more. The secret for improving any skill is practice, drill, and rehearsal.

Feelings of Power

The third of the four sources of self-esteem posited by Coopersmith[42] is a feeling of power, defined as "the ability to influence and control others." He believes that an individual who has positive self-esteem believes she can have an effect, a meaningful impact, on other people and on her environment. High self-esteem implies feelings of control, of self-determination, and of autonomy. We have considered this aspect of attitude development under our earlier analysis of locus of control in Chapter 2. Indeed, these two areas are synergistically connected so that as persons come to feel more significant and gain a sense of mastery and competence, they will be empowered to assume responsibility for themselves and establish positive relations with others. It is for this reason that the suggested activities at the end of this chapter are not listed separately. Each activity may bring about either or all of the empowerment attitudes.

Feelings of Virtue

The final facet of high self-esteem according to Coopersmith[42] is a feeling of virtue. Virtuousness is usually defined as adherence to moral and ethical standards. Virtue, as a source of self-esteem, is best experienced by attaining what is a higher standard, that of being genuinely and actively helpful and nurturing to others. Coopersmith believes, and we agree, that only by achieving this higher standard will individuals obtain sufficient feelings of virtue to produce significant self-esteem. We have found it helpful to understand this dimension of virtue in terms of leadership and assertiveness. Our clients who have reached out to assist those who stutter have not only been a help to others but they have gained a great deal of inner strength themselves. Such opportunities for leadership experiences—speaking to a parent group, addressing classes of graduate students, appearing on radio and TV—are an important area of therapy that has proven effective in increasing self-esteem and developing assertiveness. Successfully confronting the fears about speaking while at the same time helping someone understand stuttering brings a visible and valuable growth to those who accept this challenge. As Manning[21] has written:

> Self-esteem is not something that can be given to you. Nonetheless, the stage can be set by loving parents and friends as well as by a competent clinician. As the clinician provides a secure and stable therapeutic environment, growth will be likely to occur. When the client experiences success in the self-management of surface and intrinsic aspects of his fluency disorder, self-esteem and self-confidence begin to shift in a positive direction.

Clemes[45] has identified the following as characteristic of those with low self-esteem:

> They demean their own talents. "I can't."
> They feel others don't value them or give them negative feelings.
> They feel powerless and lack self confidence.
> They are easily influenced by others and are often manipulated.
> They may express a narrow range of predictable feelings.
> They will avoid situations that provoke anxiety and have a very low tolerance for stress.
> They are very defensive, easily frustrated, and "thin skinned."
> They will blame others for their own weaknesses and will rarely admit to any mistakes or weaknesses.

On the other hand, those with high self-esteem have the following characteristics:

> They will act independently in making choices and decisions.
> They assume responsibility and will act promptly and confidently.
> They are proud of their accomplishments and will acknowledge their achievements.

They approach new challenges with enthusiasm, interest, and confidence.
They exhibit a broad range of emotions and feelings without self-consciousness.
They tolerate frustrations well, and meet and deal with them effectively.
They feel special to those they love, play, and work.
They feel capable of influencing others' confidence.

In reviewing the major components of self-esteem, we recognize that ours must truly be an individual, client-centered approach. Although there is no failsafe method for helping people who stutter improve their self-esteem, we know that it has been estimated that 80 percent of this population has to struggle with this issue. In addition, in order to recognize, provide, and reinforce opportunities for a client's growth in significance, mastery, competence, power and leadership, a clinician must first have identified her own potential areas of strength as well as her limitations. With this increased self-understanding, a clinician will have the needed insight to recognize the successes in a client's life and help him to accept failures as challenges to be overcome.

Locus of Control

In Chapter 2 we defined and explored the concept of locus of control as it applies to stuttering. Depending on outside factors such as luck or chance to improve one's situation (external locus of control) is very limiting. It has been shown that people with an internal locus of control feel that they have more control over what happens to them. Research[46,47] has found that internals are more assertive, effective, and competent people. They are people who are positive and active in taking responsibility for improving their lives. Bandura's[48] self-efficacy theory is important to note in this connection. This theory proposes that people change their behavior when they alter their expectations of personal efficacy. They come to believe that they are able to execute appropriate responses because they have had experiences of mastery that arose from successful performance.

This is an integral part of the concept of locus of control and is the foundation for our therapeutic approach. People who stutter experience a history of loss of control in their ability to express their thoughts and feelings at the moment that they wish to. Stutterers often describe themselves as "powerless." As was stated in Chapter 2, we believe that the measurement of internal and external locus of control can provide clinicians with valuable information for purposes of both diagnosis and treatment efficacy. In reporting on their behavioral program for fluency, Craig and Howie[49] stressed that the results of a behavioral program should give evidence of a reduced frequency of dysfluency as well as a Locus of Control of Behavior (LCB) Score toward the internal dimension. However, Manning[21] referred to the work of other researchers[50,51] who have asserted that the predictive value of locus of control is likely to be significantly affected by the nature of the treatment program used: "If for the client to assume control of his speech is a major focus of treatment (regardless of the individual's fluency level),

LCB measures are more likely to change in their direction of internality. In addition, an intensive three-week period of treatment may not allow sufficient time for the internalization of control."

We believe that teaching targets of speech production is an important aspect of a synergistic program. In Chapter 5 we defined the Speech and Language targets that must be used when practicing some of the exercises for treating attitudinal issues such as locus of control. It is the combination of the fluency shaping techniques and the stuttering modification techniques (Chapter 1) that brings success. The successful accomplishment of these therapeutic speech targets provides the sense of mastery and competence that allows clients to develop a positive view of themselves as they take control of their fluency (fluency shaping). It is then necessary to talk about the feelings and attitudes connected with both the successes and failures in speech communication (stuttering modification).

This process of choosing responsibility for your speech (locus of control) is synergistically related to both self-esteem and assertiveness. As one takes charge of his own life, faithfully using the fluency enhancing skills they have been taught, one develops a higher self-esteem and assertiveness. The development of these empowerment attitudes is interwoven with successful improvement in the speech-language techniques (Chapter 5), which brings about an increase in motivation that is essential for success.

Application of Locus of Control to Fluency Therapy

Here we will summarize techniques that one might use in a synergistic approach to fluency therapy. It should be noted at the outset that more research is needed in this area. Studies have been done in other areas of health care, but only a few have been carried out with dysfluent clients. The general principles and activities that have increased our awareness and guided our approach to the development of internal locus of control and motivation (self-efficacy) are included in the section at the end of this chapter.

In examining the literature, we find that there are two groups of exercises and techniques that are useful in structuring the therapeutic approach for a fluency client: awareness exercises and cognitive therapy techniques. We will consider each of these in turn.

Awareness Techniques

An early goal of therapy at the identification stage has always been to increase a client's awareness of his stuttering pattern. Certainly, the awareness and evaluation of one's stuttering pattern is one of the most observable areas of fluency awareness. Although it is the easiest of the awareness techniques, it is nonetheless very important and is the cornerstone of a fluency program. However, we believe that awareness of attitudes is equally important. We agree with Ham[5] when he wrote:

Self-analysis encompasses the awareness of each stuttering occurrence when it happens; cognizance of the type, severity, and physical location(s) of the stuttering; descriptions of the struggle, overflow, and the associated behavior patterns; understanding of the attitudes concerning stuttering in particular and speech in general; and a perception of the environmental reactions to moments of stuttering, as they occur. Further, to varying degrees, self-analysis encompasses the characteristics of nonstuttered speech of the stutterer and of other speakers. These elements of self-analysis should be available as part of the stutterer's own knowledge and be functional during any situation in which he participates.

In addition to the stuttering patterns and attitudes, we believe that it is necessary to directly work with the awareness of one's own ability to make choices about speech. Every choice moves us either closer to or farther away from good communication patterns and fluent speech. We have the ability to react or to respond. If we simply react, we continue the automatic behavior that we have used for most of our lives. When one is in a difficult speaking situation, one stutters as habit dictates. If we respond, however, we choose a new behavior. Between every stimulus and response there is "pause time" during which a person can take control of his behavior and change. Allenbaugh[52] has written: "Conscious accountability empowers your internal resources to be of service in experiencing life at a more fulfilling level. Internal resources, especially when they are nurtured, frequently have more power than outside sources." Two options that clients are faced with when they are in pause time are (1) a victimized position ("Why does this always happen to me?" "I have no control over my speech. I always stuttered and I always will") or (2) a position of choice ("What are my thoughts, feelings and behaviors in this situation?" "What do I have to change?" "What can I do to make the necessary change?").

We know that all meaningful change comes from within. It is an important aspect of internal control to facilitate a position of choice with our clients. Allenbaugh[52] illustrates this phenomenon in Figure 7.1. Those who continue to react unconsciously and automatically have been described by Adams[53] as people who do not want to change their stuttering behavior. Their disinterest is genuine and strong. For many of these people, their lack of motivation comes from the believe that they cannot change their behavior. The clinical term for this is "conditioned helplessness." Seligman[54] felt that many individuals learn that the important aspects of one's life and actions are simply beyond control. When they feel this way they act helpless and they are incapable of doing anything to change their behavior. Adams[53] wrote:

Among these more helpless patients there is a strong tendency to indulge in self-pity and to complain about how fate has held them back or done them in. Once treatment begins, tardiness, a failure to keep clinic appointments, and feeble excuses for poor performance all increase as the patient is asked to assume more responsibility for controlling and changing his behavior.

In response to this behavior, Adams constructed a four-point strategy: (1) During initial evaluations look for and take special note of those who exhibit

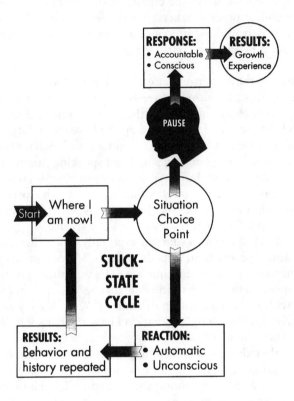

EVERY SITUATION IS BRAND-NEW!
CHOICE: Grow or repeat history

Figure 7.1 Stuck-state cycle. (Reprinted with permission from Allenbaugh, E. *Wake-Up Calls*. New York: Simon and Schuster, 1992, p. 43.)

signs of conditioned helplessness. (2) When such a patient is identified, structure treatment so as to ease the individual very gradually into accepting small and then progressively larger amounts of responsibility for the control of his speech behavior. (3) Set more readily obtainable speech goals. (4) Reward the attainment of these goals with comments that emphasize the achievement of conscious control of fluency—"You did it!" "You made it happen!" "You were really in control then!" The intent is to maximize the occurrence of successes and positive feedback so as to provide the patient with behavioral evidence that he is not a helpless victim but rather a person who can consciously organize and execute motor speech behaviors that are integral to fluency.

It is our position that many people who stutter can and do change their automatic and unconscious speech responses to responses that are conscious and accountable. The first step in any kind of change is awareness. Clients need to grow in the awareness of what their choices really are. Will they choose to stutter? Will they choose to avoid situations that could bring them happiness? Will they choose to use their speech targets? Will they choose to reach out to get involved in a new but difficulty situation? Each choice brings a direct result. We are our choices. All growth in life comes from our power to choose. Letting go of the past habit of stuttering and the past feelings and attitudes about communication demand that the person is aware, committed, and responsible. He must be actively engaged in the process. Allenbaugh[52] has encouraged the acceptance of responsibility by using the following strategies:

> Teach yourself to pause at the choice point and tap into your inner resources. The answers are within.
>
> Determine what you want to create in your life, and set specific written behavioral goals.
>
> Clarify your values and principles that can serve as guides in decision making at the choice point.
>
> Share your goals with a trusted friend and ask for assistance and periodic feedback related to behavioral progess.
>
> Maintain a confidential journal on your stuck-state choices. Your mind processes written information differently from just thinking about available choices. Your journal can be an important resource in tracking progress.
>
> Replace "This is the way I am" with "Up until now . . ." or "I am now choosing. . . ." This reflective process reinforces pausing at the choice point and encourages self-awareness.
>
> Once a week, review your choices in order to celebrate successes and take appropriate corrective action. Be gentle with yourself; this process is about correction not perfection.

We are a product of our choices, not of our circumstances. The whole course of our life is linked to the decisions that we have made in the past. Not all of our choices are made out of full awareness. Sometimes clients believe that stuttering is something that "happens to them." When this happens, a person is acting without awareness and has an increased external locus of control. Schutz[55] expressed the belief that the unconscious part of us is simply those things of which we choose not to be aware. When we accept the responsibility of becoming aware and choosing our response to life situations, we empower internal locus of control rather than external control.

This understanding is also expressed by Montgomery,[56,57] whose holistic approach to the treatment of stuttering stresses, as we do with our speech-language factors, the client's ability to feel the motor movements of the speech mechanism and to enter into as many situations as possible, accepting responsibility for the outcome. In addition , she encourages clients to accept whatever happens as feedback for learning inner control:

> If the client speaks with the new sense of control and coordination in some situations . . . great. If he has difficulty in other situations . . . fine. If he chooses not to use any new skills in a situation . . . o.k. Its all part of the learning process and "mistakes" are an essential part of it. We learn from all of it. This is now the time when he begins to take over more and more as his own coach and learns to analyze and troubleshoot. These are the critical experiences that give the client a "gut level" knowing that he can do it . . . that he can speak fluently with focus on his muscles and that he can "fix" his dysfluencies if and when they occur.[56]

We believe that this sort of awareness brings the power of internal control that we have been describing. As a person who stutters becomes more aware of and takes control of his feelings, attitudes, and behaviors, increased internality will increase and bring with it a sense of freedom and growth. Another way to nurture this growth is to be aware of and change one's cognitive self-talk. This, too, is synergistically related to a growth in self-esteem and assertiveness.

Cognitive Therapy Techniques

Either with or without a heightened self-awareness, most people carry on a silent conversation with themselves each day. This self-talk can actually direct the way they think and feel about themselves and influence the way that they behave. Sometimes this self-talk becomes a self-fullfilling prophecy: we think so much about something that we in the end act to make it come true. Cognitive theorists have addressed this problem and believe that human problems are often an identify problem of distorted thinking.[21,58] In addition, we are often in denial and unaware of our own negative thoughts and behaviors. It is important that we become aware of these negative thoughts and counter them with a realization of positive possiblities. Once again, clinicians must examine their own beliefs and self-talk before they can effectively work with their clients.

Ellis[58] developed the theory of Rational Emotive Therapy (RET) as a framework for uncovering and considering negative—or "irrational"—thoughts. Manning[21] compiled a list of these irrational ideas that all people tend to have. He believes, as do we, that changing the type of thinking represented by negative thoughts would result in our being happier and healthier. In addition, we believe that these irrational thoughts need to be explored with our clients who stutter.

> It is a dire necessity for an adult human to be loved or approved of by virtually every "significant other" in his community.
> A person should be thoroughly competent, adequate, and successful in all possible respects if he is to consider himself worthwhile, and he is utterly worthless if he is incompetent in any way.
> Certain people can be labeled bad, wicked, or villainous, and they deserve severe blame or punishment for their sins.
> It is awful or catastrophic when things are not the way an individual would very much like them to be.

Human unhappiness is externally caused, and individuals have little or no ability to control their sorrows and disturbances.

If something is or may be dangerous or fearsome, one should be terribly concerned about it and should keep dwelling on the possibility of its occurance.

It is easier to avoid certain life difficulties and self-responsibilities than to face them.

An individual should be dependent on others and needs someone stronger than himself on whom to rely.

A person's past history is an all-important determinant of his present behavior, and because something once strongly affected his life, it should continue to do so.

An individual should become quite upset over other people's problems and disturbances.

There is invariably a correct, precise, and perfect solution to human problems, and it is catastrophic if this perfect solution is not found.

Ellis[58] insisted that that these irrational thoughts must be disputed and developed a process for doing so called the "ABC's of RET":

A. Activating event—something unpleasant happens to us.
B. Belief system—we interpret the event.
C. Consequences—we get upset. We "awfulize" the situation.
D. Disputing irrational beliefs. You question and change your thinking about the event.
E. Changing irrational beliefs to rational beliefs.

An example of applying the ABC approach to stuttering is the following:

A. A person wants to make a good impression on his audience and he stutters throughout his entire talk.
B. He believes that he was a failure because he wasn't fluent.
C. He then feels incompetent and worthless.
D. He chooses to dispute these irrational thoughts: "Why is it so awful?" "Why shouldn't it be awful?" "What are the positive aspects of my talk?" He tells himself: " I don't have to speak perfectly to be good." "It's definitely disappointing but it's not a disaster."
E. Changing irrational to rational beliefs: "I would like things to be different but that doesn't mean that everything has to be the way I want it. My talk was good and I can work harder at using my targets the next time. This was a big step in the right direction."

Clients can be encouraged to make the critical move from irrational to rational beliefs. Corey[59] cites Ellis' encouragement to teach the following:

Teach clients that they are not bad people when they do not achieve their goals.

Teach clients that perfection is not required to be a worthwhile person.

Teach clients that popularity and achievement are not necessarily related and being a worthwhile person does not require 100 percent popularity.

Teach clients not to take themselves nor their situations too seriously by turning minor setbacks into catastrophies.

Although more research is needed on the application of RET to fluency therapy, we have adapted aspects of this cognitive therapy in working with our clients and they have found it helpful in assuming more control of their thinking. In turn, it enables them to grow in their recognition of their internal ability to control themselves and their speech. We have used and recommend Burns' *The Feeling Good Handbook*[60] for some practical approaches, which has a helpful checklist of cognitive distortions:

1. All-or-nothing thinking: You look at things in absolute, black and white categories.
2. Overgeneralization: You view a negative event as a never-ending pattern of defeat.
3. Mental filter: You dwell on the negatives and ignore the positives.
4. Discounting the positives: You insist that your accomplishments and positive qualities don't count.
5. Jumping to conclusions: (A) Mind reading—you assume that people are reacting negatively to you when there's no definite evidence of this. (B) Fortune-telling—You predict that things will turn out badly.
6. Magnification or minimization: You blow things way out of proportion or you shrink their importance.
7. Emotional reasoning: You reason how you feel—" I feel like an idiot, so I must be one."
8. "Should" statements: You criticize yourself or other people with "shoulds," "shouldn'ts," "must," "oughts," and "have-tos."
9. Labeling: Instead of saying "I made a mistake," you tell yourself "I'm a jerk" or "a loser."
10. Blame: You blame yourself for something you weren't entirely responsible for, or you blame other people and overlook ways that you contributed to a problem.

We incorporated Burns' steps for changing these negative thoughts in the following way:

1. Identify the upsetting event. Write a brief description of the speech problem that is bothering you. Be specific. When did it happen? What time of day?
2. Record you negative feelings. Use words like sad, frustrated, discouraged, angry, hurt, anxious, embarrassed, upset, or guilty.

3. Use the Triple-Column technique: In Column 1, record your negative thoughts (the way that you interpret the event). In Column 2, identify the distorted (irrational) thinking. In Column 3, substitute more realistic thoughts.

Some responses from our clients using this scheme were as follows:

1. I was unable to say what I actually meant on the phone, so I substituted some of the words I wanted to say. I was a failure.
2. I was very embarrassed and discouraged.
3. Apply the triple-column technique:

Negative Thoughts	Distortions	Positive Thoughts
I will never speak right. I am unable to control speech.	Labeling, over-generalization	This was a momentary lapse of a good speaking day. No one is perfect. I am making good progress in speech.

1. I was not considered for promotion because of my speech.
2. I was frustrated and angry.
3. Apply the triple-column technique:

Negative Thoughts	Distortions	Positive Thoughts
I'll never be able to support my family. I'll never be able to get a job as long as I stutter.	Fortune-telling Over-generalizing	It might not be because of my speech that I didn't get the job. I've had jobs. I will again. I can work on my speech.

In addition to using this technique with our clients, we have used it with our student therapists. They were given the same directions as our clients. Their responses were varied and reportedly helpful to the students completing the assignment. Some were as follows:

1. I failed a test.
2. I felt insecure and afraid. I was embarrassed and angry.
3. Apply the triple-column technique:

Negative Thoughts	Distortions	Positive Thoughts
I'll never be an SLP. I'm not good enough for this field.	All-or-nothing magnifications Jumping to conclusions	I have passed many other tests. I got an A in clinic.

1. My fluency client was having a bad day. I said as much as I could, as much as I knew how to say.
2. I was nervous. I was afraid that I didn't help him. I thought someone else could do it better.
3. Apply the triple-column technique:

Negative Thoughts	Distortions	Positive Thoughts
He would like another therapist. He would do better with someone else.	Mind reading Mental filter Emotional reasoning	I'm doing fine for a 1st yr. student. I need to have a class in counseling. I will sign up for one. My client said he enjoyed the class. I will be easier on myself.

We believe that the active practice of identifying distorted thoughts, feelings, and behaviors can have a positive effect on a person who stutters. It can be another way of teaching them that they have control of both the physical and attitudinal dimensions of stuttering. One should carry a small pad to record one's thoughts and feelings as soon as possible after a disturbing event. This homework is essential to the practice. Our own research has led us to encourage others to employ this strategy for changing negative to positive thoughts and for assuming greater autonomy. This, in turn, leads to becoming more assertive. Clearly, locus of control is synergistically connected with assertiveness, which we will consider next.

Assertiveness

Assertive behavior, nonassertive behavior, and aggressive behavior were defined in Chapter 2. We have found that many people who stutter come to us as people who use nonassertive interpersonal behavior—that is, they allow their own rights to be violated. Often this happens from their reluctance to speak, from their lack of self-esteem, and from the fact that they have never owned or taken control of their basic rights in life. Although the goal of communication is to engage in assertive behavior that is honest, direct, and appropriate, we find that many people who stutter move from nonassertive behavior to aggressive behavior—that is, they stand up for their own rights but do not recognize the other person's rights. Once fluency is gained and the person experiences the power of speaking, they may express this new sense of power in ways that are uncharacteristic of them and that are offensive to those around them. We have discussed this issue with several spouses, parents, and friends of people who stutter. However, there is little in the way of formal research on this issue, and we recommend that future studies be conducted on the role of assertiveness training in fluency therapy.

Schloss[61] examined the effect of assertiveness training on the communicative ability of people who stutter in employment interviews. The study provided skill training for clients who stutter in the following areas: giving corrective feedback to employers following employer interruptions, responding to pejorative statements, and making statements to set the employer at ease. This study was carried out with three people who stutter. Changes in behaviors, as evaluated by a multiple baseline design, showed training to be effective. "It is apparent from this data that individuals who stutter can be trained to behave assertively in interview situations. Tentative evidence suggests that assertive behavior may produce a collateral benefit of enhancing fluency. Future studies may be conducted to support this contention."[62] We believe that developing a repertoire of assertive behaviors will help clients achieve their desired communication goals and will enhance not only their fluency skills but will interact with their feeling of self-worth and internal perception of control.

Beaty[62] used Lazarus'[63] Multimodal Behavior Model to evaluate a client's personality across seven separate but interrelated modalities. Of these seven categories, three of them relate to the attitudes we have correlated with empowerment—self-esteem, locus of control, and assertiveness—and hence can be aligned with our focus on speech-language behaviors. They isolated the following modalities and suggest the following treatments,[62] which support the synergistic approach:

Cognitions:	Irrational self-talk. I am abnormal. I am inferior.	Training: Rational-emotive training. Challenge internal sentences in which he puts himself down.
Imagery:	Seeing himself laughed at. Seeing himself turn red when speaking.	Training: Thought stopping. Think praise, reward self.
Interpersonal Relations:	Little social contact.	Training: Assertion training, role plays of interpersonal encounters.

Lazarus[63] has argued that the major advantage of a multimodal orientation is that it provides a systematic framework for conceptualizing presenting complaints within a meaning framework. We concur and agree with Beaty[62] that this study assesses important aspects of empowerment and, although not worked out, provides evidence of their synergistic interaction.

McWhirter and colleagues[64] isolated five basic skill strengths or skill deficits that mark a critical difference between children who will succeed and children who will not. Four of these competencies are included in our approach: self-esteem, communication skills, control, and coping ability, which includes assertiveness training. "When students learn and use these skills, they become more calm in learning and social situations. They gain approval from adults and peers, improve their attention span, increase control over their lives, and become more responsible for their behavior."[64]

Continued research is needed to better understand the role and interaction of these competencies in the field of fluency. Below is a proposed model for assertiveness training that we use with our clients. In addition, we believe that those who profit from assertiveness training often become leaders in their fluency groups and within their fields. Therefore, in addition to assertiveness training, we will present aspects we consider to be important for assertiveness and leadership training.

ASSERTIVENESS TRAINING: AN INTRODUCTION TO LEADERSHIP

Assertive behavior enables you to interact in social situations in a manner that protects your best interests, to stand up for yourself without undue anxiety, and to exercise your rights without denying the rights of others. When this behavior becomes part of you, you enter into relationships and professional situations with evidence of inner strength. Manning[21] noted that with a decrease in avoidance behavior there is likely to be an increase in assertive behavior:

> It is a distinctive indicator of progress when the speaker begins to decrease his reflexive censorship and begins to consider many speaking situations that he once considered unimaginable This is not to say that he will now take part in these situations with ease or idyllic fluency, but choosing to take part nonetheless and thus to consider new opportunities is a significant measure of progress.

As a person practices this assertive behavior, he or she moves from passivity in a group to a leadership role. In order to achieve these results, we provide our clients with the following summary of the components of assertive behavior:

I. Content
    A. A specific goal is considered
        1. Establish a relationship with someone
        2. Express your feelings, beliefs, or opinions
        3. State an objection or point of view in opposition to another
        4. Set limits on another in regard to what can be expected or demanded of you
        5. Obtain something that you want
    B. Usually there are three components in the content
        1. Recognition of the other's feelings and rights
        2. Expressions of your own feelings and rights
        3. Description of desired action

   II. Communication Skills
      A. Good eye contact
      B. Relaxed body posture
      C. Confident voice
      D. Use of "I" statements instead of "you" statements
  III. Development of Self-Esteem

It should be clear that assertiveness is synergistically related to both self-esteem and communication skills. In addition, we believe that implementation of assertiveness both enhances and depends on an internal locus of control. These interactions are embodied in Le Mon's[65] "Rights of the Assertive Person":

> The right to be human and take full responsibility for your decisions and actions.
> The right to be wrong.
> The right to tell others what you are thinking and feeling.
> The right to change your mind.
> The right to stand in judgment of your thoughts and actions.
> The right to feel and express anger.
> The right to be independent.
> The right to make mistakes.

Many people who stutter often find that the expression of assertive behavior is not something that they have practiced because of their difficulty in basic expression. As a first step in developing assertiveness, they must understand the difference between nonassertive, assertive, and aggressive behavior.[66]

Assertive Behavior   In this type of interpersonal behavior, a person stands up for his legitimate rights in such a way that the rights of others are not violated. It is an honest, direct, and appropriate type of behavior conveying respect for the other person, although not necessarily agreement with that person's ideas or behaviors. The feelings that one has when engaging in this behavior are confidence and self-respect. The other person feels valued and respected and also respects the assertive person for his strength. The verbal behaviors of the assertive person include statements of wants, honest statements of feelings, objective words, direct statements that say what is meant, and use of "I" statements—e.g., "I know that you would like me to do fluency homework every night, however, I have little time for myself and I feel that this is not realistic."

Nonassertive Behavior   This type of behavior enables the person's rights to be violated by another. Such behavior inhibits honest, spontaneous reactions and often leaves the nonassertive person feeling hurt, anxious, and angry. The other person often feels personally guilty or superior and is irritated with the nonassertive person. The nonassertive person's verbal messages usually include apologetic words, veiled meanings, hedging, failure to come to the point or to say what is really meant.

Aggressive Behavior   In this type of behavior, a person stands up for his rights in such a way that the rights of others are violated. The behavior is often viewed as an attack on the other person rather than an expression of disagreement with the other's ideas. When engaged in aggressive behavior, a person generally feels righteous or superior, but often later feels guilty. The other person usually feels hurt or humiliated and becomes angry at the aggressor. The aggressive person often uses accusations, superior words, and "You" messages—e.g., "You are very unrealistic in your fluency homework expectations. You expect me to do the impossible!" Such exchanges cause and deepen conflicts.

How one opts to behave is a choice each person must make. After one becomes aware of the differences among the types of behavior, some hard questions must be answered:

1. What do I gain from staying nonassertive?
    a. Praise for conforming to another's expectations
    b. Maintenance of a familiar behavior pattern
    c. Avoidance of confronting difficulty situations
    d. Avoidance of stuttering in difficult situations
2. What do I lose by being nonassertive?
    a. Honesty in human relations
    b. Other's respect for my rights and wishes
    c. Relaxation and inner tranquility
    d. My ability to influence others' decisions, demands, and expectations
    e. The satisfaction of initiating and carrying out plans
    f. The freedom to use fluency techniques even in difficult situations

If a person who stutters decides to change her behavior, she must necessarily grow in internal locus of control. Maintaining control is at the heart of assertiveness. The person who asserts herself not only refuses to be controlled by others but also refuses to be controlled by negative emotions. Assertive behavior is a choice and a skill. Le Mon[64] identified the major assertiveness skills that must be used regularly: fogging, negative assertion, negative inquiry, broken record, and squeaky wheel techniques.

Fogging   The practice of resisting manipulation without giving the other person an opportunity for a direct counterattack. Fogging can take the form of agreeing with the truth in the manipulation or agreeing with the possibility of truth in the manipulation. For example:

Supervisor: "Well, your speech won again. You didn't contribute anything at the meeting today."
Client: "Yes, I did let my speech control my behavior today."

Fogging accomplishes two things: It forces both parties to focus on the real issue, in this case stuttering, and it forces the manipulator to think of other possibilities. Maybe his aggressive attacks won't work. Maybe a discussion about the impact of stuttering would result in more understanding.

Negative Assertion   Some people just wait for you to make a mistake and then let you and the rest of the world know about it. Negative assertion involves not only agreeing with your adversary but using exaggeration to further emphasize that you were wrong. For example:

> *Supervisor:* "You never speak up at meetings. I don't even know you are there. Where is your commitment?"
>
> *Client:* "You're right again. My silence creates a huge hole! I keep letting my speech rule me. What is wrong with me?"

The assumption behind negative assertion is that the criticism is legitimate and you will dwell on the real issue.

These first two techniques are useful in handling criticism that has a factual basis. Other ways to assist you in using these techniques are as follows[66]:

> Agree with the truth or generalities in the critic's statement. Remember no one can make you feel inferior unless you let them.
>
> Respond in a calm, conversational, matter-of-fact way.
>
> Don't defend yourself or attack the other person.
>
> If you want to apologize for a mistake, keep it simple. Don't make a case out of it.

Negative Inquiry   When a person criticizes another and there does not seem to be any factual basis for the criticism, you can try another assertive skill called "negative inquiry." Instead of being confrontational, one asks the other person to elaborate on what is being done wrong.

> *Client:* "I was quiet at the meeting. When did you think I might have responded?"

Negative inquiry does not confront the other person in a defensive way. One continues to ask the person to define the specific issue. The main thing is to keep delving for the real reason for the criticism. The result of this process is to identify areas where one needs improvement. Some ways to implement this technique are the following[66]:

> When there is vague criticism, probe to find out specifically what you're doing wrong.
>
> Keep probing until the critic comes up with the real reasons for the dissatisfaction.
>
> No matter what the person says, don't act defensive or hurt. This criticism may be useful information that can help improve the situation.

When trying to get feedback from a passive, timid person, remember to remain sympathetic and keep any sarcasm and accusations out of your voice.

Broken Record   Often people ignore our rights and feelings and persist in the attempt to manipulate us. They might use guilt, power, and embarrassment in order to force us to agree with them. An assertive person doesn't have to apologize for his thoughts or feelings, and there is no reason to give in to manipulation. One of the best ways to end a manipulative conversation is to try the broken record technique. Once you have given your assertive response, continue to repeat yourself even if the manipulator's tactics change:

> *Client:* "I just don't have time to do my fluency homework. There are too many important things to do."
> *Therapist:* "I can only help you if you, also, work. How can you find time?"
> *Client:* "I don't know. I have to work, go to school, go to the store for my mom, and see my friends. There is no more time."
> *Therapist:* "I can only help you if you, also, work. How can you find time?"

Some ways to assist you in using this technique are as follows[66]:

> Speak in a calm, conversational, but firm voice. No matter what the other person says, don't become excited or angry.
> Keep repeating the message.
> Don't let yourself be sidetracked by excuses, accusations, other issues.
> Follow up to make sure the person is doing what you asked him/her to do. Come back as many times as necessary until it's done.

Squeaky Wheel Technique   When using this technique, one communicates the message and then leaves. The natural inclination is to push a person until the response required is received. In effect, you may reinforce the avoidance because the issue becomes the confrontation, not what you want done. For example:

> *Client:* "I wasn't able to do my homework. My tape recorder broke."
> *Clinician:* "Here is a tape recorder, instead of going to the group you can do your homework, now. It will give you good practice time. I will be back in ten minutes."

[Ten minutes later:]

> *Client:* "I didn't have time and I got talking to Joe. I understand what to do."
> *Clinician:* "You continue to work here on your homework. I will be back in another ten minutes. The practice is good for you."

Some suggestions to assist you in implementing this technique include the following[66]:

First, state your wants clearly.

Persist in your original demand until you feel you are past the other person's excuses.

When you want something, ask for it in a direct, positive way. Back up your requests with benefits, reasons, and a plan.

When you get what you wanted, or something close to it, thank the person responsible for your getting it.

Some people are naturally self-assertive and self-confident. Becoming assertive is something that can be accomplished by all people. We use our group practice as a means for people to practice difficult interactions. After many experiences, we find that clients gain confidence in speaking in small and large groups. They are willing to assume offices and they speak on the radio, in classes, and on TV. They assume roles of leadership. We see how assertiveness is the result of moving from self-awareness to self-esteem. Both of these qualities lead to an increase in self-confidence and enable one to grow in an internal locus of control. Once again, we should recognize the synergistic aspects of each of these empowerment attitudes. We next present activities to increase each of these components.

SUMMARY

Attitudes and feelings have long been a part of fluency therapy. After acknowledging the important history of the research that supports the necessity for including attitudinal aspects of stuttering in both diagnostic and remediation, we have highlighted three specific attitudes that we believe interact synergistically—self-esteem, locus of control, and assertiveness. As clinicians strive to include goals for therapy that targets these empowerment attitudes, we hope that further research will support our clients increased confidence, assertiveness, and leadership. We close this chapter with some activities that help to increase clients' functioning in each of these areas.

ACTIVITIES TO INCREASE SELF-ESTEEM, LOCUS OF CONTROL, AND ASSERTIVENESS

Since these three dimensions of the developmental self are interconnected, activity to foster any one of them will necessarily affect the other two. As a person develops self-esteem through gaining significance, mastery, and competence, that person will gain the necessary awareness of the importance of taking control of his own life and will be willing to reach out, assertively, to help others. We list here a variety of activities that might be used with clients who stutter. They are divided into two parts: (1) the internal principles for providing a climate where self-esteem, control, and assertiveness can grow, and (2) specific activities that can be included in therapy.

Internal Principles—The Soil from Which the Self Can Grow

A. Because we see others in the light of our own self attitudes, perhaps the most important activity we can recommend for clinicians is self-examination. Briggs[66] encourages us to: "Answer the question: 'Who am I?' Write out your personal feelings about yourself. What kind of person are you? What qualities do you see yourself as having, and how do you feel about them? Do you basically enjoy being yourself or would you rather be someone else? If you don't like yourself keep in mind that this attitude is learned." Remember: low self-esteem is not a commentary on your value but rather a reflection of the judgments and experiences you have had. YOU HOLD THE POWER OF CHOICE TO DO SOMETHING ABOUT YOUR LOW SELF-ESTEEM. The way you work on your own issues will be a great determiner of how well you can assist your client in attaining a feeling of esteem, power and assertiveness.

B. Create a climate in your therapy interactions that provides focused attention on the client. A genuine sense of interest in your client will strongly communicate your respect for her. Rather than focusing on what you can do for your client, you focus on her as a person. We believe that it is important for a clinician to be trained in the basic listening skills, which we present in the Chapter 9. From this stance, one can determine the individual needs, thoughts, and behaviors of the client that need to be addressed.

C. Nathanial Brandon,[68] renowned in the area of self-esteem, encourages us to live consciously rather than unconsciously. Brandon believes this to be the foundation for healthy self-esteem. He presented the following examples that we believe are important for clinicians working with people who stutter:

- Thinking, even when thinking is difficult, versus nonthinking.
- Awareness, even when awareness is challenging, versus nonawareness.
- Clarity, whether or not it comes easily, versus obscurity or vagueness
- Respect for reality, whether pleasant or painful, versus avoidance of reality
- Respect for truth versus rejection of truth
- Independence versus dependence
- Active orientation versus passive orientation
- Willingness to take appropriate risks, even in the face of fear, versus unwillingness
- Honesty with self versus dishonesty
- Living in and being responsible to the present versus retreating into fantasy
- Self-confrontation versus self-avoidance
- Willingness to see and correct mistakes versus perseverance in error
- Reason versus irrationalism

These principles become an integral part of life for those who focus on personal growth and development. As we continue to incorporate these principles into our own life, we will be better able to provide the same rich soil for our clients.

D. Recommend that people who have a healthy self-esteem and an internal locus of control take full responsibility for the attainment of their goals. "To the extent that we shift from a passive to an active orientation, we like ourselves more, trust ourselves more, and feel more competent to live and deserving of happiness."[68] Brandon further stated that self-responsibility entails such realizations as the following:

- I am responsible for my choices and actions.
- I am responsible for the way I prioritize my time.
- I am responsible for the level of consciousness I bring to my work.
- I am responsible for the care or lack of care with which I treat my body.
- I am responsible for being in the relationships I choose to enter or to remain in.
- I am responsible for the way I treat other people—my spouse, my children, my parents, my friends, my associates, my boss, my subordinates, the sales clerk in the store.
- I am responsible for the meaning I give or fail to give to my existence.
- I am responsible for my happiness.
- I am responsible for my life—materially, emotionally, intellectually, spiritually.

Of course, we would extend this list to include:

- I am responsible for improving my communication skills.

External Activities

1. Help your client to look at the positive sides of failure. Have a discussion with him about the value of directly facing failure and discovering ways to overcome obstacles to success. Daly[44] presented some examples of the world's biggest "failures":
- Colonel Sanders tried to sell his chicken recipe to restaurants. He was rejected 1,009 times before someone finally said yes.
- Walt Disney was turned down 302 times before he got financing for his dream of creating "The Happiest Place on Earth." Today millions of people around the world derive pleasure from that dream.
- Theodore Geisel was rejected 23 times before his children's book was finally accepted by a publisher. His pen name was Dr. Seuss.
- Tom Watson was fired from the NCR company before he decided to start his own company, IBM.
- Richard Hooker received rejections 21 times before his story about his experiences in an army medical unit was finally accepted. His story was called *M*A*S*H*.

2. A clinician's language can aid in the increased development of the self. When a client is struggling to learn something new, you might say:

- "You can do it yourself. You just did part of it."
- "You are really keeping at it. It makes me proud to see you work so hard."
- "Making mistakes is the best way to learn. Now you know you will practice harder."
- "That was an excellent gentle onset or target production. Do you realize how you did it yourself? What did you do?"
- "What are the goals that you want to set? I will support you as you carry them out."
- "Stuttering isn't just something that happens to you. It is also something that you are doing. Tell me what you are doing."

3. Decide which methods of coping with difficult situations is best for her clients. Present the client with the following options. Thoroughly discuss and plan appropriate goals around the needed methods.

Successful Affective Methods

- Learn about yourself. Recognize strengths and weaknesses. Highlight positives.
- Listen to your thoughts and feelings. Are you a positive or a negative person?
- Be self-affirming. Tell yourself when you do a good job.
- Be conscious about the details of how you are producing speech and what situations are most difficult. Be conscious of the feelings associated with speaking.
- Admit your feelings about your speech.
- Cry . . . release your feelings about past or present hurts.
- Motivate yourself to follow an action plan for speech improvement.
- Laugh at your mistakes. Revisit the scene of past mistakes and practice fluency enhancing techniques. See the humor in difficulties.
- Forgive yourself and others. Remember that we all make mistakes. We don't have to be perfect.
- Create courage. Actively enter into your most feared situations.
- Be humorous. Humor helps us to change and to gain a balance in life.
- Express your feelings to others.
- Create positive feelings through self-affirmations.

Successful Relationship Methods

- Talk out conflicts; don't "stuff" them.
- Treat yourself and others with respect.
- Tell others your story about growing up as a person who stuttered.
- Be assertive in expressing your feelings and needs.

- Communicate for yourself. Don't allow others to speak for you.
- Be patient but not passive in your relationships.
- Take risks. Overcome your fear—see it as a challenge.
- Be verbally appreciative.
- Call a person that you have been avoiding speaking to.

Successful Verbal Methods

- Use "I" statements when speaking to others.
- State your opinions. Know that they are important.
- Contribute to a group discussion, even if it is difficult.
- Remember the more you talk, using targets, the more potential fluency will be yours.
- Remember the more you talk, using stuttering, the more you are practicing stuttering.
- Praise yourself. Internalize a positive self-image.
- Practice speaking in your more difficult hierarchies, using your most feared sounds.
- Create positive self-talk. If you think "I know I can do the job," you'll have a better chance at success.
- Eliminate negative self-talk. If you think "I'll never get hired for that position," you probably won't.

Successful Behavioral Methods

- Make a list of your prioritized goals. Be certain to include an increase in responsibility for speech as an important goal..
- Work a minimum of 15 minutes every day on your speech targets. Expand this time when possible.
- Practice your targets as you drive to work. Practice every time you make a phone call.
- Determine strategies that will be helpful for you to carry out your speech goals.
- Take control of your speech improvement. Bring a tape recorder with you to school or work. Tape your speech. Analyze your performance at a later date.
- Listen to a tape of yourself speaking fluently. Highlight the fluent words. How did you make them? What did you do differently than when you stutter?
- Bring a small card that will remind you to slow down and use your targets: "Slow and easy!" Stop and look at that before you speak.
- Volunteer to head a committee; talk to others about stuttering. Exercise leadership.
- Use assertive rather than aggressive techniques in your everyday life.
- Make your world bigger. Don't meet all of your needs through one thing.

- Evaluate speakers in your environment: Do they speak very fast, very slow, very loud, very soft, with a high or low pitch, or with easy or hard onsets?

Successful Cognitive Methods

- Recognize your irrational fears about speaking.
- Dispute your irrational fears and replace them with positive thoughts.
- Study the specifics of the fluency enhancing techniques that are most helpful to you.
- Repeat often: "Stuttering is not something that happens to me. It is something that I DO and I can change the way I speak."
- Challenge the way you look at success: Feel good about trying. Realize that the process, not the product, is most important. Accept that CHANGE is a SLOW process. Don't always interpret failure as a negative experience.
- Learn about yourself. Recognize your strengths and weakness.
- Praise yourself. Internalize a positive self image. Be self affirming.

REFERENCES

1. Conture EG. *Stuttering* (2nd ed). Englewood Cliffs, NJ: Prentice Hall, 1990.
2. Drever J. *A Dictionary of Psychology*. London: Penguin, 1952.
3. Guitar B, Peters J. *Stuttering: An Integrated Approach to Its Nature and Treatment*. Baltimore: Williams and Wilkins, 1991.
4. Riley GD, Riley J. A component model for treating stuttering in children. In M Peins (ed), *Contemporary Approaches in Stuttering Therapy*. Boston: Little, Brown, 1984.
5. Ham R. *Therapy of Stuttering*. Englewood Cliffs, NJ: Prentice Hall, 1990.
6. Bloodstein O. The development of stuttering: I. Changes in nine basic features. *J Speech Hear Disord*. 1960;25:219–237.
7. Cooper E, Cooper C. Clinician's attitude toward stuttering; a decade of change (1973–1983). *J Fluency Disord* 1985;10:19–33.
8. Sheehan J. Principles of therapy. In J Gruss (ed), *Counseling Stutterers*. Memphis: Speech Foundation of America, 1982.
9. Watson J, Gregory H, Kistler D. Development and evaluation of an inventory to assess adult stutterers' communication attitudes. *J Fluency Disord* 1987;12;429–450.
10. Leith W, Mahr G, Miller L. *The Assessment of Speech Related Attitudes and Beliefs of People Who Stutter*. Baltimore: ASHA, 1993;29.
11. Ammons R, Johnson W. Studies in the psychology of stuttering: XVIII The construction and application of a test of attitudes toward stuttering. *J Speech Hear Disord* 1944;9:39–44.
12. Bloodstein O. *A Handbook on Stuttering* (5th ed). San Diego: Singular Publishing Group, 1993.
13. Lanyon RI. The measurement of stuttering severity. *J Speech Lang Hear Res* 1967;10:836–843.
14. Lanyon RI, Goldsworthy RJ, Langon BP. Dimensions of stuttering and relationship to psychopathology. *J Fluency Disord* 1978;3:103–113.
15. Woolf G. The assessment of stuttering as struggle, avoidance and expectancy. *Br J Disord Commun* 1967;2:158–171.

16. Erikson RL. Assessing communication attitudes among stutterers. *J Speech Lang Hear Res* 1969;12:711–724.
17. Guitar B. Pretreatment factors associated with the outcome of stuttering therapy. *J Speech Lang Hear Res* 1976;19:590–600.
18. Guitar B, Bass C. Stuttering therapy: the relation between attitude change and long-term outcome. *J Speech Hear Disord* 1978;43:392–400.
19. Bandura A. Toward a unifying theory of behavior change. *Psychol Rev* 1977;1: 191–215.
20. Ornstein A, Manning W. Self-efficacy scaling by adult stutterers. *J Commun Disord* 18:313–320.
21. Manning W. *Clinical Decision Making in the Diagnosis and Treatment of Fluency Disorders.* Albany: Delmar, 1996.
22. Silverman FH. The stuttering problem profile; a task that assists both client and clinician in defining therapy goals. *J Speech Hear Disord* 1980;45:119–123.
23. Watson JB. Profiles of stutterers' and nonstutterers' affective, cognitive and behavioral communication attitudes. *J Fluency Disord* 1987;12:389–405.
24. Watson JB. A comparison of stutterers' and nonstutterers' affective, cognitive and behavioral self reports. *J Speech Lang Hear Res* 1988;31:377–385.
25. Watson J, Gregory H, Kistler D. Development and evaluation of an instrument to assess adult stutterers' communication attitudes. *J Fluency Disord* 1987;12: 429–450.
26. Costello J. Treatment of the young chronic stutterer. In RF Curlee, WH Perkins (eds), *Nature and Management of Stuttering.* San Diego: College Hill Press, 1984; 88.
27. Silverman FH. Concern of elementary school stutterers about their stuttering. *J Speech Hear Disord* 1970;35:361–363.
28. Culatta R, Brader J, McCaslin A., Thomason N. Primary school stutterers. Have attitudes changed? *J Fluency Disord* 1985;10:87–91.
29. Devore JE, Manning WH. Protective drawings and children who stutter. *J Fluency Disord* 1984;9:217–226.
30. Brutten GJ, Dunham SL. The communication attitude test: a normative study of grade school children. *J Fluency Disord* 1989;14:371–377.
31. De Nil L, Brutten GJ. Speech associated attitudes of stuttering and nonstuttering children. *J Speech Lang Hear Res* 1991;34:60–66.
32. Vanryckeghem N, Brutten G. The communication attitude test: a test-retest reliability investigation. *J Fluency Disord* 1992;17:177–190.
33. Vanrckeghem M. The communication attitude test: a concordancy investigation of stuttering and nonstuttering children and their parents. *J Fluency Disord* 1995;20: 191–203.
34. Riley G, Riley J. Evaluating stuttering problems in children. *J Child Commun Disord* 1982;6(l):15–25.
35. Silverman EM, Zimmer CH. Demographic characteristics and treatment experiences of women and men who stutter. *J Fluency Disord* 1982;7:273–275.
36. Culatta R, Goldberg S. *Stuttering Therapy: An Integrated Approach to Theory and Practice.* Needham Heights, MA: Allyn & Bacon, 1995.
37. Bloom C, Cooperman D. *The Clinical Interview: A Guide for the Speech-Language Pathologist and Audiologist.* Rockville, MD: NSSLHA, 1992.
38. Prutting C. Battle for the light. *NSSLHA J* 1992;13:5–9.
39. Maslow AM. Some basic propositions of a growth and self-actualizing psychology. In *Association for Supervision and Curriculum Development Yearbook* 1962: 34–39.

40. Combs AW. What can man become? In D Avela, A Combs, W Pruskey (eds), *The Helping Relationship Sourcebook*. Boston: Allyn and Bacon, 1982.

41. Frey D, Carlock CJ. *Enhancing Self-Esteem*. Bristol, PA: Accelerated Development, 1989.

42. Coopersmith S. *The Antecedants of Self-Esteem*. San Francisco: W. H. Freeman, 1967.

43. Rogers C. A note on the nature of man. *J Counseling Psych* 1957;4:199–203.

44. Daly D. *The Source for Stuttering and Cluttering*. Moline, IL: Linguisystems, Inc., 1996.

45. Briggs D. *Your Child's Self Esteem*. New York: Doubleday, 1975.

46. Lefcourt H. *Research with the Locus of Control Construct*. Vols. I, II, III. New York: Academic Press, 1981–1984.

47. Rotter JB. Generalized expectancies for internal versus external control of reinforcement. *Psychol Monographs* 1966;80:609.

48. Bandura A. *Principles of Behavior Modification*. New York: Holt, Rinehart & Winston, 1969.

49. Craig AR, Howie P. Locus of control and maintenance behavioral therapy skills. *Br J Clin Psychol* 1987;21:67–68.

50. De Nil LF, Kroll RM. The relationship between locus of control and long-term stuttering treatment outcome in adult stutterers. *J Fluency Disord* 1995;20:345–364.

51. Ladoceur R, Carm C, Carm G. Stuttering severity and treatment outcome. *J Behav Ther Exp Psychiatry* 1989;20:49–56.

52. Allenbaugh E. *Wake Up Calls*. New York: Fireside, 1994.

53. Adams M. Learning from negative outcomes in stuttering therapy: I. Getting off on the wrong foot. *J Fluency Dis* 1983;8:147–153.

54. Seligman M. *On Depression, Development and Death*. San Francisco: W. H. Freeman, 1975.

55. Schutz W. *The Human Element*. Mirer Beach, CA: Will Schutz Association, 1988.

56. Montgomery CO. Paper delivered at the First World Congress on Fluency Disorders. International Fluency Association. San Francisco, June 1994.

57. Montgomery CO. Paper delivered at the Second World Congress on Fluency Disorders. International Fluency Association. San Francisco, June 1997.

58. Ellis A. The basic clinical theory of rational-emotive therapy. In A Ellis, R Greiger (eds), *Handbook of Rational Emotive Therapy*. New York: Springer, 1977.

59. Corey G. *Theory and Practice of Counseling and Psychotherapy* (3rd ed). Monterey, CA: Brooks/Cole, 1986.

60. Burns D. *The Feeling Good Handbook*. New York: Penguin, 1990.

61. Schloss P. Developing assertiveness during employment interviews with young adults who stutter. *J Speech Hear Disord* 1987;52:30–36.

62. Beaty D. Multimodal approach to elimination of stuttering. *Percept Mot Skills* 1980;50:51–55.

63. Lazarus A. *Multimodal Behavior Therapy*. New York: Springer, 1976.

64. McWhirter J. High and low risk characteristics of youth: the five C's of competency. *Elementary Guidance Counseling* 1994;28(3):188–196.

65. Le Mon C. *Assertiveness: Get What You Want Without Being Pushy*. Shawnee Mission, KS: National Press Publications, 1990.

66. Taetzsch L, Beasm E. *Taking Charge on the Job!* New York: Executive Enterprises, 1978.

67. Briggs M. *Your Child's Self-Esteem*. New York: Doubleday, 1975.

68. Brandon N. *How to Raise Your Self Esteem*. New York: Bantam, 1987.

8

Environmental Aspects of Fluency Disorders

Problems that we encounter in our everyday life are usually the result of the interaction of the personal, interpersonal, and environmental systems with which we are involved. People with fluency disorders tend to react to these interacting factors with heightened emotion. Researching in fluency disorders has long established, with some disagreement, that environmental factors play an important role in stuttering.

Bloodstein[1] described the involvement of environmental factors when he noted that there is a higher prevalence of stuttering in the cultures that are more achievement oriented. It has also been observed that certain stressors increase stuttering and when these stressors are removed, stuttering stops. Guitar and Peters[2] list some of the stressors that influence a child's fluency:

1. The child's family moves to a new house, a new neighborhood, or a new city.
2. The child's parents separate or divorce.
3 A family member dies.
4 A family member is hospitalized.
5 The child is hospitalized.
6. A parent loses his or her job.
7. A baby is born or another child is adopted.
8. An additional person comes to live in the house.
9. One or both parents go away frequently or for a long period of time.
10. Holidays or visits occur, which cause a change in routine, excitement, or anxiety.

Indeed, when any of these stressors appear in a child's life, it is important to be aware of and responsive to the child's needs. The stuttering symptom can actually alert us more quickly to these underlying environmental issues.

Starkweather[3-6] has described in detail the interaction of the physical and environmental aspects of fluency development. As noted in Chapter 6, physiologic demands are related to those noted in our first spiral as depicted in Figure 1.1. Starkweather contributed greatly to our understanding when he described both the internal and external environment of the child. We believe that our second spiral in Figure 1.1 embodying attitudes—self-esteem, locus of control, and assertiveness—is comparable to the internal environment of people who stutter. This has been expanded in Chapter 7. The external environment that is defined by Starkweather involves the demands made by the parents: rapid questioning, complex statements, impatience with stuttering, and demand for high level performance.

While the case for recognizing the environmental issues involved in stuttering has long been recognized, we are grateful for Starkweather's work and join with him in emphasizing that it is the synergistic interaction of the physiologic, attitudinal (internal environment), and the external environment that influences stuttering behavior. This approach has been supported by the work of different researchers[7-9] presented in Chapter 2. In this chapter we will isolate some of the specific environmental aspects that are important in the synergistic approach and necessary to be included as part of any therapy program that hopes to work with the whole person. The aspects of the external environment to consider are the communication environment, the family, and the cultural environment. These are separate but interacting aspects of each fluency client's environment that are essential to target in fluency therapy.

THE COMMUNICATION ENVIRONMENT

Starkweather and Givens-Ackerman[10] described the communicative environment of the person who stutters as "any stimuli, events or ongoing characteristics that have an effect on the person's fluency level. The communicative environment can be either demanding or facilitating of fluency." Children's communication demands come from parents, siblings, babysitters, and teachers. Adults who stutter have communication demands from family, work, and social settings. In Chapter 2, we highlighted the relationship of language and communication to fluency disorders and the research to support this. In this chapter we will discuss aspects of the communication environment that are important to the clients, clinicians, and the parents. We believe that communication for all persons can be increased through a knowledge and practice of specific communication skills. A thorough understanding of these skills can help us work with our clients and also help clients and families to communicate with each other. However, as we examine these skills, it is important to realize that skills alone are not sufficient for successful interaction with the environment. There must be a balanced focus on the person and the environment. Hepworth and Larson[11] presented a number of important environmental needs: (1) having sufficient opportunities for social relationships, (2) having sufficient opportunities to express feelings, (3) having sufficient sources of emotional support, (4) being able to fulfill responsibilities, (5) having opportunities to engage in interesting and productive activities and to achieve goals, and (6) having the means to maintain physical mobility. These are the contexts within which skills can be developed and it appears to us that this basic environmental balance is clearly related to the development of the empowerment attitudes discussed in Chapter 7. With this in mind, we will now examine the listening skills that are important in working with clients. In addition, we believe that these communication skills can also be taught to more advanced fluency clients to improve their communication.

Communication Skills

Many clinicians possess a gift for interpersonal communication. However, that is not true for all clinicians and it is certainly an area of difficulty for people who stutter. Certain communication skills can be taught to greatly enrich our communication experiences. In Chapter 9, these skills are represented as an aspect of the counseling triangle. Since they provide the tangible vehicle for interacting with the environment, we chose to illustrate several of these skills in this chapter. Virginia Satir, a renowned psychologist, has pointed out the importance of developing effective communication skills:

> I see communication as a huge umbrella that covers and affects all that goes on between human beings. Once a human being has arrived on this earth, communication is the largest single factor determining what kinds of relationships she or he makes with others. How we develop intimacy, how productive we are, how we connect—all depend largely on our communication skills.[12]

Overview of Microskills

Ivey[13] has outlined and researched the skills necessary to facilitate one's own and another person's growth. He called these the "microskills of communication" (Figure 8.1). He provides a person with a range of communication alternatives so that each person can develop her own style of listening and interacting with another individual. This is a precision system that enables one to enter the clinical arena with specific skills and competencies and yet provides enough flexibility that one is encouraged to develop her own style while using these skills. Scheuerle[14] noted that Ivey searched for attending behaviors that could be demonstrated, observed, identified, taught, practiced, videotaped, and counted. Others have expanded on this work and Scheuerle presented these behaviors in alphabetical order as shown in Table 8.1.

These helping behaviors are familiar to most people. They are the behaviors that can occur in daily interactions and in social communication. We are all involved in the use of these techniques whether we are aware of it or not. For those who have not developed these skills they can be learned. For clinicians who wish to grow in the conscious awareness of behaviors that facilitate change, these skills can provide this awareness. For clients who desire to improve communica-

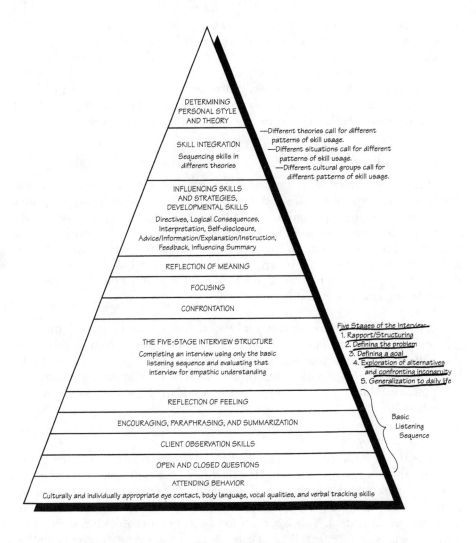

Figure 8.1 Microskills of Comunication. (Reprinted with permission from Ivey A. *Intentional Interviewing and Counseling.* Belmont, CA: Brooks/Cole, 1994, p. 16.)

tion, these skills are invaluable. Schuerle further stated: "We need to consider these identified helping skills as part of the treatment of communicatively handicapped clients and their families. The clinician must recognize the need for selective application of helping skills as being quite different from their casual use in social interaction."[14]

It seems particularly important for fluency clinicians to have a conscious awareness of these skills in order to best facilitate the growth of their clients. Use of the microskills becomes an integral part of the ongoing diagnostic and therapeutic process. Since one of the goals of fluency therapy is to assist the person to take responsibility for his stuttering behavior and life generally, these skills enable a clinician to be client-centered and maximize the therapeutic time. In order to do this, clinicians must practice, practice, and practice. At first the use of these skills seems unnatural. But when one understands the client-centered nature of the interaction, it makes the use of the microskills more natural. It is recommended that clinicians observe, audiotape, and videotape their interactions with friends, colleagues, and family members. We encourage fluency clinicians to become active learners of these skills through reading, workshops, and everyday practice. A thorough understanding of both the principles involved and the specifics of the skills themselves will enrich communication personally and clinically. Moreover, when the clinician has integrated the skills into her own life it becomes easier to teach the aspects of the skills that are important for our fluency clients.

Table 8.1   Three Examples of the Basic Listening Sequence

Skill	*Counseling*	*Management*	*Medicine*
Open question	"Could you tell me what you'd like to talk to me about . . ."		
Closed question	"Did you graduate from high school?" "What specific careers have you looked at?"	"Who was involved with the production line problem?" "Did you check the main belt?"	"Is the headache on the left side or on the right side? How long have you had it?"
Encouragers	Repetition of key words and restatement of longer phrases.		
Paraphrases	"So you're considering returning to college."	"Sounds like you've consulted with almost everyone."	"It looks like you feel it's on the left side and may be a result of the car accident."
Reflection of feeling	"You feel confident of your ability but worry about getting in."	"I sense you're upset and troubled by Hank's reaction."	"It appears you've been feeling very anxious and tense lately."
Summarization	In each case the effective counselor, manager, or physician summarizes the story from the client's point of view *before* bringing in the interviewer's point of view.		

Reprinted with permission from Schuerle J. *Counseling in Speech-Language Pathology and Audiology.* New York: Macmillan, 1992, p. 157.

We focus, again, on the purpose of communication skills in the therapy process and note that as clinician-counselors, our goal is to help the client *change his thoughts , feelings, and behaviors* related to the dysfluency. The way to work with each of these components is to integrate the microskills into each phase of the helping process (Chapter 9). We must gain an accurate account of what the client *thinks, feels, and does in regard to stuttering.* The use of these skills in all stages of the process has been termed "active listening" and can provide insights into the client's "story," which is necessary to know if goals are to be actualized.

We have found and our students have reported that learning the skills makes a significant difference in everyday life. They are surprised by their own habits of communication that are contrary to the newly learned skills. Hutchins and Cole[15] reported that everyday observation demonstrates that instead of using communication skills with each other, we often find the following:

- People talk in rapid succession, one person quickly following another.
- Each person contributes his or her own two cents worth of the conversation.
- There are practically no periods of silence. If too much silence occurs, individuals move to other groups in search of more active or more interesting conversations.
- Comments and questions frequently do not relate to the subject being discussed.
- People interrupt others who are speaking.
- Frequent shifts in content occur, depending who is talking.
- The content of the topic falters from one person to another.
- More than one person speaks at a time, perhaps several speak at the same time.
- One person may dominate conversation, giving others little opportunity for input.

In eac of these examples, no true listening is possible. At the heart of communication skills is active listening. Luterman[16] quoted the following anonymous poem to sum up the importance of listening:

When I ask you to listen to me and you start giving advice you have not
    done what I asked.
When I ask you to listen to me
    and you begin to tell me why I shouldn't feel that way you are
    trampling on my feelings.
When I ask you to listen to me
    and you feel that you have to do something to solve my problem,
    you have failed me, strange as that may seem.
Listen! All I asked, was that you listen
    not talk or do—just hear me.

Advice is cheap. 10 cents will get you both Dear Abby and Billy
   Graham in the same newspaper.
And I can do for myself; I'm not helpless.
Maybe discouraged and faltering, but not helpless.
When you do something for me that I can and need to do for myself,
   you contribute to my fear and weakness.
But when you accept as a simple fact that I do feel what I feel, no matter
   how irrational, then I can quit trying to convince you and can get about
   the business of understanding what's behind this irrational feeling. And
   when that's clear, the answers are obvious and I don't need advice.

When the basic listening skills, as outlined by Ivey[13], Eagen,[17] and Bloom
and Cooperman[18] are utilized, the negative behaviors noted in this poem are not
part of the communication interaction. We will summarize these skills using
Ivey's format: attending; open and closed questions; client observation skills; encouraging, paraphrasing, and summarizing; and reflecting of feelings. These
skills are integrated throughout all phases of therapy to ensure a client-centered
approach.

Basic Listening Skills

Attending   Ivey teaches that attending behaviors encourage the client to
talk more freely and openly; the clinician talks less and the client has the opportunity to examine concrete issues in detail. Physical attending conveys caring, understanding, and respect. Attending means that you are really "tuned in" to all
the signals that are coming from the client.

Eagen[17] summarized the microskills of attending in the acronym SOLER:

S: Face the client squarely: Adopt a posture that indicates involvement. It
   usually says "I'm here with you; I'm available to you."
O: Adopt an open posture. Crossed arms and crossed legs can be signs of
   lessened involvement with or availability to others.
L: At times, lean toward the client. Leaning toward is a natural form of
   involvement. In our culture, a slight inclination toward a person is often seen as saying "I'm with you, and I'm interested in what you have
   to say."
E: Maintain good eye contact.
R: Try to be relatively relaxed or natural in these behaviors.

Eagen cautioned us to recognize that different *cultures* demonstrate attentiveness in various ways. What is important is that an internal mindset of open,
attentive, availability be communicated to your client. It is important that these
skills not be used rigidly. They are only guidelines to facilitate communication
with others.

Ivey[13] listed four ways to facilitate attending behavior:

- Eye Contact: If you are going to talk to people, look at them.
- Attentive Body Language: Clients know you are interested if you face them squarely and lean slightly forward, have an expressive face, and use facilitative, encouraging gestures.
- Vocal Qualities: Your vocal tone and speech rate also indicate clearly how you feel about another person. Think of how many ways you can say: " I am really interested in what you have to say," just by altering your vocal tone and speech rate.
- Verbal Tracking: The client has come to you with a topic of concern; don't change the subject. Keep to the topic indicated by the client.

Attending demonstrates to clients that they are important to you and you are carefully listening to their story. If you attend, your clients will usually talk more. As you integrate this skill with the others, you will find that you will be better able to assist your clients in finding their own answers.

Open and Closed Questions   Questioning in a helping relationship can help to direct the process. There are two types of questions that facilitate the client's telling of his story: open questions and closed questions. Open questions are an invitation for clients to describe how they think, feel, and behave in relationship to their fluency disorder. Closed questions are questions that could, but do not have to be, answered with a yes or no response.

Open Questions   These ask who, what, where, could and how. (Why questions are not generally used, because they can put a person on the defensive. Moreover, it is often difficult to assess one's own motivation, which is what the why question asks!)

Who are the people you feel comfortable speaking with?
What motivated you to practice your targets of speech?
Where were you when you experienced increased disfluency?
When do you feel most stressed about speaking?
How do you react when someone criticizes your speaking?
Could you tell me more about what is bothering you?

Ivey[13] states that one of the most useful open questions asks the client to be specific in describing his situation: "Could you give me a specific example." Questions are the heart of the interview process and they can be used effectively throughout the entire therapeutic process in order to ascertain if we are meeting the true needs of the client.

Closed Questions   These help to provide additional factual information that the clinician thinks is important:

Were you able to do your homework?
Are you currently working?
Is there a history of stuttering in your family?
Have you had therapy before?

The skill of questioning involves alternating open and closed questioning. Using questions can be systematic. In acquiring information about the client's thoughts, feelings, and behaviors, Hutchins and Cole[15] recommended that one ask:

- Thinking questions: "What?" These explore factual information about the client, and ideas, concepts, data, and cognitive aspects.
- Feeling questions:. "How?" These illuminate the client's feelings, emotions, and other affective aspects.
- Action questions: "Could?" These reveal things the client does, such as physical activity, homework, and carry-over of targets.

Some examples of these questions, which can elicit a great deal of information about the client's fluency, are the following:

- "Could you tell me more about . . ? "
- "Can you tell me something about . . ? "
- "How does (did) that affect you?"
- "What will that mean to you?"
- "What was the significance of that event for you?"
- "Tell me how you feel (felt or expect to feel) about that?"
- "What impact did that have on you?"
- "What do you imagine that will be like for you?"
- "I'm wondering what did that mean to you?"

Although questioning is an important part of the therapeutic process, clinicians must use it wisely. Skillful questioning involves open-ended questions that enable a client to explore their own situation. Questions are not used just to satisfy one's curiosity. They are used to elicit elaborated responses, which lead to a choice to change. These questions are also alternated with reflective feeling responses, to be explained later.

In summary, Murphy and Dillan[19] listed the following principles regarding the use of questioning:

- Questions should be intentional.
- Clinicians need to be sensitive to cultural attitudes toward questioning.
- Questions should be well timed.
- Too much questioning makes the clinician the director.
- Questions can interrupt concentration.
- Good questions can be supportive and therapeutic; as well as useful for gathering data.
- Difficult questions should be introduced carefully.
- Too little questioning can make for drift, or leave the client at a loss for direction.
- Follow-up questions are often necessary.
- Answer to questions can be both verbal and nonverbal.
- Clinicians need to be aware of what they are not asking.

Client Observation Skills　　Clients send messages to us through verbal and nonverbal communication. The skilled clinician needs to interpret these messages with knowledge, understanding, and care. It is important that they not be distorted or overinterpreted. There are so many ways that client's nonverbal and verbal messages can be interpreted. Our goal is to enter into the world of our client and see that world as if it were our own.

Ivey[13] listed three aspects of clients' behavior to help understand their messages:

1. Client nonverbal behavior: Some authorities have claimed that 85 percent of client communication of meaning is nonverbal. Client eye contact patterns, body language, and vocal qualities should be observed.
2. Client verbal behavior: Words form the basis of most therapeutic sessions. Clients tend to focus on certain key words and constructs Through selective attention and verbal tracking, you can better enter clients' worlds and understand their pattern of thinking.
3. Client discrepancies: Incongruities; mixed messages, contradictions, and conflict are often the reason clients come to us. Careful observation of client verbal and nonverbal behavior will provide the clinician with extensive data on conflict and discrepancies in the client's world. It is often these data that provide the framework for attacking the problem.

In addition to these areas of observation noted by Ivey, other specific areas that can be observed when working with a fluency client are the following:

1. *Opening and Closing Sentences*　　The manner in which clients present their problems is usually significant. They may say, "I don't think you can help me, but . . ." or "I'm only here because . . ." or some other statement that typically provides helpful insight for future work. A person's closing remarks also can be important. Clinicians can note how clients feel about the session and how much their own forces have been mobilized for proceeding with work on the problem. Many fluency clients are not motivated for therapy and this can be identified early on in the process.

2. *Themes*　　Very often, clients will continue to repeat certain ideas, subjects, or stated difficulties. These are usually areas that need to be targeted as goals or included in the treatment plan. Sometimes clients are unaware of how much these areas have been influencing all of their communication and their life. Very often fluency clients don't realize that what they are tell themselves about their inability to speak has a direct influence on their behavior. We look for the themes in their thinking, feeling and behavior.

3. *Inconsistencies and Gaps*　　Clinicians must listen for patterns in their clients' stories. They also must note when a story is not unified. It is important to listen carefully for times when clients contradict themselves or when the meaning of what they say is unclear. These inconsistencies must be clarified and explored. Very often these spots contain valuable information or represent areas in which

clients can work. Clients also may provide a straightforward story with some identifiable gaps that the clinician may note. These, too, must be explored. Often, the gaps provide information necessary for understanding a client's problems, although the client may not even be clear about their significance.

4. *Concealed Meaning* It is important that clinicians hear all that their clients say, not just the words that are most obvious. The tone, posture, facial expressions, and behavior of our clients might give much additional meaning to their stories. Slips of the tongue, attitudes, and casual references also might carry a great deal of importance. Clinicians need to listen and probe the meaning of these for their clients. Sometimes clinicians will not pursue these immediately but will note the possibility for future exploration.

5. *Client Strengths* Clients are often discouraged with their lives, relationships, and with their stuttering. They are unaware of the strengths they possess and their self-esteem is low. Clinicians who are good listeners not only will lighten the load of discouragement by listening acceptingly but will also reflect back the resources they see within their clients. Ivey[13] called this a "positive asset" search:

> Even when working with the most complex case, it is wise to focus on client strengths and assets from time to time. Including the question "Talk about something you feel good about" is ideally part of every interview. The focus on positive assets is necessary to combat the tendency to search constantly for problems and difficulties. People solve problems with their strengths, not with their weaknesses.

Encouraging, Paraphrasing, and Summarization Although some clients have no difficulty "telling their story" to the clinician, this is not usually the case. It is most often necessary to prompt, probe, encourage, paraphrase, and summarize so the client can explore and communicate their own experience. Eagen[20] wrote: "The ability to use prompts and probes well is an important skill. They are verbal tactics for helping clients talk about themselves and define their problems more concretely in terms of specific experiences, behaviors and feelings. As such they can be used in all stages of the helping process." We would like to look at each of these skills separately.

1. *Prompts and Probes* Two valuable prompts and probes used in the clinical process are open-ended questions and statements. We have explained these above, but these questions can also be used whenever the clinician wishes to focus the interaction. Some examples of focusing through questioning are:

> "You've discussed many topics during the last half hour. Could you choose the most important one and tell me more about it?"
> "When you talked about Mary's fluency problem, your voice trembled. Could you talk about what was happening to you then?"
> "Can you give me some examples of that?"
> "What are some good things about using your fluency targets?"

These prompts can help move the session from the general to the specific. Clinicians who ask "closed questions" (that is, those that require a "yes" or "no" answer) find that they have to ask a greater number of questions.

Statements can also be used as probes. These are usually indirect questions that prompt clients to expand their discussion of their experiences and feelings. By encouraging clients to talk more about what they have said, clinicians can lead them to a greater awareness of their feelings and motivations. For example:

"I know that you get upset when Mary stutters, but I'm not sure how you show that to Mary."

Here, the clinician offers the client the opportunity to provide more information about her behavior.

If probes are to be effective, they should provide clinicians with rich information that needs to be heard, understood, and reflected. After probes are used, therefore, clinicians should find themselves using empathetic responses. The use of probes and empathetic responses together is called "blending." Hepworth and Larsen[11] provided the following example of blending:

Clinician: As you were speaking about your son, I sensed some pain and reluctance on your part to talk about him. I'd like to understand more about what you are feeling. Could you share with me what you are experiencing right now?

The blended response usually enables the client to move forward with important information.

2. *Encouragers* Ivey[13] defined encouragers as "head nods, open gestures, and positive facial expressions that encourage the client to keep talking." Minimal verbal utterances such as "Ummm" and "Uh-huh" have the same effect. Silence accompanied by appropriate nonverbal communication can be another type of encourager. Encouragers indicate that the clinician is listening attentively and encourage the client to say more. Another valuable encourager is for the clinician to accent the responses made by the client by repeating in a questioning tone or emphasizing a word that the client used. For example, a client says, "It's a real pain to have to come to speech class!" The clinician might use the short, accented speech response, "A pain?" All of these encouragers facilitate client growth unless they are not used well. As we all know, excessive parroting, head nodding, or gestures can be annoying. These encouragers must be economically used and integrated with the other techniques.

3. *Paraphrasing* Hepworth and Larsen[11] defined paraphrasing as using fresh words to restate the client's message concisely. Responses that paraphrase are more apt to draw heavily on the cognitive aspects of client messages (i.e., emphasize situations, ideas, objects, persons) than to focus on the client's affective state. Once again, these responses must be carefully used with other facilitating responses lest they sound too mimicking. The art of paraphrasing is successfully

used when the clinician transforms the client's statement into a succinct and meaningful statement. The statement must be true to the words that the client said, but need not repeat them verbatim. A paraphrase is longer than an encourager, but not quite as long as a summary. Schuerle[14] provided the framework for the following paraphrasing by the clinician:

> *Client:* I don't know where to turn. When I was little, I could just be quiet and watch what was going on. But now I'm growing up. Being a person who stutters and 16 are the worst possible combination.
>
> *Clinician:* Your stuttering is interfering with things you care a great deal about.
>
> *Client:* Yeah. My friends talk a lot faster and I can't keep up with the group discussion.
>
> *Clinician:* You feel like you miss a lot even if you are part of the group.

4. *Summarization* In a summarization, the clinician pulls together the major ideas, themes, and concepts that have been expressed by the client and reflects them back to the client. When a topic has been completed, a session ended, or the initial assessment completed, clinicians can provide closure by summarizing their perceptions. The summary may consist of one thought brought out in the session or more: "From what you have said so far, your stuttering has affected all of your relationships." It also may be a general statement of what has taken place: "To sum up, you seem very anxious to improve your speech, but you don't feel as if you can spend the time or money involved."

Summaries may also be used to provide a focus when clients get stuck and the session seems to be going nowhere. A good summary will bring together the relevant data that has been presented in the session. When clients have not put together the pieces for themselves, the summarization can be clarifying for them.

At the completion of the assessment phase and throughout the therapy session, the clinician might want to periodically summarize how the problem seems to be produced by the interplay of several synergistic factors: physiologic, attitudinal, and environmental. The summary would be individual, citing the primary factors in each client's "story."

Noting and Reflecting Feelings The fifth basic listening skill is one that is at the heart of the process. The art of good listening involves paying attention to what the client is saying, both verbally and nonverbally. Our aim is to hear the content of the client's experiences related to their fluency problems as well as to the feelings that have accompanied them. Listening on all levels of response requires stepping into the shoes of the other person. The clinician must try to perceive the world of the client without losing her own perspective or taking on the emotions of the client. This understanding of the person is both demonstrated and extended with empathetic listening responses. Empathetic responding involves reporting back to the client on both the content and the feeling level of what has been expressed.

Luterman[16] has called this the "affect response" and wrote:

On the surface, the affect response appears risky, but actually it is responding to what Rogers in a lecture called "the faint knocking." By listening
very carefully and trying to see the world as the client sees it and reflecting
the feelings back, the counselor can help to open up the relationship, sometimes very dramatically. The appropriate affect response greatly increases
the intimacy level in a relationship. I have found that not even an inaccu-
rate response is harmful. It generally forces people to clarify further their
feelings, and in the process of clarification, we both can generally understand the feelings better."[16]

Hepworth and Larsen[11] stated: "Empathetic responding involves understanding the other person's feelings and experiences without taking that person's
position (e.g., "I sense that you're feeling . . ." or "You seem to be saying . . .")."
Thus, the clinician retains separateness and objectivity—a critical dimension in
the helping process, for when clinicians take on the client's feelings and positions
they lose not only vital perspective but the ability to be helpful as well. When the
clinician remains separate yet reflects the client's experiences and feelings, the clinician provides a mirror for the clients to both hear what they have said and to
get in touch with how they are feeling about it. In this process of both being mir-
rored and being understood, the client comes to a greater understanding of the
problem and a clearer awareness of what must be done to solve it.

When speech-language pathologists are first introduced to the skill of empathetic responding, they often react negatively. Again, it seems too mechanical
and artificial at first. However, that impression passes with practice. When the
skill is used accurately, the client's sense of being truly understood will become a
freeing experience, and their feedback will demonstrate this to the clinician. If
you have ever had anyone listen to you wholeheartedly, you, too, can appreciate
the value of this skill.

It is not ordinarily difficult for a clinician to respond in a way that reflects
the *content* of the client's message. It is, however, more difficult to verbalize the
feeling. There are literally hundreds of words that can be used to capture feelings, yet clinicians often limit themselves to just a few (e.g., "upset" or "frustrated"). If a client is expressing rage at a person's treatment of him, a reflection
of how "upset" he seems will not further your understanding of the story. When
you accurately reflect the client's feelings, the client will probably respond with
an enthusiastic "yes" or "right!" Therefore, it is important that we hear the different levels of feeling and acquire words that will capture this potential variety
of feeling states. Hutchins and Cole[15] have provided examples of a variety of feeling words (Table 8.2).

Eagen[17] encouraged the clinician to listen for the "core message" expressed
in feelings and for the experiences and behaviors that underlie these feelings.
Once you feel that you have identified the core message, use the formula: "You

feel _____ because _____." (E.g., "You *feel* that no one likes you *because* they make fun of your speech.") With practice, a clinician can use this formula in an individual way, one that becomes part of her style.

Various levels of empathetic listening can be practiced by a clinician. On the higher levels of listening, the clinician's responses convey an understanding of what the client has said as well as what the client might only imply. Through this type of reflecting, the clinician can better understand the client's deeper feelings and unexplored meanings and, after attending and listening, may connect current feelings to previously expressed experiences or feelings. This may help the client to identify patterns, themes, or purposes. This careful listening and reflecting may also help clients to identify the goals that will lead to their own growth. These kinds of responses build a basis of trust and understanding, both of which help to facilitate a successful treatment program.

Bolton[21] proposed these guidelines for improved empathetic listening:

- Don't fake understanding.
- Don't tell the speaker you know how she feels.
- Vary your responses.
- Focus on the person's feelings.
- Choose the most accurate feeling word.
- Develop vocal empathy.
- Strive for concreteness and relevance.
- Provide nondogmatic but firm responses.

As we have already noted, one might feel awkward when first using this technique, but with practice it will seem natural. Although it is indeed a technique, when one understands its purpose to identify the feelings and the underlying meaning behind the feeling, it is easier to practice.

The "because" element in the reflection statement encourages the expression of the experiences and feelings that underlie the client's feelings. "You feel angry *because* you didn't use your targets and you stuttered in front of the other children." Some additional examples are as follows:

- "You feel sad because you were afraid to speak up in class and you didn't get to play on the team."
- "You're worried because you might stutter when you make your presentation for your promotion."

Although the formula provides a framework for understanding what is happening, we encourage clinicians to use the words that sound best and most natural to them. In this way, they have the formula as a background: "You feel . . . because . . . ," but they vary their responses that elicit the feelings, experiences, and behaviors. Some common errors in using empathetic responses have been compiled by Brammer[22]:

Table 8.2 Feeling Words

Relative Intensity of Words	Feeling Category				
	Anger	*Conflict*	*Fear*	*Happiness*	*Sadness*
Mild Feeling	Annoyed	Blocked	Apprehensive	Amused	Apathetic
	Bothered	Bound	Concerned	Anticipating	Bored
	Bugged	Caught	Tense	Comfortable	Confused
	Irked	Caught in	Tight	Confident	Disappointed
	Irritated	a bind	Uneasy	Contended	Disconnected
	Peeved	Pulled		Glad	Mixed up
	Ticked			Pleased	Resigned
				Relieved	Unsure
Moderate Feeling	Disgusted	Locked	Afraid	Delighted	Abandoned
	Hacked	Pressured	Alarmed	Eager	Burdened
	Harassed	Torn	Anxious	Happy	Discouraged
	Mad		Fearful	Hopeful	Distressed
	Provoked		Frightened	Joyful	Down
	Put upon		Shook	Surprised	Drained
	Resentful		Threatened	Up	Empty
	Set up		Worried		Hurt
	Spiteful				Lonely
	Used				Lost
					Sad
					Unhappy
					Weighted
Intense Feeling	Angry	Ripped	Desperate	Bursting	Anguished
	Boiled	Wrenched	Overwhelmed	Ecstatic	Crushed
	Burned		Panicky	Elated	Deadened
	Contemptful		Petrified	Enthusiastic	Despairing
	Enraged		Scared	Enthralled	Helpless
	Fuming		Terrified	Excited	Hopeless
	Furious		Terror-	Free	Humiliated
	Hateful		stricken	Fulfilled	Miserable
	Hot		Tortured	Moved	Overwhelmed
	Infuriated			Proud	Smothered
	Pissed			Terrific	Tortured
	Smoldering			Thrilled	
	Steamed			Turned on	

Note: The context in which words such as these are used may result in shifting their intensity as well as changing the category in which they are used. Words are listed here only to suggest the range of options available to the helper seeking to identify feelings of the client.

Source: Reprinted with permission from Hutchins D, Cole C. *Helping Relationships and Strategies.* Belmont, CA: Brooks/Cole, 1992, p. 60.

- Stereotyping your responses. This means that helpers tend to begin their re-flections in the same monotonous way: "You feel," "You think," and "It seems to you." This repetitive style gives the impression of insincerity or an impoverished word supply.
- Timing: Beginning helpers get into a pattern of reflecting every statement. It is not necessary to reflect every statement, and it can be effective to inter-rupt the client occasionally if he/she is in a long monologue.
- Overshooting with too much depth of feeling.
- The language must be appropriate to the cultural experience and educational levels of the client.

As important as the empathetic response is, it must be integrated with the other basic listening skills. Ivey[13] pointed out that these basic listening skills provide a helper with an array of skills to ensure her understanding of the client's thinking, feeling, and behaving. A special advantage of mastering these skills is that they can be used in a variety of situations (Table 8.3).

Goal Setting

The basic listening skills are tools that increase our knowledge of our client's world and that help us to be of assistance in the goal setting and implementation process of treatment. It is important that the client and clinician mutually identify goals that the client wants to work on. This communication is essential if we are to build up the empowerment attitudes (Chapter 7) and encourage growth in the client's responsibility. The listening skills are the means to achieving successful goal setting. The clinician can ask the client to identify behaviors the client has discussed and would like to change. This becomes the primary goal. In order to bring about change, however, additional goals may be targeted. When goals occur to the clinician that were overlooked by the client, it is important to offer these to the client. If these goals were taken from the client's own story, clients will usually agree to work on them.

Hutchins and Cole[15] have stressed that "[t]o resolve a problem, the client must change behavior." Goals relate to what the client will be doing in the future to overcome, reduce, or eliminate concerns or problems he currently has. This means that the client will deliberately change combinations of behavior in the following ways:

- *Change thoughts:* The client changes from irrational, unproductive, self-destructive, negative thinking to more positive thinking about self and others. The client learns to accept self and aspects of situations that cannot be changed.
- *Change feelings:* The client changes worrisome, hostile, depressive, angry, or negative feelings to more positive feelings and emotions about self and others.

Table 8.3 Basic Listening Skills

Accept without judgment	Identify incongruities	Restatements
Active listening	Interpretation	Self-disclosure
Adjust tense/time of language to here and now	Minimal encourages	Sharing oneself
Attend selectively to positive aspects of client	Minimal verbalization	Silence
Body language	Movement	Target client reference to "first person"
Challenge incongruities	Paraphrasing	Touches client
Constructed/closed questions	Position	Unstructured/open questions
Eye contact	Posture	Verbal and nonverbal matching of client messages
Facial expression	Promptness—timely action	Verbal clarifying
Facial scanning	Recall previous content	Verbal elaboration
Find and verbalize assets of client	Recall previous interaction	Verbal following
Give directions	Reflection of client's feelings	
Give instructions	Refrain from interrupting client	

Reprinted with permission from Ivey A. *Intentional Interviewing and Counseling*. Belmont, CA: Brooks/Cole, 1994, p. 35.

- *Change actions:* The client changes from displaying destructive, inappropriate, spontaneous, or counterproductive actions to more positive, constructive, socially appropriate, and thoughtful goal actions.

In order to accomplish these changes, clinicians must assist clients to make their goals specific. One must narrow the breadth of the goal and describe what the client will be doing in relationship to improving his stuttering. When will the behavior occur? Where will the practice take place? What are the specific target productions one will aim for? What are the positive and negative consequences of using these goals? One uses listening skills to help the client set individual goals. In addition, it is important to teach the clients some of these rules of communication.

Summary   The specifics of communication skills seem important for both fluency clinicians and fluency clients. It has been demonstrated that these skills can be taught and can improve the quality of therapeutic intervention (Ivy[13]).

The basic skills explored were based on Ivy's microskills: attending, open and closed questioning, client observation skills, encouraging, paraphrasing, noting and reflecting feelings, and goal setting. The next aspects of the communication environment that are important for both the clinician and client to be aware of are the social and pragmatic aspects of communication.

Social and Pragmatic Aspects of Communication

Whitmire[23] noted that language is the principal means of social adaptation in our educational system. To become integrated into the social culture, peer relationships contribute to the development of social skills that reduce the likelihood of social isolation.[24] For individuals who stutter, the avoidance of people, situations, and experiences that would expose them as people who stutter has been central to their behavior. Nelson[25] highlighted the need for a person to know the rules of communication in order to succeed in areas beyond the overt curriculum. He outlined six curricula the student must master to succeed in school, two of which are the following:

- *School Culture Curriculum:* The set of spoken and unspoken rules about communication and behavior in classroom interactions. Includes expectations for metapragmatic awareness of rules about such things as when to talk, when not to talk, and how to request a turn.
- *Underground Curriculum:* The rules for social interaction among peers that determine who will be accepted and who will not. Includes expectations for using the latest slang and pragmatic rules of social interaction discourse as diverse as bragging and peer tutoring.

The importance and the subtle difficulty of learning the social and pragmatic rules of interaction are apparent to all who work in the field of communication disorders. We have already noted the synergistic involvement of language. Here we would like to cite some of the specific social and pragmatic interactional skills one might target in a therapy program.

We have found that one of the most difficult aspects of therapy for people who stutter is transfer of skills to the everyday environment. We also realize that the pragmatic aspects of language are essential for the learning of language and for social interaction. Some clients may have a pragmatic language disorder based on additional physiologic concomitants. Others who stutter have simply avoided the necessary interactions to acquire these rules. Tanner et al.[26] pointed out:

> One of the major limitations of many of the stuttering programs currently in use is that the pragmatic aspects of communication receive little or no attention. It often is assumed that the client will be able to communicate effectively once he/she overcomes his/her fluency disorder. Because of the anxiety caused by stuttering and the individual's efforts to avoid speaking

in various contexts, some clients fail to acquire the conversational skills necessary for them to effectively make use of language. The improvements in fluency that occur during the course of the stuttering intervention program are not necessarily accompanied by improvements in the client's functional communication skills. Therefore, the functional aspects of communication need to be addressed in treatment.

We agree with this outlook and use in our therapy both assessment and treatment recommendations made by Tanner:

- *Greets others:* To what extent does the individual greet others? When others greet the individual, does he return the greeting: Is greeting others considered stressful by the client?
- *Initiates conversations:* To what extent does the individual approach others to initiate conversations? Would the client find it abnormally stressful to ask someone for a date? Would he avoid a major school/work activity because of the fear of initiating a conversation? Does the client feel that he is abnormally shy about initiating interactions in specific situations? How effectively is the individual able to start a conversation with a friend, stranger, or an authority figure?
- *Asks questions:* To what extent does the individual ask questions when information is needed? If the client is having difficulty finding a particular office in a large building, would he ask an employee for directions? Would the client be more comfortable asking a stranger, acquaintance, or friend for information? Is the asking of questions during class or at work a particularly stressful event?
- *Gives complete answers when asked for information:* To what extent does the individual verbalize information when asked? Is he unusually tense or evasive about giving verbal information? Does the client volunteer information other than the specific information that is being requested?
- *Requests assistance when help is needed:* Does the client avoid asking for assistance because of the fluency disorder? How effectively does the client ask family members, friends, and strangers for help? What situations create a level of high anxiety and make it more difficult to ask for help?
- *Offers suggestions to others:* To what extent does the client offer suggestions to others when needed? Does the client voluntarily offer verbal suggestions? Does the client feel anxiety when giving suggestions to specific individuals?
- *Volunteers information during discussions:* To what extent does the client volunteer information or ideas during a discussion? Does the client feel comfortable volunteering information in a one-to-one situation? Does the client feel comfortable volunteering information to a group of friends during a discussion? Is a formal discussion uncomfortable for the client? Does an informal social discussion cause the client to experience anxiety? Whom

does the client direct comments to when participating in group discussions? Whom does he avoid?

- *Describes events accurately and in sufficient detail:* To what extent does the client describe events accurately with detail? Does the client leave out sequences of events that he may not want to discuss or describe? Does the client fail to mention certain details because of a fear that stuttering might occur on specific sounds, words, or phrases? When describing an event in detail, does the client exhibit circumlocutions in an effort to avoid feared words?

- *Maintains a topic over a series of utterances:* Do certain topics create anxiety or fear for the client? How long can the client maintain the same topic? When the client becomes uncomfortable or starts to stutter, does he change the topic immediately? Does the client's ability to maintain a topic vary depending on the nature of the subject matter? For example, a client who is able to maintain a topic of general interest might experience difficulty maintaining a discussion in which information of a personal nature must be expressed.

- *Describes personal experiences:* How effectively does the client describe personal experiences? Do certain situations/memories create high levels of anxiety? When the individual feels anxious about describing personal experiences, how is fluency affected?

- *Takes turns appropriately during conversation:* To what extent does the client take turns appropriately during conversation: Does the client put off taking a turn until asked to respond to a question? Does the client talk without pausing to let others speak because of a fear that stuttering will occur when future utterances are initiated?

- *Participates verbally during group activities:* How often is the client an active verbal participant during activities in which several individuals are working on the same task? Does the client give verbal input or ideas? Does the client resist contributing information when members of the group ask for opinions or ideas? Does the client resist contributing information when members of the group ask for opinions or ideas?

- *Expresses needs:* Is the individual able to express needs? Do inhibitions increase when assistance from a stranger or an authority figure is needed to fulfill these needs? How effectively does the individual express needs when interacting with close friends or family members?

- *Shares feelings:* To what extent is the individual able to share personal feelings? In what situations does the person have difficulty expressing feelings? Do certain topics create high levels of anxiety? Is it easier to share feelings with friends than with strangers?

- *Expresses viewpoints:* To what extent does the client express opinions, beliefs, and ideas in various speaking contexts? Are withdrawal behaviors observed because of a fear of disfluency? Does the individual react defensively when confronted with topics that are sensitive in nature?

- *Expresses feelings of disagreement:* How does the individual express feelings of disagreement? Does anger create anxiety levels that result in increased disfluency? Does the client withdraw from communication when confronted with opposition? Is it easier to disagree with friends than with strangers?

We believe that these questions and the techniques based on them pull together the basic aspects of the social and pragmatic needs of the fluency client. Tanner et al.[26] integrated activities for increasing self-esteem, social and pragmatic skills, and other empowerment attitudes. Although not naming the synergistic interaction of these areas, it is clear that language, communication skills, social/pragmatic skills and empowerment attitudes are interacting

Summary   Since language is a principle means of both education and personal growth, we have highlighted some specific goals of pragmatic intervention. We agree with Nippold[27] that there is a need for research in this area of treatment and we encourage fluency specialists to examine it with us.

FAMILY INFLUENCE

When working with fluency clients in a synergistic approach, one knows that it is not sufficient to work with the fluency problem in isolation. In Chapter 2, we defined the basic components of family inclusion and family-based therapy. We have noted that it is important to expand the traditional view of counseling parents of children who have a fluency disorder and work toward incorporating counseling skills and family therapy techniques in working with the whole family. Counseling skills will be presented in Chapter 9. In this chapter, we will examine more completely the techniques of family therapy that are helpful in treating fluency disorders.

Families of Fluency Clients

When one member of the family has a fluency disorder, the entire family is affected. Most parents find disability to be the great spoiler of their dreams because most dreams require an unimpaired child.[28] The fluency disorder may be new to the family, or the family may be all too familiar with the effects of stuttering behavior. In all cases, we are dealing with a family system that has special and individual needs. Gordon[29] states that when dealing with disabilities, the needs of the child are great, but the needs of the family are greater. The needs of the children are frequently met, but the needs of the family are too seldom recognized or satisfied.

Speech-language pathologists may be the first and only professionals to come into contact with the needs of the families of people who stutter. We are the ones who can respond to these needs by incorporating them into our treatment programs. Moses[28] wrote:

You—the special educator, audiologist, speech-language pathologist—are the ones who deal firsthand with people who are under stress in a circumstance that is most appropriately dealt with by you rather than by psychologists, social workers, or psychiatrists. You are the people who can take a truly holistic approach in the treatment of the child and deal with the emotional impact upon the parents of having an impaired child within a nonpathology-oriented environment.

Luterman[16] states:

Our job as professionals in working with persons with communicative disorders is to help the family become optimal, or as close to it as possible. We can teach parents, mainly by modeling, how to manage conflict, how to communicate openly, and how to display their affection and caring for their children. In effect, what we do is parent the parents and create for them in our relationship, an optimal family. The parents then can take from our optimal clinical family the information and skills necessary for their own home situation.

In order to maximize the success of our work with family members, it is important to look at the traditional approach to the families of people who stutter and then to look at possible ways our interactive approach can offer improvements. Clinicians who wish to expand their concepts of family interaction will draw heavily on the counseling skills presented in Chapter 9 as well as the family therapy principles discussed in this chapter.

Traditional Approaches to Families with Dysfluent Children

In Chapter 2, we provided background research related to families of people who stutter and the way that we have examined stuttering within the family. Myers and Freeman,[30-32] Riley and Riley,[33] Conture and Caruso,[34] and Kelly and Conture[35] have studied parent-child interaction and provided us with valuable information about how to create a verbal environment that can assist in facilitating fluency. Zebrowski and Schum[36] summed up this research by saying:

Regardless of the age of the children or the nature of the stuttering, much of the information and counsel that speech-language pathologists provide to parents is directed toward helping them modify the verbal interactions they have with the children so as to increase the probability that the children that the children will speak more fluently.

To accomplish this, parents are advised, among other things, to model a slowed speech rate when talking to or in the presence of the children,[35,37] to increase the duration of the pauses they produce before responding to the children's utterance,[35,38] and to avoid interrupting the children in conversation.[39-41]

Table 8.4 Techniques to Facilitate Parent-Child Interactions

Mirroring	The adult observes and then reflects the child's nonverbal and motor expression
Self-Talk	The adult talks out his or her own participation during a joint activity with the child
Parallel Talk	The adult talks out the child's participation during a joint activity
Reflecting	The adult listens to the child and then repeats nonpunitively what the child has said
Expansion	The adult listens to the child's utterance and expands it by adding relevant grammatical, semantic, and/or phonological details
Speech Pattern Modification	The adult deliberately slows down his or her speech rate to about 160–190 syllables per minute and uses 5–6 word utterances

Source: Reprinted with permission from Langlois A, Long S. A model for teaching parents to facilitate fluent speech. *J of Fluency Disord* 1988;13:165.

The traditional approaches have provided us with valuable techniques for increasing communication skills within the family. Below, we summarize some of the techniques that have proven to be most helpful.

Langlois and Long[37] focused on teaching facilitative techniques to parents to increase the positive interactions with their child and contribute to the increases in the child's fluency. These techniques are presented in Table 8.4.

Peter Ramig[42] identified three stages of partnership for the parents of children who stutter, their children, and the clinician:

1. Educating with respect to the myths and realities about stuttering.
2. Facilitating parent awareness of communicative interaction styles and other environmental stresses such as interpersonal interaction. Parent and child interactive styles are noted: parent speaking rates, the amount of time parents take between the time a child ends his utterance and the beginning of the parent's utterance, and parent interruptions as the child is talking. Parents learn how to modify these styles and ways for dealing with the interpersonal stress are not offered.
3. Encouraging parents' involvement as observers and participants in therapy sessions: Parents are gradually incorporated into the therapy for their child. They assume the roles of observer and participant, and accept responsibility for facilitating fluency in the home environment.

Guitar and Peters[2] identified the objectives of a family-counseling program as:

1. Explaining the treatment program and the parents' role in it.
2. Discussing the possible causes of stuttering.

3. Identifying and reducing fluency disrupters.
4. Identifying and increasing fluency enhancing situations.

Guitar and Peters see this as an ongoing dynamic process.

All of these approaches highlight the primary importance of increased awareness of communication skills by the parents and integrate the parents in a positive, productive, and essential manner. The programs are absolutely essential for parental involvement and are synergistically interrelated with the communication skills and physiologic skills presented in this text. However, in addition to the interactive communication style of the family members, we believe that it is important to assess and work with the interactive thoughts, feelings, and behaviors related to the fluency disorder of the primary people in the client's environment. Several programs have begun to include this aspect of family interaction. In the next section, we highlight some of the leading work in the expansion of the families' role with the fluency client.

Expansion of the Role of Families with Dysfluent Children

Ham[43] has provided several forms to assist the parent in observing the environmental factors noted above (see Table 8.5). In addition to outlining these various communication interactions, Ham noted that parents are surprised to discover how stuttering is related to the various situations one encounters each day. Ham also proposed that while general family life cannot be so easily measured on a chart, it is important for us to include it in our remediation. He stated: "Topics in this section (general family life) are covered best by the clinician's ability to establish good relationships, be an uncritical listener, avoid judgements, piece together scattered comments and information, encourage without pressing, and guide conversation without being obvious." In other words, the clinician must know and practice listening and counseling skills not only with the individual client but also with the family members.

Ham[43] listed the following areas of general concern for families of children with fluency disorders:

- Spouses' marital relationship and attitudes and behaviors toward each other.
- Availability and responsiveness of each parent in terms of work schedules and other demands.
- Spouses' separate philosophies of child rearing and how these interact.
- Parents' attitudes in general toward their children. Conture[38] noted: "We never cease to be amazed at how some parents can continually and consistently selectively attend only to the negative aspects of their child's behavior."
- Disciplinary practices in the home. Who is punished for what, differences in punishment for different behaviors, and so on. Particular interest in child's reactions to punishment. If there are siblings, review their punishment and reactions.

Table 8.5 Parent Observation of Environmental Factors

Item	Areas				
	Person	Person	Person	Home	Outside
1. Rapid speech rate.					
2. High vocabulary rate.					
3. Bilingual pressures.					
4. Perfectionistic demands on pronunciation, articulation, vocabulary, etc.					
5. Quiet, nontalkative.					
6. Very talkative.					
7. Dysfluency reactions: Interruption, stoppage Say things for child Helpful advice Express concern Criticism, comment Scolding Imitation, teasing Punishment					

Instruction: Identify and specific persons. Rate the behaviors, Put a 3 if behavior is frequent or strong; put a 2 if occurrence is occasional or mild; and put a 1 if occurrence is rare or absent.

Source: Reprinted with permission from Ham R. *Therapy of Stuttering*. Englewood Cliffs, NJ: Prentice Hall, 1990, p. 186.

- Repeat the previous item, more or less, replacing punishment with reward, attention, love and so on.
- What kind of family? Closely knit or open, quiet or noisy, talkative or nontalkative, reasonable or argumentative, emotional or balanced, and so on.

These are excellent areas to explore when working with fluency clients. The skills one would use to explore these attitudes are discussed in Chapter 9 and in the above section on communication skills. Since we believe that dealing with a fluency problem requires a systemic approach, we encourage clinicians to become familiar with these necessary skills and to incorporate our gleanings from the family therapy literature that we present later.

Family Therapy Literature

In order to increase maintenance and carry-over, Mallard[44] patterned a program after Rustin's[45-47] that involved the entire family in therapy. One of the present authors was able to serve as a consultant to this program and found it to be an excellent approach to therapy with children and their families. The opportunity to implement Rustin's program in the United States was a valuable one that has provided many insights into the functioning of the family around dysfluency. Major targets of this therapeutic approach include talk time, turn taking, interruption patterns, listening patterns, strategy for discipline, and problem-solving.

The programs begin with a detailed assessment. During this time the clinician learns about the child's difficulties and the siblings' and parents' attitudes toward the stuttering behavior. An effort is made to assess the family structure. Clinicians are asked to pursue all behavioral, social, and emotional aspects of the families' functioning. The evaluation is comprehensive and includes a multi-dimensional assessment aimed at the many important aspects of fluency. This assessment is one of the few diagnostic tools for fluency that systematically expand the broader scope of family concepts that are important. For example, some factors that are involved in the assessment are:

- *Recent behavior and emotional health:* general health; eating, sleeping, and elimination; muscular system and concentration; speech, tics, and mannerisms; attack disorders; emotions; peer relationships; relationships with siblings; relationships with adults; antisocial trends; sex education; schooling.
- *Family structure and history:* personal background; parents' family background; the child's grandparents and extended family issues; home circumstances; finances and neighborhood.
- *Family life and relationships:* parental relationships; parent-child interaction; child's participation in family activities and discipline.
- *Temperamental or personality attributes:* meeting new people; new situations; emotional expression; sensitivity.

Although this assessment is a time-consuming process, it is from this breadth of understanding that the treatment program is developed. We heartily endorse this direction for fluency assessment and think it important to highlight those strategies of remediation that are most helpful for including the thoughts, feelings, and behaviors related to changing the fluency behaviors of the client within the environment of the family—talk time, strategies for discipline, and problem solving.

Talk Time   After the interview, parents are given an assignment to set aside a specific period of time (four minutes, twice a week) to do nothing but talk with their children. All the person's energies are to be devoted to listening and then they fill out a task sheet to send to the clinician. Mallard and Rustin believe that this provides the foundation on which all future home management can be conducted. During this time, interaction styles are focused upon and often important feelings are expressed.

Strategies for Discipline   This is a crucial aspect of the program and one arrives at individual strategies for individual families through problem-solving techniques.

Problem-Solving Techniques   Mallard[44] recommended that the following instructions be read verbatim to parents:

> Problem solving is one of the most important skills that you will learn in this course. This technique can be used to solve all types of problems, not just stuttering. The steps are as follows: First, identify the problem. This can be very difficult. You must, however, be specific about what the exact problem is. Write the problem in the middle of the paper and draw a circle around it. Second, list all possible options around the circle, no matter how far out or silly. Third, erase the ones that are really not options for your family. Fourth, list the options in order of their likelihood of happening for you. Fifth, discuss the consequences of the options that you listed. Sixth, put into practice the option that you wish. Seventh, be satisfied with your decision. Be happy that you are calling your own shots. If other people don't like what you have decided, then it is their problem, not yours. Eighth, reevaluate this process and your decision after a short period of time.

We believe that these techniques provide a valuable framework for interaction among family members and we encourage these techniques to become a part of therapy with children and with families. In order to most effectively carry out this process, we urge clinicians to practice and improve their listening skills and to incorporate aspects of the counseling process (Chapter 9) as they progress through these steps.

It is clear that fluency therapy has grown to include both the communication skills and the interpersonal skills within the family setting. This underscores our belief that the environmental aspects of fluency must include these components.

Contemporary Family Therapy

The traditional idea of the family as comprising father, mother, and children is no longer the norm. We must extend our view of the family to include single parent families, blended families (children of one or both parents who have been previously married), multigenerational families, and other nontraditional types of families. At present, the culturally pluralistic population challenges us to become sensitive to many diverse family groups. As we noted in Chapter 2, these nontraditional and traditional families operate as a system and replace the unidimensional view of individual therapy that has guided us in the past. Andrews and Andrews[48,49] called the shift in thinking about families a "paradigm shift" away from the individual model of service delivery to the systemic. They stated that the individual model is characterized by four features: (1) the interaction system is the client and the clinician, (2) change is looked for only in the client, (3) the primary intervention is with the child, and (4) change occurs during the session. On the other hand, the systemic approach contrasts with the individual approach in the following ways: (1) the interactive system is the child and a circumscribed group of people who interact with the child, have influence on the child, and are concerned about the problem, (2) change is expected in the individual and the interactive system, (3) change occurs in the natural environment, and (4) the primary intervention is with the interactive systems.[48]

Donohue-Kilburg[50] has quoted with approval Virginia Satir's view of family:

> The family is a factory where people are made, and parents are people-makers. The family provides self-worth, communication, rules and a link to society. These factors are dealt with differently in each family. Some families are "nurturing" families in which members experience (1) high self-worth, (2) direct, clear, specific, and honest communication, (3) flexible, human, appropriate, and changeable rules, and (4) an open and hopeful link to society. Other families are "troubled" and their members experience (1) low self-worth, (2) indirect, vague, or dishonest communication, (3) rigid, inhuman, and non-negotiable rules, and (4) a fearful, placating, or blaming link to society. In reality, all families exist on a continuum somewhere between nurturing and troubled, and probably change position on that continuum frequently.[50]

Ylvisaker and Feeney[52, 53] contended that the best way to serve our clients is by incorporating the help of the "everyday people" in the client's environment. We know that "everyday people" may include the nuclear family (Mom, Dad, and children), the extended family (grandparents, cousins, aunts, and uncles who have a strong relationship with the nuclear family), and the "selected family" (close friends and other persons such as teachers, mentors, therapists, or social group leaders who may at times fulfill the role of family members). Ylvisaker and Feeney highlighted the following reasons that "everyday people" can be a help to communication disorder specialists in delivering services:

- Respect for everyday people, their insights, and their potential contribution
- A likely increase in the intensity, consistency, and duration of intervention
- Facilitation of generalization, and maintenance of learned skills
- Support for a long-term focus in rehabilitation
- Cost effectiveness of intervention[53]

Maintenance for fluency is an issue of major concern that is best addressed by including the family (nuclear, extended, and or selected) in the planning of our assessment and rehabilitation programs. Although Andrews and Andrews[48] noted that change from an individual to a systemic approach has been slow, our work is part of that "paradigm shift," and we are encouraged to continue to include goals for family assessment and treatment in our synergistic approach.

Family-Based Assessment

Part of a systemic approach to therapy is the understanding that not only the client but the family must be included in the assessment process. Counseling and listening skills are part of this process; however, there are additional considerations related to family interaction. We need to observe and evaluate not only the client's speech problem but also the interactive patterns of all the participants. In fact, this approach is in keeping with our expanded knowledge of the communication process itself. Lund[54] noted that the pragmatic view of communication disorders departs from the traditional view and calls us to look at interactive patterns. When communication breaks down, it is a problem for all participants. Using the basic listening skills of attending, observation, encouragement and paraphrasing, reflection, and summarization can help explore that family interaction. There are additional skills that are family oriented:

Joining

In order to join a family, clinicians must learn and accept the organizational style of the families and blend with them. They must experience the interactional patterns within the family and sense the pain of those who are scapegoated or the joy of those who are loved. They must join the culture that they are assessing.[55] As clinicians become joined with each of the family members, communication and interaction become more open.

Joining can be accomplished by becoming aware of the family's strengths and by affirming the self-worth of each of the family members. Some of the behaviors recommended by Andrews[56] that facilitate joining are:

- Socializing (briefly) about everyday issues
- Mirroring the posture of the person being listened to
- Using everyday language and terminology that matches the family's level of understanding
- Matching affect (smiling, frowning, looking puzzled)
- Sharing common experiences

Minuchin and Fishman, who believe that joining is the basis of family change brought about in the family system, wrote:

How does the therapist join the system? Like the family members, the therapist is more human than otherwise. Somewhere inside, he has resonating chords that can respond to a human frequency. In forming the therapeutic system, aspects of himself that facilitate the building of common ground with the family members will be elicited. And the therapist will deliberately activate self-segments that are congruent with the family.[57]

The purpose of joining is to connect and engage each of the family members in the process. Each person needs to feel the clinician's warmth and concern. As in all skill use, we must act out of our own personal style. Virginia Satir[12] begins a family meeting by making contact with each member of the family. She shakes hands with each in turn; establishing eye contact, touching them, and calling each by name. Her style is one of warm and intimate informality. She reported a first session with a family in which the grandmother, a woman in her late seventies, participated. As introductions were taking place, a family spokesman said, "And this is Grandma." Satir, after asking Grandma what her first name was, took the elderly woman's hand and said, " Hello, Mildred, I'm glad to meet you." Mildred's response, as her individuality was thus validated, was touching. Her eyes filled with tears, and taking Satir's hand in both of hers she said, "No one has called me that for years." Clearly, a strong connection had been made. We believe that joining behaviors evolve quite naturally when the clinician is committed to an appreciation of the family member's point of view. However, joining is also a skill that can be cultivated.

Tracking

An important way to gain information about the family relationships and interactions is to track behavioral or action sequences. In its simplest form, the clinician follows the content of the family's communication and behavior and encourages them to continue speaking. Tracking operations are nonintrusive, but they elicit information, pursue clarification, and seek expansion of content from all of the family members. In tracking, it is important to discover the facts that occurred before, during, and after the behavior being discussed. As clinicians attend to descriptions of family interaction and communication sequences, they acquire information about the structure of the family itself and also about the interactive communication patterns. Hartman and Laird have observed:

> To repeat an essential point, in family systems interviewing, innate or intrinsic characteristics of individuals are not the focus of our exploration; rather we are always seeking information about relationships. When we hear, for example, that Ann is "quiet," the questions that immediately come to mind are: "Compared to whom?" "Was she more quiet before Dan went to college or after?" " In what circumstances is Ann most quiet?" The behavior Ann is showing us is not seen as a characteristic which "belongs to" Ann, but as an aspect of a relationship system set in the context of and interacting with a series of people and events.[58]

Minuchin[55] also asks the family to enact certain interactions as part of his tracking procedure. He asks the family to show him what it is like when they are planning a family outing. "Don't tell me about it. Show me." This very often provides clear information about the family interactional system.

The Eco Map

In addition to the skills of joining and tracking, there are visual ways to learn about the client's family relationships. One of these is the Eco map, which depicts the major systems that are part of the family's life and that help to describe the nature of the family's relationship. An Eco map portrays the family's "life space." It shows all the elements of their social and physical environment, which can help the fluency clinician learn more about aspects of transfer and resources that could be utilized in carry-over activities. An Eco map can also point out the important nurturing or conflict-laden connections between the family and the world. According to Hartman and Laird, "The Eco-map, in portraying the flow of resources and the nature of family-environment exchanges, highlights any lacks or deprivations which erode family strength. As it is completed, then, family and clinician should be able to identify conflicts to be mediated, bridges to be built, and resources to be sought and mobilized."[58] Figure 8.2 depicts a blank Eco map as used by Hartman and Laird. It is helpful if the clinician has empty maps available when doing an assessment.

In the center of the map, the nuclear family is drawn. It is common practice to depict males with squares and females with circles. The person's age is put in the center. Drawing lines between the family and those systems indicates connections between the family and the various systems. The nature of the connection is represented by the type of line used—an important connection is a solid line; a dotted line is a tenuous connection; jagged lines suggest a stressful connection. Arrows can demonstrate the flow of energy or interest. Significant words can be written on the map as the client provides the information (Figure 8.3).

It is easy to use an Eco map, but clinicians should have some practice with it before using it with a client. It is suggested that clinicians do their own Eco maps and practice on friends before attempting to use it clinically.

After completing the map, a clinician will see that its primary value is its ability to organize and display factual and relational information for understanding the family dynamics. Compton and Galway[59] found that the family connections, themes, and quality of life seem to jump off the page after doing an Eco map. They feel that this leads to a more holistic and integrative perception of the system. A 12-year-old client, after seeing her map, said, "Gee, I never saw myself like that before!"

We believe that the Eco map can serve as a tool to help families plan for change in their lives. They make it possible to identify problem areas, resources needed, and potential strengths, as well as to plan actions needed to bring about change. Research is needed to bear out this application to fluency disorders, which we are in the process of pursuing.

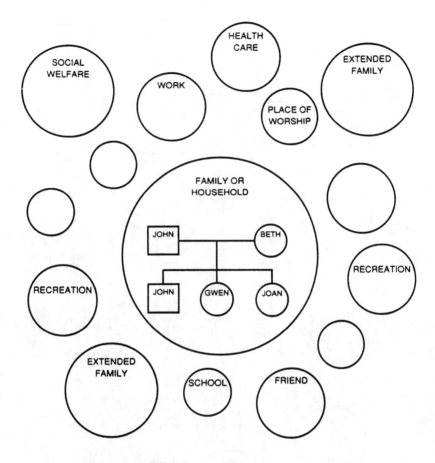

Fill in the connections where they exist.
Indicate nature of connections with a descriptive word or by drawing
    different kinds of lines; _____ for strong, ---- for tenuous, - - - for
    stressful.
Draw arrows along lines to signify flow of energy, resources, etc.
>>>> Identify significant people and fill in empty circles as needed.

Figure 8.2 Blank Eco Map by A. Hartman and J. Laird. (Reprinted with permission from Hartman A, Laird J. *Family Centered Social Work Practice*. New York: Free Press, 1983, p. 160.)

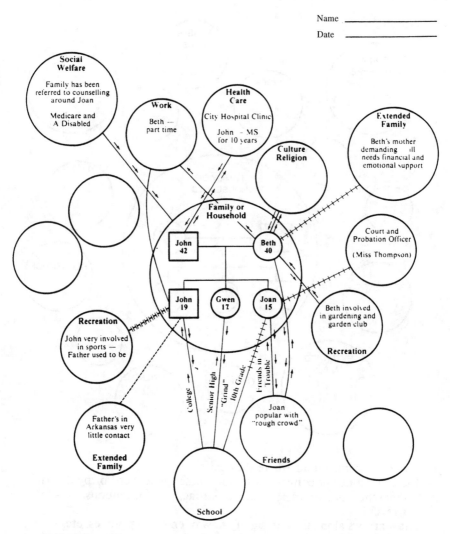

Name _____

Date _____

Fill in connections where they exist.
Indicate nature of connections with a descriptive word or by drawing different kinds of lines:
————————— for strong, – – – – – – – – for tenuous, +++++++ for stressful.
Draw arrows along lines to signify flow of energy, resources, etc. → → → →
Identify significant people and fill in empty circles as needed.

Figure 8.3 Completed Eco Map by A. Hartman and J. Laird. (Reprinted with permission from Hartman A, Laird J. *Family Centered Social Work Practice*. New York: Free Press, 1983, p. 195.)

The Genogram

Another visual aid for understanding the family is the Genogram. Hayhow and Levy[60] have used the Genogram in their work with people who stutter and have found it helpful in assessing client interactions. This visual map depicts the family in both spatial and temporal relationships. Each family is seen as part of a complicated system that has developed over many generations. Compton and Galway found that this intergenerational history has transmitted powerful commands, role assignments, events, and patterns of living and relating. If we, as fluency clinicians, believe that stuttering is embedded in the environment of our clients, we need to know something about their family relationships and intergenerational family history. Genograms graphically display family information in a way that provides a quick gestalt of complex family patterns and a rich source of hypotheses about how a specific problem may be connected to the context. Although this tool is used widely among family therapists, its use in the field of communication disorders is minimal. We have begun to incorporate the use of the Genogram in our assessment and, again, encourage fluency clinicians to explore the many possibilities of this assessment tool.

Compton and Galway defined the Genogram as a "map of genealogical relationships, major family events, occupations, losses, family migrations and dispersals, identifications and role assignments, and information about alignments and communication patterns."[60] On the basis of our own theoretical assumptions about communication disorders, we can use this to gather any and all of the information we feel would be helpful in working with our clients. Ivey[13] and Hayhow and Levy[60] pointed out that developing a Genogram with the client allows the clinician to focus not only on the individual but also on the family history and culture. Hayhow and Levy[60] have used genograms with fluency clients (Figure 8.4).

In order to construct a Genogram, guidelines were provided by Ivey[13], which we expanded as follows:

- List the names of family members for at least three generations with ages and dates of births and deaths. List occupations, significant illnesses, and cause of death, as appropriate. Note any issues with communication patterns, communication styles, and communication breakdowns.
- List important cultural, environmental,and contextual issues. These may include ethnic identity, religion, economic, and social class considerations. In addition, pay special attention to significant life events such as trauma or environmental issues.
- As you develop the Genogram with your client, use the basic listening sequence (Chapter 9) to draw out the client's thoughts, feelings, and behaviors. You will find out that considerable insight into one's personal life issues, related to the communication disorder, may be generated this way.

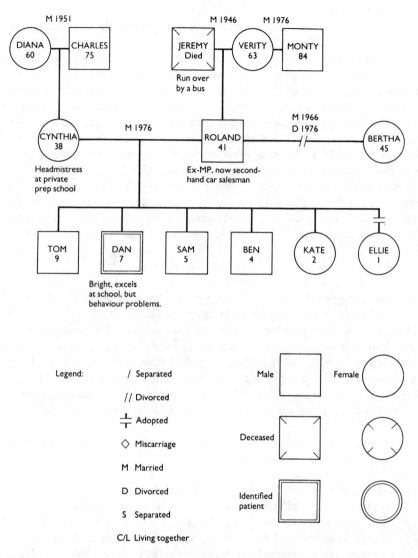

Figure 8.4   Genogram by R. Hayhow and C. Levy. (Reprinted with permission from Hayhow R, Levy C. *Working with Stuttering*. Bricester, UK: Winslow Press, 1989, p. 54.)

When constructing a new Genogram, a marriage is indicated by drawing a line from a square (man) to a circle (woman); the marital date is added to the line. Children are added according to age, beginning with the oldest on the left. A divorce generally is portrayed by a dotted line, and, again, it helps to include dates. Drawing an "X" through the figure and dating it indicates a death. Some of the information that can be gleaned through the use of the Genogram includes naming patterns, birth order, major family losses, relationships, educational backgrounds, family functioning, and communication patterns. Although the information on the genogram generally is collected in the initial interview, the clinician can continue to add to it throughout the helping process. When depicting the relationships of the members of the family, symbols are used as shown in Figure 8.5. The relationships reported by the family and observed by the clinician can be visually represented and provide fluency clinicians with a view of the family interactions and communication patterns that make up the everyday life of the family. These relationships have a direct influence on the emotional life of our client and are usually found to influence the stuttering behavior as well. Gathering the information in this way serves not only as informational, but also as a way to engage the family system.

As with the Eco map, it is recommended that clinicians first work with their own genograms so that they become familiar and comfortable with the process and so that they can gain some understanding of their own place within their families. McGoldrick and Gerson[61] believe that a clinician tends to get blocked with the families that they work with in the same way that they get blocked with their own families. Bowen,[62] whose family therapy theory is the basis for Genograms, observed that family therapists have the very same problems in their own families that are present in the families that they see professionally. We, too, believe that it is important for clinicians to work through the histories of their own family of origin. For this reason, we recommend that all university training programs include a course in counseling techniques that enable one to understand this relationship between personal growth and professional competence.

Family Interactions: What to Look For

During the initial assessment and then throughout all stages of the treatment process, the clinician will analyze the behaviors of her clients as they interact with the operations of their respective family groups. The following are salient aspects of the family relationship to observe:

Interaction Patterns
Consider the following questions:

1. Does one member of the family do all the talking?
2. Does one person always speak for another person?
3. Are messages given and received clearly?

PART 1: GENOGRAM FORMAT

A. Symbols to describe basic family membership and structure (include on genogram significant others who lived with or cared for family members – place them on the right side of the genogram with a notation about who they are.)

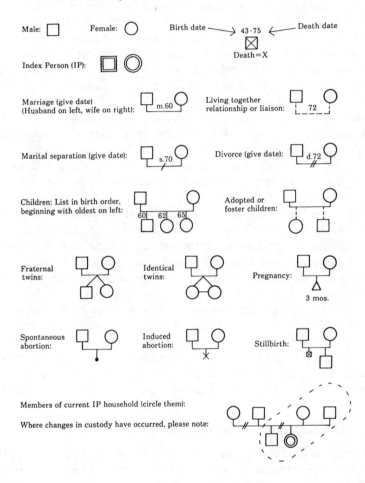

Figure 8.5 (This page and opposite) Symbols depicting relationships between family members. (Reprinted with permission from Compton B, Galaway B. *Social Work Processes* (4th ed). Belmont, CA: Wadsworth, 1989, p. 154.)

B. Family interaction patterns. The following symbols are optional. The clinician may prefer to note them on a separate sheet. They are among the least precise information on the genogram, but may be key indicators of relationship patterns the clinician wants to remember:

Very close relationship:

Distant relationship:

Fused and conflictual:

Conflictual relationship:

Estrangement or cut off (give dates if possible):
Cut off 62–78

C. Medical history. Since the genogram is meant to be an orienting map of the family, there is room to indicate only the most important factors. Thus, list only major or chronic illnesses and problems. Include dates in parentheses where feasible or applicable. Use DSM-III categories or recognized abbreviations where available (e.g., cancer: CA; stroke: CVA).

D. Other family information of special importance may also be noted on the genogram:

1) Ethnic background and migration date
2) Religion or religious change
3) Education
4) Occupation or unemployment
5) Military service
6) Retirement
7) Trouble with law
8) Physical abuse or incest
9) Obesity
10) Alcohol or Drug abuse (symbol= ▢ ◖)
11) Smoking
12) Dates when family members left home: LH '74.
13) Current location of family members

It is useful to have a space at the bottom of the genogram for notes on *other key information*: This would include critical events, changes in the family structure since the genogram was made, hypotheses and other notations of major family issues or changes. These notations should always be dated, and should be kept to a minimum, since every extra piece of information on a genogram complicates it and therefore diminishes its readability.

PART 2: GENOGRAM FORM

FAMILY NAME _____
Date Filled In _____
Filled In By _____
Family Address _____

Key Hypotheses &
Life Events

Significant Others

G1

G2

G3 (IP)

Sequences of interaction also may yield important information about family functioning. Hepworth and Larsen[63] cited some categorical responses of family members that obstruct open communication and that prevent genuine encounters in relationships. We believe that these can have a negative influence on a person with a fluency problem and can be explored in the process of fluency therapy. Some of these responses are:

- prematurely shifting the subject
- avoiding topics
- asking excessive questions
- underresponding
- directing, ordering, threatening, or admonishing
- agreeing or disagreeing excessively
- giving advice frequently
- negatively evaluating, blaming, name-calling, or criticizing

These responses reflect the synergistic integration of pragmatic language issues and communication skills, as well as the underlying emotional issues discussed in Chapter 6.

Bonding and Support

Adequate support plays a crucial role in determining the level of social functioning of human beings. A nurturing, healthy environment is important for a change in communication patterns to occur. Consider the following questions:

1. How do family members express their needs to one another?
2. How do family members enjoy one another?
3. How do members support one another?
4. Is this support seen and acknowledged?
5. How do families support the fluency therapy program?

Roles

The roles of each family member are significant for family interaction. Some important questions when assessing the role each person plays are as follows:

1. How is power distributed in the family?
2. Who is in charge? How does that person relate to the fluency client?
3. What role does each member play in this family?
4. Does the client with the fluency disorder covertly hold the power, or has he become powerless?
5. How does everyone feel about these roles—especially their own?

Rules and Regulations

Very often the rules of the family are both written and unwritten. Each family member knows how far they can go with each person.

1. What are the rules of behavior for each family member?
2. Are there different rules?
3. Why?
4. Who makes the rules?
5. How are they communicated?
6. Why are these rules important to the family?
7. How are rules enforced?
8. Who handles discipline? How?
9. What are the rules for discussion of fluency?

If the rules in a family are "functional," they enable each member of the family to respond to their environment and their needs. Examples of functional rules are:

- Everyone's input into this family is important.
- It's important to talk about your feelings (hurts, disappointments, anger, criticism, joy, or achievements).
- It's important to work out disagreements.
- It's ok to make mistakes.
- It's ok to be different.

If the rules are dysfunctional, they may be destructive to a family and interfere with the client's progress. Changing the rules might be an appropriate treatment goal. Some examples of dysfunctional rules are:

- Don't do things differently from other family members.
- Don't take responsibility for your own behavior. Always put the blame on someone else.
- Don't feel.
- Be perfect.

Boundaries

The clinician needs to consider the role that boundaries play within the family.

1. Are people allowed to be separate, different, and independent?
2. What are the boundaries within and without this family?
3. How do family members feel about these boundaries?

Some boundaries or problems with boundaries that a clinician might look for include the following:

- *Enmeshment:* an acute togetherness and interaction between family members. It is usually at the expense of personal autonomy and interaction with people outside the family.
- *Disengagement:* a lack of closeness, sharing, cooperation, and/or togetherness. Acute individuality and lack of "connectedness" tend to accompany this.

- *Differentiation:* Individuals are seen as unique and different from one another. Difference and disagreement are allowed and not seen as dangerous.

As we pursue an understanding of the synergistic components of fluency
therapy with each client and his family, it is helpful to remember the following
observation by Shapiro:

Some may ask why an understanding of a family life cycle is important to
working with people who stutter. We have underscored the point that anything happening to one person affects and is affected by other members of
the family system. For this reason alone, it is foolhardy to direct our clinical
efforts to the person who stutters without consideration of the others with
whom this person communicates regularly. The needs of all involved must
be taken into account for treatment to be effective and generalized.

Summary   While we are not family therapists, we are clinicians with a
broad view of helping others. This includes our astute observation and assessment of clients and our design of rehabilitation procedures to include family
members. We have presented techniques for family-based assessment, the Eco
map, the Genogram, and what to look for in family interactions. Use of these
suggestions for working with clients and their families will assist in furthering
transfer of our client's fluency goals.

MULTICULTURAL ISSUES AND FLUENCY DISORDERS

The definition of multicultural disorders and the history of our profession's
growing involvement with people who are culturally and linguistically diverse
were presented in Chapter 2. Based on this earlier overview of the issue, we will
examine the salient issues that have been applied to fluency disorders.

Stuttering Among Indian Tribes

Although a limited amount of research has been devoted to cultural groups
and stuttering, it has long been known that cultural factors have an influence on
stuttering behaviors. Van Riper[65] reported much of the detail of Johnson's study,
which found that the Native Americans had no name for stuttering. This lack of
stuttering was often assumed to be because of the cultural differences among the
Indians and their lack of stress and pressure in daily living. However, this debate
was not easily resolved. Conrad and Seymour have summarized some of the early
research that attempted to determine the effect of culture on stuttering:

A limited amount of research has been conducted regarding stuttering
among minority groups in North America. Early investigators, interested in
documenting the influence of environment on the development of stuttering, were eager to locate American cultures in which stuttering was absent

or low in incidence. These early studies focused on Native American tribes and are indicative of the nature of early research in the field of stuttering among minority cultures, in that they lacked quantitative data and relied upon interviews collected with the help of a translator.[65]

Studies of the Shoshone and Bannock tribes of the northwestern United States; the Salish, Kwatkiutl, and Nootka tribes of British Columbia and Vancouver; and the Ute and Cowichan tribes[67-69] indicated that the prevalence of stuttering was influenced by the type of child-rearing practices and the attitudes of the tribes toward disabled speech. A later study refuted the findings of these early investigators. Zimmerman and colleagues[70] were able to obtain more direct information from the Bannock and Shoshone because one of the researchers spoke the language of these Native Americans and was himself a stutterer.

These studies found that the coastal Indians of the Northwest stuttered and the Bannock and Shoshone did not. Much of this research was used to support Johnson's Diagnosogenic Theory of stuttering,[71,72] which held that stuttering in the child was related to parental perceptions and standards. Johnson found that parents of children who stutter tended to be more dominating, anxious, and perfectionistic. He also found them to have high expectations of their children and to be discontented with their spouse, children, and social and economic status. Lemert[69] helped to support Johnson's research by finding that the members of tribes in the Northwest demonstrated exacting educational practices for their children and rejection of those with perceived disabilities: left-handedness, lameness, obesity, smallness, and speech defects. Among the Bannock and Shoshone Indians, such perceived disabilities were accepted and child rearing practices were lax. Johnson's Diagnosogenic Theory was widely accepted for many years, and it was supported by this cultural research. However, there was no room in this theory for the components of a physiologic approach to stuttering, and in the 1970s Johnson's theory began to be seen as limited. Cooper and Cooper[73] nevertheless believe that this research has provided us with a valuable model for cross-cultural research and demonstrates that fluency disorders are common to all cultures.

Stuttering Among African-Americans

In 1975, Leith and Mims[74] did a study that tested the following three-part hypothesis: (1) black teens who stutter are basically behaviorally different from white teens who stutter with regard to their stuttering patterns; (2) the behavioral differences in stuttering patterns are the result of cultural differences; (3) these cultural differences will result in stutterers who are black reacting differently to treatment than stutterers who are white. The data showed that stuttering behavior in adolescent African-American males was qualitatively different from young, adolescent white males. Based on a profile rating system, it was found that the white teen-agers exhibited overt stuttering behaviors (prolongations and repetitions). Black males, however, tended to hide the core stuttering behaviors and to generally avoid speech, which brought about stuttering behaviors such as eye blinks, head jerks, and bodily movements. The authors attributed these findings to the difference in cultural expectations. In the African-American culture, there is a great emphasis on the oral tradition. Verbal fluency is a high value as seen in black preaching, rapping, and the ability to be "cool":

> Cool? No one ever hears him speak above a whisper. Always calm. I mean never in a hurry. Slow and steady. Always seeming to know his next move in advance. Talking cool and being fluent would appear to be directly related. The black stutterers whose culture places a particular premium on being fluent and cool would appear to have a handicap that deprives them of a culturally unique source of prestige among their peers.[75]

Leith and Mims[74] further proposed that in order to deal with these clients one must be clinically aware and respond to the cultural expectations, even if it means asking the client to be "counter-cultural," in order to face and accept the stuttering behavior.

Conrad and Seymour[65] noted that two studies of the prevalence of stuttering among African-Americans indicated a difference in the gender of people who stutter. A higher prevalence of stuttering among African-American women has been reported.[76,77] They believe that the ratio of two boys to one girl (versus four boys to one girl for the general population) could result from environmental stress on the women.

Stuttering Among Other Cultural Groups

Bloodstein[78] wrote: "Fragmentary as they are, the research findings on the anthropology of stuttering have made it clear that the problem occurs in a very wide variety of cultural settings. Some workers have expressed doubt that it is absent from any ethnic group at all." Bebout and Bradford[79] surveyed the attitudes toward four disorders (cleft palate, dysfluency, hearing impairment, and misarticulation) among 166 university students representing English-speaking and several other cultures—Chinese, Southeast Asian, and Hispanic. The data revealed two conclusions important for clinicians:

- People born outside of North America are more likely to consider people with disordered speech to be emotionally disturbed.
- Foreign born (especially Asian) subjects were more likely to state that the speech disordered person could improve the speech if he "tried hard."

Conrad and Seymour pointed out the sparsity of research among minority groups. They stated that perhaps the lack of research is related to the limited number of minority speech-language pathologists and researchers. "Fewer than 6% of the members of the American Association of Speech-Language Pathology and Audiology are members of minority groups. Further research of stuttering in minority persons would enhance the knowledge base and help to improve treatment of stuttering in minorities."[66]

Issues of Multicultural Assessment

Aware of the need for research, as well as the need for increased sensitivity to fluency clients who are bicultural and bilingual, we have been assisted in our work by that of Watson and Kayser.[80] In addition to the assessment procedures noted in Chapter 3, we would like to summarize here some of the aspects of the assessment process highlighted by their research:

- Monolingual speech-language pathologists might profit from using a team approach when assessing bilingual stutterers. Use of the client's community members, as well as trained observers within the culture, is recommended when available.
- Stuttering behaviors may be first identified in English and then in the second language. Language samples need to be taken within different contexts of the community and with different linguistic partners.
- Before meeting the client, the clinician should prepare for the meeting by learning as much as possible about the client's culture and language.
- Areas to probe during case history include: reason left native country, reason members of cultural group settled in local community, generation first to move from homeland, intentions to return to homeland, family members remaining in homeland, occupation prior to moving to this country, current occupation, cultural status of family, concept of majority and subculture, structure of the community, typical family size, roles of individual family members, customs, values, beliefs about children, child-rearing practices, medical practices, interpersonal relationships, concept of self, social functions and leisure activities, cultural group's view of handicap and handicapped individuals, and cultural group's view of stuttering and stutterers.
- Attitudes toward communication in both languages, toward stuttering and other handicapping conditions, toward one's self as a person, and as a communicator, and toward therapy must be assessed.

This approach to multicultural assessment demonstrates the components of a synergistic model of stuttering and provides useful leads for completing the assessment. One can note the importance of family issues, communication issues, and issues of self-esteem and locus of control within the battery of cultural sensitivities. Indeed, while highlighted here, these are integrated throughout the assessment process. Additional interviewing techniques might be obtained from Westby's "Ethnographic interviewing."[81] Watson and Kayser concluded:

> The challenge for monolingual clinicians in working with individuals of the New America is both formidable and exciting, but when met, will enhance

both services and sensitivities when working with clients. Each client seeking services brings to therapy his or her own unique culture that deserves careful attention and respect.[80]

This underscores the entire purpose of a synergistic approach.

Issues of Multicultural Treatment

Cooper and Cooper[73] caution against the development of potentially detrimental stereotypes by focusing only on differences within a culture. They urge us to assess the individual's affective, behavioral, and cognitive components of stuttering (the ABCs of stuttering) across cultures. Focusing on the universality of these behaviors in treatment can help us to collect valuable data across cultures. We agree and note that these ABCs are included in our synergistic approach. Nevertheless, Leith[82] provided examples of cultural differences that a clinician should be aware of:

- Time factors. Different cultures have different perceptions of time. It could be disrespectful to arrive either early or late.
- Rate of speech. Some cultures value fast speaking and others slow.
- Gender issues. In some cultures, the female is subservient to the male. If the female is the clinician, it may be difficult for the client to adjust.
- Parent's beliefs about treatment.
- Eye contact. Stuttering therapy often focuses on eye contact as a goal. One must be sensitive to the fact that in some cultures eye contact is perceived as invasive and negative.

Leith[82] also presented valuable recommendations for speech clinicians who work with clients whose culture is different than their own. In this regard, members who attended a three-day conference on "Cultural Influences in Communication Disorders" at Wayne State University (1994) also compiled a list of helpful recommendations. After overviews of Arabic, African-American, Indian, Hispanic, and Oriental cultures, the participants discussed the application of culture to articulation, language, and stuttering disorders. The following are highlights of conclusions that emerged from that discussion:

- It is extremely important for speech-language clinicians to recognize that there is no standard cultural group. Each group represents a wide variety of subcultures, depending on the degree of assimilation into the general American culture, the socioeconomic level of the subculture, the geographic location of the subculture, and so forth. The awareness of variability will prevent stereotyping on the part of the clinician.
- Some cultures are extremely private about their family and personal lives. The clinician should respect this privacy and not discuss such matters if the client is from such a culture.

- Some cultures protect their children to the point where the child has great difficulty in adjusting to the school setting. It may be generally difficult for the child to interact with adults, other than family members, on a one-to-one basis.
- Within some cultures it is impolite to speak in a "loud" voice. A child from one of these cultures might speak very softly, to the point where it is difficult to understand what is being said. This may not be shyness but rather a cultural influence carried over from the home.
- Since various cultures respond to the handicapped in different ways, it is very important for the clinician to know the response of the client's culture to handicapped persons.
- Establishing rapport with the family may be difficult if the clinician is female and the culture of the family does not accept the female in this type of role. There may also be problems if the clinician is from another culture. Both of these factors may be compounded by the fact that the clinician represents a "figure of authority."
- The role of the child within the family unit varies from culture to culture. If the cultural family is child oriented, a home program may be able to be instituted since the parents are involved with their children. However, if the cultural family unit is not child oriented, parental cooperation is not likely to occur, regardless of attempts on the part of the clinician.
- In some cultures, the female rarely comes in contact with people in other cultures, relating only with people of her own culture. This can create problems both in terms of home visits by the clinician and the establishment of home programs.
- There may be instances where a child is unwilling to communicate with a person of another culture. The clinician should be sensitive to this possibility.
- Failure on the part of a child to maintain eye contact with the clinician may be a cultural factor. It should not be misinterpreted as an attitudinal sign or a secondary mannerism associated with stuttering.
- Depending on the culture, it may not be appropriate for the clinician to touch the child. This is particularly true for some Indian tribes where the hair is considered sacred. A pat on the head would be most inappropriate with a child from such a tribe.
- If the family is required to sign forms or other documents for the testing of a child, this may, depending on the culture, embarrass or shame the family. If this is the case, the parents may not sign the forms or documents.
- Mannerisms used by a bilingual child to cover up his lack of English proficiency may be misinterpreted as secondary mannerisms associated with stuttering. The clinician should check to see if the mannerisms occur when the child is speaking his native language. If not, there is still a possibility that the child is stuttering while speaking English. This factor should be carefully assessed and appropriate action taken if the child is stuttering.

- If a child is demonstrating some stuttering in his or her native language, it would be advisable to remedy the stuttering problem before enrolling the child in a program for English as a second language. Communication stress is an important factor in the development and maintenance of stuttering, and the demands for learning and speaking English would create even more communication stress on the child and make the problem worse.
- Communicative stress can often be found within the culture itself if oral ability is a source of peer recognition and status. Various cultures view oral ability as an important factor for status within the community. This cultural attitude can have a profound effect on the treatment of stuttering. The clinician should be aware of this factor and determine its influence on the particular child she is working with.
- Various cultures have different attitudes toward stuttering, and it is important that the clinician determine the attitude of the family. In some cultures it is viewed as a curse or has some religious overtones. The family's attitude will have a direct influence on the treatment of the problem.

As clinicians examine clients from various cultures, they must remember that there are no "right," "wrong," "good," "bad" or "pure" cultures. There are only "different" cultures.

SUMMARY

In conclusion, the environmental aspects of a fluency disorder are an integral part of the assessment and treatment program for a fluency client. The complexity of stuttering requires that clinicians assess a client's interactive communication style, the involvement of family members, and the cultural components of that client's individual community. In order to draw on the resources necessary for understanding the subtle implications of each of these areas, clinicians must be open to pursue and adapt aspects of both communication theory and family therapy procedures as they pertain to fluency treatment. Further research on multicultural treatment is needed.

REFERENCES

1. Bloodstein O. *A Handbook on Stuttering* (5th ed). San Diego, CA: Singular Publishing Group, 1995.
2. Guitar B, Peters TJ. *Stuttering: An Integrated Approach to Its Nature and Treatment.* Baltimore: Williams and Wilkins, 1998:69.
3. Starkweather CW. The development of fluency in normal children. In Speech Foundation of America (ed), *Stuttering Therapy: Prevention and Intervention with Children.* Memphis: Speech Foundation of America, 1985.
4. Starkweather CW. *Fluency and Stuttering.* Englewood Cliffs, NJ: Prentice Hall, 1987.
5. Starkweather CW, Gottwald SR. The demands and capacities model II: Clinical applications. *J Fluency Disord* 1990;15:143–157.

6. Starkweather CW, Gottwald SR, Halfond MH. *Stuttering Prevention: A Clinical Method.* Englewood Cliffs, NJ: Prentice Hall, 1990.
7. Kidd KK. Stuttering as a genetic disorder. In RF Curlee, WH Perkins (eds), *Nature and Treatment of Stuttering: New Directions.* San Diego, CA: College-Hill Press, 1984.
8. Howie PM. Concordance for stuttering in monozygotic and dyzygotic twin pairs. *J Speech Hrng Res* 1981;24:317–321.
9. Ham RE. *Therapy of Stuttering.* Englewood Cliffs, NJ: Prentice Hall, 1990.
10. Starkweather CW, Givens-Ackerman J. *Stuttering.* Austin, TX: Pro-Ed, 1997:89.
11. Hepworth D, Larsen J. *Direct Social Work Practice.* Chicago: Dorsey Press, 1988: 102–219.
12. Satir V. *The New Peoplemaking.* Mountain View, CA: Science and Behavior Books, 1988:5.
13. Ivey A. *Intentional Interviewing and Counseling.* Belmont, CA: Brooks/Cole, 1994: 24–103.
14. Schuerle J. *Counseling in Speech Language Pathology and Audiology.* New York: Macmillan, 1992:60.
15. Hutchins D, Cole C. *Helping Relationships and Strategies.* Belmont, CA: Brooks/Cole, 1992:56–136.
16. Luterman D. *Counseling Persons with Communication Disorders and Their Families* (3rd ed). Austin, TX: Pro-Ed, 1996:91–109,161.
17. Eagen G. *The Skilled Helper: A Systematic Approach to Effective Helping* (4th ed). Pacific Grove, CA: Brooks/Cole, 1990:91.
18. Bloom C, Cooperman D. *The Clinical Interview: A Guide for Speech Language Pathologists and Audiologists* (2nd ed). Rockville, MD: NSSLHA, 1992.
19. Murphy B, Dillon C. *Interviewing in Action.* Pacific Grove, CA: Brooks/Cole, 1998:111–114.
20. Eagen G. *The Skilled Helper* (3rd ed). Monterey, CA: Brooks/Cole, 1986:141.
21. Bolton R. *People Skills.* Englewood Cliffs, NJ: Prentice Hall, 1979.
22. Brammer LM. *The Helping Relationship: Process and Skills* (6th ed). Needham Heights, MA: Simon and Schuster, 1996.
23. Whitmire K. Social integration of mainstream students. Presentation to the Berne-Knox-Westerlo Schools, Berne, NY, May 1996.
24. Stinson MS, Whitmire K. Students' views of their social relationships. In TV Kwin, DK Moores, MG Gausted (eds), *Toward Effective Public School Programs for Deaf Students.* New York: Teachers College Press, 1992:149–174.
25. Nelson NW. Curriculum based language assessment and intervention across the grades. In GP Wallach, KG Butler (eds), *Language Learning Disability in School Age Children and Adolescents: Some Principles and Applications.* New York: Macmillan, 1994:104–131.
26. Tanner D, Belliveau W, Seibert G. *Pragmatic Stuttering Intervention.* Oceanside, CA: Academic Communication Associates, 1995.
27. Nippold MA. Concomitant speech and language disorders in stuttering children: A critique of the literature. *J Speech Hear Disord* 1990;55:51–60.
28. Moses K. Dynamic intervention with families. In E Cheron (ed), *Hearing Impaired Children and Youth with Developmental Disabilities: An Interdisciplinary Foundation for Service.* Washington, DC: Gallaudet College Press, 1985:82–100.
29. Gordon R. Special needs of multi-handicapped children under six and their families: One opinion. In E Sontag (ed), *Educational Programming for the Severely and Profoundly Handicapped.* Reston, VA: Council for Exceptional Children, 1977: 61–71.

30. Myers SC, Freeman FJ. Interruptions as a variable in stuttering and disfluency. *J Speech Hrng Res* 1985;28:428–435.
31. Myers SC, Freeman FJ. Mother and child speech roles as a variable in stuttering and disfluency. *J Speech Hrng Res* 1985;28:436–444.
32. Myers SC, Freeman FJ. Are mothers of stutterers different? An investigation of social-communicative interaction. *J Fluency Disord* 1985;10:193–209.
33. Riley GD, Riley J. Evaluation as a basis for intervention. In D Prins, RJ Ingham (eds), *Treatment of Stuttering in Early Childhood: Methods and Issues.* San Diego, CA: College-Hill Press, 1983.
34. Conture EH, Caruso AJ. Assessment and diagnosis of childhood disfluency. In L Rustin, H Purser, D Rowley (eds), *Progress in the Treatment of Fluency Disorders.* London: Whurr, 1987.
35. Kelly CM, Conture EG. Speaking rates, response time latencies, and interrupting behaviors of young stutterers, nonstutterers, and their mothers. *J Speech Hear Res* 1992;35:1256–1267.
36. Zebrowski PM, Schum RL. Counseling parents of children who stutter. *Am J Speech-Language Pathol* 1993;2:65–73.
37. Langlois A, Long S. A model for teaching parents to facilitate fluent speech. *J of Fluency Disord* 1988;13:162–172.
38. Conture EG. *Stuttering* (2nd ed). Englewood Cliffs, NJ: Prentice Hall, 1990.
39. Myers SC, Freeman FJ. Mother and child speech rates as a variable in stuttering and disfluency. *J Speech Hrng Res* 1985;28:436–444.
40. Starkweather CW, Gottwald SR, Halford MM. *Stuttering Prevention: A Clinical Method.* Englewood Cliffs, NJ: Prentice Hall, 1990.
41. Richardson M, Oyler ME. *Stuttering: Vulnerability, Demands and Capacity Model and Treatment.* Workshop Sponsored by the International Fluency Association. San Fransisco, CA, 1997.
42. Ramig P. Parent-clinican-child partnership in the therapeutic process of the preschool- and elementary-aged child who stutters. *Seminars in Speech & Language* 1993;14(3):226–237.
43. Ham R. *Therapy of Stuttering.* Englewood Cliffs, NJ: Prentice Hall, Inc., 1990.
44. Mallard AR. Family intervention in stuttering therapy. In RF Curlee (ed), *Seminars in Speech and Language* (vol. 12). New York: Thieme Medical Publishers, 1991: 265–278.
45. Rustin L. The treatment of childhood fluency through active parental involvement. In L Rustin, H Purser, D Rowley, (eds), *Progress in the Treatment of Fluency Disorders.* London: Taylor and Francis, 1987.
46. Rustin L (ed). *Parents, Families and the Stuttering Child.* San Diego, CA: Singular Publishing Group, 1991.
47. Rustin L, Purser H. Child development, families and the problem of stuttering. In L Rustin (ed). *Parents, Families and the Stuttering Child.* San Diego, CA: Singular Publishing Group, 1991:1–24.
48. Andrews J, Andrews M. Family systems and treatment: Understanding the systemic perspective. Short course presented at the ASHA Convention, St. Louis, MO, November 1989.
49. Andrews J, Andrews M. *Family Based Treatment in Communication Disorders: A Systemic Approach.* Sandwich, IL: Janelle, 1990.
50. Donahue-Kilburg K. *Family-Centered Early Intervention for Communication Disorders.* Gaithersburg, MD: Aspen, 1992.
51. Satir V. *Peoplemaking.* Palo Alto, CA: Science and Behavior Books, 1972.

52. Ylvisaker M, Feeney T. Everyday people as supports: developing competencies through collaboration. In M Ylvisaker (ed). *Rehabilitation Following Traumatic Brain Injury in Children and Adolescents*. Boston: Butterworth-Heinemann, 1996.
53. Ylvisaker M, Feeney T, Urbanczyk B. Developing a positive communication culture for rehabilitation. In C Durgan, J Fryer, N Schmidt (eds), *Brain Injury Rehabilitation: Clinical Intervention and Staff Development Techniques*. Gaithersburg, MD: Aspen, 1992.
54. Lund N. Family events and relationships: Implications for language assessment and intervention. *Semin Speech Lang* 1986;7:347–357.
55. Minuchin S. *Families and Family Therapy*. Cambridge, MA: Harvard University Press, 1974.
56. Andrews MA. Application of family therapy techniques to the treatment of language disorders. *Semin Speech Lang* 1986;7:347–357.
57. Minuchin S, Fishman HC. *Family Therapy Techniques*. Cambridge, MA: Harvard University Press, 1981.
58. Hartman A, Laird J. *Family Centered Social Work Practice*. New York: Free Press, 1983.
59. Compton B, Galaway B. *Social Work Processes* (4th ed). Belmont, CA: Wadsworth, 1989;169.
60. Hayhow R, Levy C. *Working with Stuttering*. Bricester, UK: Winslow Press, 1989.
61. McGoldrick M, Gerson R. *Genograms in Family Assessment*. New York: W. W. Norton, 1985:154–155.
62. Bowen M. *Family Therapy in Clinical Practice*. New York: Jason and Aronson, 1978.
63. Hepworth D, Larsen J. *Direct Social Work Practice*. Chicago: Dorsey Press, 1986: 257.
64. Shapiro DA. *Stuttering Intervention: A Collaborative Journey to Fluency Freedom*. Austin, TX: Pro-Ed, 1999.
65. Van Riper C. *The Nature of Stuttering* (2nd ed). New York: Prentice Hall, 1982.
66. Conrad C, Seymour C. Stuttering. In C Seymour, EH Nober (eds), *An Introduction to Communication Disorders: A Multicultural Approach*. Boston: Butterworth-Heinemann, 1998:165–184.
67. Sindecor JC. Why the Indian doesn't stutter. *Q J Speech* 1947:33–49.
68. Stewart JK. The problem of stuttering in certain North American Indian societies. *J Speech Hear Disord* 1960;6:1.
69. Lemert E. Some Indians who stutter. *J Speech Hear Disord* 1983;26:168–174.
70. Zimmerman G, Liljeblad S, Frank A, Cluland C. The Indians have many terms for it: Stuttering among the Bannock-Shoshone. *J Speech Hrng Res* 1983;26:315–318.
71. Johnson W. The Indians have no word for it. *Q J Speech* 1944;30:330–337.
72. Johnson W, Leutenegger RR (eds). A study of the onset and development of stuttering. *J Speech Disord* 1942;7:251–257.
73. Cooper E, Cooper C. Fluency disorders. In D Battle (ed), *Communication Disorders in Multicultural Populations*. Stoneham, MA: Andover Medical Publishers/Butterworth-Heinemann, 1993:189–211.
74. Leith W, Nims H. Cultural influences in the development and treatment of stuttering.: A preliminary report on the black stutterer. *J Speech Hear Disord* 1975;4: 459–466.
75. Cole JB. Culture: Negro, black, nigger. *Black Scholar* 1970;I:40–44.
76. Conrad C. An incidence study of stuttering among black adults. Dissertation, Northwestern University, 1985.

77. Goldman R. Cultural influences in the sex ratio in the incidence of stuttering. *American Anthropologist* 1967;69:69–78.
78. Bloodstein O. *Stuttering: The Search for the Cure.* Needham Heights, MA: Allyn and Bacon, 1993.
79. Bebout L, Bradford A. Cross cultural attitudes toward speech disorders. *J Speech Hear Disord* 1992;35:45–52.
80. Watson JB, Kayser H. Assessment of bilingual/bicultural children and adults who stutter. *Semin Speech Lang* 1994;15(2):149–163.
81. Westby CE. Ethnographic interviewing: Asking the right questions, to the right people, in the right ways. *J Childhood Commun Disord* 1990;13:101–111.
82. Leith W. Treating the stutterer with atypical cultural influences. In K St. Louis (ed), *The Atypical Stutterer: Principles and Practices of Rehabilitation.* Orlando, FL: Academic Press, 1996.

9

Counseling

Although "counseling" has evolved over the years to become a catchall term, its meaning is not universally agreed upon. Brammer[1] noted two opposing views about counseling. One view emphasizes helping as a specialized enterprise based on a firm foundation in the behavioral and medical sciences. The other view sees helping as a broad human function using the helping skills possessed by most people. In a recent text by Crowe,[2] these views were integrated as counseling was presented as both an art and a science, and as a clinical process applicable to many disciplines. This recent description and interpretation of counseling is the one that is most applicable to a Synergistic Model of fluency and one that will be considered in this chapter.

DEFINITION OF COUNSELING

The following definitions of counseling embody some of the essential components of the process of counseling that are useful in the practice of fluency therapy and all therapy within the field of communication disorders:

- Nugent[3]: "Professional counseling is a process in which a trained counselor helps an individual, groups of individuals, or family members gain self-understanding and understanding of others in order to solve problems more effectively and resolve conflicts in every day living. This process involves a professional relationship in which counselors and clients jointly participate in problem resolution for the client."
- Jones[4]: "Counseling is the establishment of an effective interpersonal relationship within which client change and growth are fostered. The process is a collaborative effort in which an attempt is made to create conditions that allow change to occur. Its usual purpose is to help those seeking assistance to become more autonomous, more self-directed, and more responsible by fostering learning and providing the tools that individuals may need to make change."
- Rollin[5]: "The counseling process is characteristically supportive, insight re-educative and usually short term. It is used to help individuals make practi-

cal changes in their lives without modifying established personality patterns. The essential task of the counselor is to help individuals work toward an understanding of themselves in order to learn new ways of coping with and adjusting to life situations."

- Thompson and Rudolph[6]: "Counseling involves a relationship between two people who meet so that one person can help the other person. We see counseling as a process in which people learn how to help themselves and, in effect, become their own counselors."

Thompson and Rudolph credit David Palmer of the Student Counseling Center at UCLA with the following definition of counseling:

I. To be listened to
   To be heard . . .
   To be supported
   While you gather your forces
   And get your bearings.
II. A fresh look at alternatives
    Some new insights
    Learning some needed skills.
III. To face your lion—your fears,
     to come to a decision—
     the courage to act on it
     to take the risks
     that living demands.

These assorted definitions stress that counseling includes an emphasis on building a relationship, problem solving, gaining control of one's behavior, and self-improvement. We believe that counseling is a process that happens as the relationship is formed between the professional and the client, parent, and family. When we consciously incorporate counseling techniques into our therapeutic process, we believe that we can help our clients to change not only their speech and language but also their views of themselves and their environment. We hope that our fluency clients can identify their strengths and weaknesses and that they can change undesirable feelings and behaviors that have resulted because of their communication disorder. We strive to empower our clients to develop unused potential, to manage problem situations, and to achieve valued outcomes. These goals are derived from our understanding of the counseling process and the role that it plays in a synergistic, holistic approach to fluency therapy.

COUNSELING AS A SCIENCE AND AN ART

Crowe stated that "the art of counseling concerns its clinical practice and the talents and skills the clinician brings to it. The science of counseling concerns the theories that support the art of practice; the formation of those theories through scientific process; and the testing, revision, and validation of theories through ongoing research. The art and science of counseling are mutually dependent, mutually enhancing dimensions."[2] We agree with this understanding of counseling and believe that the art and science of counseling are also synergistically united. In addition, in order to fully enter into the counseling process, we believe that a third dimension is important to include—namely, the personal development of the counselor. This aspect integrates the information learned from theoretical research (the science) with the knowledge and practice of the skills (the art), and provides a personal foundation for the clinician and the client when attempting to do the work that the counseling process demands. Whenever we speak of counseling, we believe that it is important to understand how these aspects of the process work together and assist the clinician in implementing the counseling aspect into fluency therapy. Therefore, clinicians benefit from understanding the theories of counseling, from practicing the skills of counseling, and from consciously working on their own personal development. The view of the counseling process is depicted in Figure 9.1.

Theories/Issues
Adlerian
Rogerian
Existention
Cognitive
Gestalt

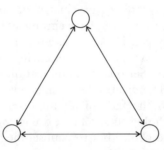

Skills	*Personal Style*
Attending behavior	Knowledge of self
Observation skills	Understanding self-esteem issues
Encouraging, paraphrasing	Understanding issues of
Summarizing, confronting	assertiveness
Reflection of feeling	Understanding inner control
Reflection of meaning	Commitment to personal growth
Personal style	Commitment to living consciously

Figure 9.1   The Counseling Triangle by C. Bloom and D. Cooperman.

These three separate components are synergistically integrated and provide the structure and guidance for one who enters into a counseling relationship with a client. As clinicians become more knowledgeable and aware of the components of the triangle and the process, their therapy, their interactions with clients, and their own personal lives become enriched. Understanding and practicing the skills, knowing the issues highlighted by theory, and committing oneself to personal growth takes the mystery out of the process of counseling and is one that many fluency specialists now recognize as essential to therapy.

COUNSELING AND THE FIELD OF COMMUNICATION DISORDERS

As speech-language pathologists and audiologists, do we counsel our clients? This is a frequent inquiry of those in our field. Crowe observed that the "question of whether counseling should be essential to the clinical practice of speech-language pathology and audiology is rhetorical. Counseling, in fact, does occur in almost every therapy encounter, whether it is intentionally employed by clinicians to achieve specific therapy goals, or whether it happens spontaneously and unguided toward any purpose."[2] We would argue that intentional counseling should be the foundation and framework for our clinical work with fluency clients.

Manning[7] also responded to this question:

Should speech-language pathologists even be dealing with counseling issues? Should issues such as affect, emotions, and cognitive change be left to the professions of psychology, psychiatry, or counseling? If we find ourselves working with clients who have chronic life-adjustment problems, the answer is most likely yes. However, as Luterman[8] notes, the vast majority of our clients are ordinary people experiencing a normal reaction to a communication disorder. Serious communication disorders create genuine stress and anxiety. He indicates that such people are generally experiencing normal emotions in the face of an important problem. Clearly, then, speech-language pathologists should be doing counseling with their clients. Actually, we have no choice but to counsel them if our goal is to provide truly comprehensive treatment.

The understanding of counseling embodied in these statements is supported by the American Speech and Hearing Association (ASHA) in its Preferred Practice Patterns[9] and Scope of Practice in Speech-Language Pathology and Audiology.[10]

ASHA's Preferred Practice Patterns

07.0 Definition of Counseling: Procedure to facilitate the patient's/client's recovery from or adjustment to a communication disorder. Specific purposes of counseling may be to provide patients/clients and their families with information and support, make appropriate referrals to other professionals, and help patients/clients to develop problem-solving strategies to enhance the (re)habilitation process.

Expected Outcome(s): Professionals assist patients/clients and their families to develop appropriate goals for recovery from, adjustment to, or prevention of a communication or related disorder by facilitating change and growth in which patients/clients become more autonomous, more self-directing, and more responsible for achieving their potential and realizing their goals to communicate more effectively.

Clinical Process: Counseling services for patients/clients and their families include:

- Assessment of counseling needs
- Provision of information
- Use of strategies to modify behavior and/or the patient's/client's environment
- Development of coping mechanisms and systems for emotional support
- Development and coordination of patient/client and family self-help and support groups

Professionals are responsible for ensuring that the patient/clients and their family receive adequate counseling. Referrals to and consultation with mental health professionals may be an integral part of counseling.

ASHA's Scope of Practice in Speech-Language Pathology and Audiology

- Speech-language pathologists and audiologists counsel individuals with the listed disorders , as well as their families, caregivers, and other service providers, related to the disorders and their management.
- Speech-language pathologists and audiologists provide consultation and counseling, and make referrals when appropriate.

Clearly, the mandate for speech-language pathologists and audiologists to become aware of and knowledgeable about their role in the counseling process is important for those in all areas of communication disorders. It is our belief that our clients with fluency disorders are particularly in need of clinicians possessing these skills.

SPEECH-LANGUAGE PATHOLOGISTS AND AUDIOLOGISTS AS CLINICIAN-COUNSELORS

As we have grown in our understanding of the need to include the counseling process in the diagnostic interview and therapy procedures, attempts have been made to identify and define our role more specifically. Scheurle[11] has traced the emergence of the fields of communication disorders and counseling as shown in Figure 9.2. She demonstrated the views of counseling that support the medical model and how these influenced the fields of human services. She also noted Carl Rogers' finding that the psychotherapeutic process is not the singular province of psychiatrists or psychotherapists. Rogers used the terms *interviewing, counseling,* and *helping* to describe the process. Indeed, friends, family members, and parents use these same skills in most professional roles. However, most use them unintentionally, and we hope that fluency clinicians will recognize that there are skills to be learned that can become intentional and affect their therapy.

Kennedy [12] has discussed this role of helper in terms of a "nonprofessional counselor." We would prefer to call ourselves "clinician-counselors"[13] as we attempt to integrate the skills of the counseling profession, the research surrounding the theoretical issues of counseling, and the work directed toward our own personal growth. We believe that the title "clinician-counselor" allows us to maintain our primary identity as speech-language pathologists and audiologists and yet adopt appropriate techniques of the counseling profession as they can assist us in a holistic approach to our clients. It is always essential to remember that any counseling that we do as clinician-counselors is always centered around the problems that arise from a communication disorder. A clinician with a clinician-counselor's orientation will be a person who is committed to her own professional growth, who has learned the skills of listening, and has understood and worked through some understanding of theoretical issues. Thus, the clinician-counselor will be sensitive to the client's thoughts, feelings, and behaviors as expressed by the client. Before a plan of therapy is decided upon, the clinician-counselor will encourage an abundance of client input, listening carefully to what is said and to what is inferred. Together the clinician-counselor and client will choose the goals that are important to therapy, and together they will assess progress. Always the clinician-counselor and client will work toward change and growth.

In order to change behavior, feelings must be expressed and understood. Luterman wrote: "I have learned that the goal of counseling is not to make people feel better, but to separate feelings from nonproductive behavior. The feelings must always be acknowledged." After exploring the thoughts, feelings, and behaviors of our clients, we hope that our empowerment of our clients will continue throughout all stages of the helping process. We believe that clients do not fully improve their fluency disorders unless such a holistic approach is utilized. Therefore, it is important that clinician-counselors understand (1) the phases of the helping process, (2) the role of the clinician-counselor, and (3) the elements of the counseling triangle.

PHASES OF THE HELPING PROCESS

The phases of the helping process have been outlined by Eagen,[14] Carkhuff,[15] Hepworth and Larson,[16] and Brammer.[17] Our own summary and overview of this process is depicted in Figure 9.3. It is important to stress that the

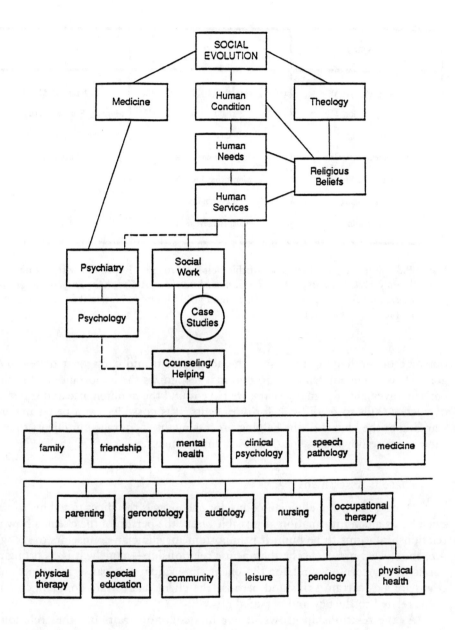

Figure 9.2 Schema of the Evolution of Counseling and Human Services by J. Scheuerle. (J Scheuerle. *Counseling in Speech-Language Pathology and Audiology.* New York: Macmillan, 1992, p. 17.)

PHASE I	PHASE II	PHASE III
Assessment	**Implementation**	**Termination**
Exploration	Partializing Goals	Mutually Planning Termination
Attending	Planning Tasks	Planning Carryover Activities
Empathetic Listening	Implementing Tasks	Conducting Follow-up
Prompts and Probes	Monitoring Progress	
Summarizing	Confronting	
Goal Setting	Goal Achievement	

Figure 9.3 Summary of the Phases of the Helping Process. (Reprinted with permission from Bloom CM, Cooperman DK. *The Clinical Interview: A Guide for Speech-Language Pathologists and Audiologists* (2nd ed), edited by BB Shulman. National Student Speech-language Hearing Association, 1992, p. 28.)

outcome of the helping process is the achievement and carry over of selected goals. This is a client-centered process that recognizes the importance of the client's involvement. For many years, we have found the maintenance and transfer of fluency skills to be difficult for our clients. It is possible that a better understanding of the phases of the helping process might encourage our clients to assume more responsibility for their own improvement.

Phase I: Assessment

During Phase I, a clinician-counselor encourages the client to tell his story. Eliciting as much information as possible about the person of the client is how a relationship begins to be built. It is important for clinician-counselors to recognize the special nature of the therapeutic relationship—namely, it is is brought about by concerns of and for the client. It originates because the clinician-counselor has certain skills and because the client has certain communication needs related to fluency and personal growth.

As the relationship grows, it exhibits common traits of other relationships—trust, respect, and honesty. However, clinician-counselors must always remember that the nature of this relationship is unique. It is enhanced as clinician-counselors strive to facilitate high levels of warmth, acceptance, caring, and empathy within a "safe environment," attempting to uncover the thoughts, feelings, and behaviors of the client in relation to fluency. Schum and Cooper wrote: "This dynamic relationship is a combination of the technical skills and personal style of the clinician, matched with the needs, abilities, style, and effort of the client." Clinicians must also recognize that many fluency clients are unmotivated for therapy. They must be encouraged to become aware of their problem and to actively work toward its solution. The therapeutic relationship is a powerful tool in this process. Through this relationship, clinicians can enhance the motivation of their clients and assist them in growing in areas of self-esteem, assertiveness and locus of control (Chapter 7). In order to accomplish this, a clinician-counselor utilizes the communication skills of attending, empathetic listening, prompts and probes, summarizing, and goal setting. Furthermore, the clinician-counselor synergistically supports and enriches her interviewing of the client during Phase I with an understanding of theories of counseling as well as the awareness that has come from commitment to personal growth.

Phase II: Implementation

In Phase II, the clinician-counselor joins with the client in implementing goals that are important to the client. After learning and understanding the thoughts, feelings, and behaviors that make up the problems of the fluency client, the clinician-counselor assists the client in naming the areas in which he would like to change.This is the action-oriented and change-orientated aspect of the process. What does a client have to do in order to change his fluency? What goals must be set in order to bring about this change? It is important that these goals be defined in terms of subgoals (partialization of goals) so the client can experience progress and personal responsibility for the change process. It is during this phase of the helping process that one draws attention to the client's strengths and affirms incremental progress toward goal attainment. It is the completion of these goals that provides the material for the attitudinal areas of the synergistic approach.

During this phase, clinician-counselors are urged to monitor the progress of their clients on a regular basis. Compton and Galway[19] stressd the following reasons for monitoring:

1. To evaluate the effectiveness of change strategies. If an approach does not produce desired effects, practitioners should determine the reasons for this and consider negotiating a different approach.
2. To guide clients' efforts toward goal attainment. Evaluating movement toward goals enhances continuity of focus and efforts and promotes efficient use of time.
3. To keep abreast of clients' reactions to progress or lack of progress. When they believe they are not progressing, clients tend to become discouraged and may lose confidence in the helping process. By evaluating progress periodically, clinician-counselors will be alerted to negative client reactions that might otherwise undermine progress.
4. To enhance clients' motivation and confidence in the helping process. Concentrating on goal attainment and evaluating progress tend to sustain clients' motivation to work on their problems. Moreover, clients

tend to respect clinicians who do not passively permit them to waste time in unproductive work not focused on the task at hand.

As the relationship continues to build during this phase, the clinician-counselor must help to maintain the focus and to confront the client when there is a discrepancy between the client's goals and behavior. Clinician-counselors facilitate assertiveness as well as practice it when working with difficult clients.

Phase III: Termination

Terminating the helping relationship with clients is an important phase for the clinician-counselor to incorporate into therapy plans. Fluency clients share significant aspects of their lives as they discuss and face fears, avoidances, and feelings of low self-esteem and low self-worth. As clinician-counselors relate with warmth and understanding, clients develop a close feeling toward them. Thinking of leaving them brings mixed feelings. On the one hand, they are grateful for their newfound ability to speak and for the help given to them by their clinician-counselor. On the other hand, some clients are relieved not to have to come to therapy anymore. Many clients put too much emphasis on the clinician-counselor and are now afraid to leave them. For these clients, emphasizing locus of control continues to be important in this phase.

Recognizing their ability to cope independently is an essential aspect of this phase. For all clients, a sense of loss also accompanies the separation from what has been ongoing and productive in their lives. Therefore, it is especially important in our therapy with fluency clients to be aware of and provide time for this phase of the helping process.

Compton and Galway[19] identified the four major components of the Termination Process: (1) assessing when individuals and group goals have been satisfactorily attained and planning termination accordingly, (2) effecting successful termination of the helping relationship, (3) planning for maintenance of change and continued growth following termination, and (4) evaluating the results of the helping process.

It is our belief that careful planning of the termination process can bring long-term benefits to our clients. Having the client participate in that planning prepares him for assuming the role of self-therapist. It also reinforces the essential responsibilities necessary if carryover is to be effective. Together, the clinician-counselor can plan, role-play, and discuss carry-over activities. It is also important to plan follow-up activities that will facilitate maintenance. We have found that connecting with weekly fluency group meetings has been a support for our clients, which provides an opportunity to focus on targets and to reestablish supportive ties. There comes a time, too, when one must plan to terminate the support group. Murphy and Dillon wrote: "An agreed upon, planned ending is the nicest way to wrap up working together, as it provides many opportunities to review, compare expectations with realities, look ahead, and both regret and celebrate concluding this cycle of work."[20]

Although these three phases have been presented separately, they actually are woven throughout the therapy process. Within each of the phases, the components of the Counseling Triangle emerge as the clinician-counselor integrates the science, the art, and the result of personal growth into a personal style of helping. We next consider more thoroughly those three major components of the Counseling Triangle: the personal development of the clinician-counselor, the theories of counseling, and the skills of counseling. It is important to note that these aspects of the Counseling Triangle interact synergistically to provide client-centered treatment for our fluency clients. Clinician-counselors integrate these three aspects of the triangle as we work with the thoughts, feelings, and behaviors that are related to the fluency disorder of our clients. Figure 9.2 demonstrates that clinician-counselors do not work with character disorders, psychological disorders, or issues not directly related to the communication disorder; we refer clients to psychologists for these.

THE COUNSELING TRIANGLE: PERSONAL DEVELOPMENT OF THE CLINICIAN-COUNSELOR

The first component of the Counseling Triangle is that the clinician-counselor grow in awareness of her own person. Indeed, we believe that the most important instrument for delivery of services is the clinician-counselor's own person. Corey[21] notes:"The human dimension is one of the most powerful determinants of the therapeutic encounter we create with clients." In our field, we have often recognized the importance of the therapeutic relationship and the qualities necessary for effective clinicians. It sometimes seems, however, that we have neglected to highlight the specifics of personal growth that are necessary for a successful clinical relationship. While these characteristics come easily to some clinicians, they can be learned by most all. Some of the general characteristics of competent professionals that have bee identified[13,20-22] are as follows:

Self-awareness	Ability to show emotion
Empathy	Acceptance
Genuineness	Ability to communicate
Compassion	Commitment
Purposefulness	Warmth
Enthusiasm	

Each of these characteristics is both essential to and an outgrowth of the clinical process. As one studies the theories of counseling and learns the listening skills, the opportunity to grow in self-knowledge is increased. As one learns and applies the other two areas of the Counseling Triangle (listening skills and theories), personal growth is furthered. In addition, the clinician-counselor is encouraged to commit herself to her practice in an ongoing manner. A knowledge of the important characteristics of the helping relationship and an attempt to increase their presence in one's own personal life is essential to personal growth and effective practice.

Core Facilitative Dimensions of the Clinician-Counselor

Scheuerle[11] cited with approval Spieberg's[23] list of characteristics necessary for an effective clinician-client relationship. Described as the 10 core facilitative dimensions of the helping relationship, they are defined as follows:

1. *Empathy:* the ability to perceive and communicate accurately what another person is feeling.
2. *Genuineness:* outward evidence of inward feelings and attitudes.
3. *Respect:* regard for the client as an individual who can make choices, grow, and change.
4. *Concreteness:* the ability to specify feelings, experiences, and actions.
5. *Confrontation:* the ability to indicate lack of consistency or congruence between verbal expressions and nonverbal behaviors.
6. *Self-disclosure:* the sharing of information about the self to facilitate self exploration by the client.
7. *Warmth:* concern and regard for the client expressed both verbally and nonverbally.
8. *Immediacy:* the sharing of feelings between client and clinician.
9. *Potency:* the ability to show confidence and have an impact on client and therapy.
10. *Self-actualization:* the state of being a fully functioning individual.

This list incorporates all three aspects of the Counseling Triangle and demonstrates how synergistically these components are integrated. The clinician's motivation to increase self-actualization is key to this process. As the clinician works on her own growth, the client is served. A client who works with one who has explored her own inner world will find strength, support, and direction for growing in self-esteem, assertiveness, and locus of control. Empowerment will be a reality, as one takes control of his speech and life. One of the key means of change for both the clinician and the client is self-awareness.

Self-Awareness

Whether we are motivated by Shakespeare's dictum "to thine own self be true" or by Hoff's[24] question "How can you get very far if you don't know who you are?," knowing yourself is a cornerstone of the counseling relationship. Accoriding to Scheuerle,[11]

Socrates, the ancient Greek philosopher, knew and taught the wisdom of self-knowledge: *Know yourself. Know your strengths and your weaknesses, your potentials and limitations. Take stock of yourself.* In doing so, mentally healthy people can accurately assess their needs, their value systems and their goals in life and realize that these change over time.

However, Rollin[5] reminded us that "one of the most difficult aspects in all of our personal relationships is to be fully aware of what we are, who we are, and what we are feeling when in the presence of others." We believe that before clinicians can respond adequately to their clients with fluency disorders, their parents, or family members, they must first have made a commitment to pursue their own personal growth. Clinician-counselors must become aware of their own strengths and limitations. We must be in touch with the choices that we have made in our personal and professional lives and be aware of the freedom that we have to make new choices if we hope to help clients change their lives. We must become aware of our thoughts, feelings and behaviors as they contribute to the therapeutic process. As Compton and Galway[19] put it: "The capacity to observe self probably requires the ability to care deeply about oneself and one's goals, to respect and believe in oneself, and yet to be able to stand back and observe oneself as an important piece of the complex activity of helping."

Motivation

One of the areas that is essential to bring into awareness is the motivation of the clinician-counselor. Most people who enter the helping professions have a deep desire to help others grow and change. This is an essential prerequisite for being an effective clinician-counselor. However, the reason for entering a helping profession is not usually unidimensional, nor is it always entirely clear to the person herself what personal needs the profession will be filling. Therefore, it is important as clinician-counselors who work with fluency clients that we become aware of our own needs, personal conflicts, and areas of unfinished business, defenses, and the vulnerabilities that motivated our career choice.

We all have certain "blind spots" that keep us from being aware of our unmet needs, our weaknesses, and vulnerabilities. Corey[21] feels that many are attracted to the helping professions in order to "'help others,' to 'teach people how to live a good life,' to 'straighten people out,' and 'to solve others' problems.'" Others may be motivated by the need to receive the respect, admiration, approval, appreciation, affection, and caring of others. The clinician-counselor soon learns that the rewards for nurturing others are great. That the helper has needs is not wrong, nor are we suggesting that all one's needs must be met before entering a therapeutic relationship. Needs can work both for and against a clinician-counselor. The key is for the clinician to be aware of what the needs are and how they might influence the therapeutic relationship as it develops. Corey[21] listed the following ethical questions related to this issue:

1. What are the dangers to the client's well being when the clinician has an exaggerated need for being nurtured by the client?
2. Can helpers distinguish between what is for the client's benefit and what is for their own gains?
3. Are clinicians sufficiently aware of their needs for approval and appreciation?

4. Do they base their perceptions of their adequacies strictly on reactions from clients?
5. What are the dangers that exist when clinicians depend too heavily on client conformation of their adequacy, worth and values as both a counselor and a person?

These questions must be asked by all clinicians who hope to work with fluency clients. Those clients who gain fluency, who work through intensive and long-term treatment programs, are deeply grateful and would often like to become personal friends with their clinician. It is flattering and fulfilling to know of the client's progress in life changing behaviors and we encourage clinicians to accept the client's praise. At the same time, clinicians need to remind the client that it is he who has done the work More importantly, the clinician must separate her own needs from the process and maintain a professional relationship, which is warm and caring but not a personal friendship.

In further examining one's motivation for helping, one might ask the following questions:

1. Am I interested in my own growth?
2. How aware am I of my own needs and motivations?
3. How do I get my own needs met?
4. Do I always put others first and myself second?

The answer to these questions may be the beginning of a clinician-counselor's inward journey. Clinicians who are not meeting their own needs outside of the clinical setting may very well seek to meet those needs through the helping relationship. When that is the case, it is difficult for clinicians to genuinely focus on the client's concerns. Clinicians who need others to feed their egos and to reinforce their sense of personal adequacy foster dependency in clients. When this situation occurs we find that the clinician is in greater need of the client than the other way around. A professional is one who may be depended on by the client, but the professional should not herself become dependent on the client. Therefore, it is important for persons who are entering into the field of communication disorders to be relatively integrated and fulfilled. They need to be open to exploring their own needs and motives if they are to foster client growth and change.

Corey and Corey[25] identified a number of attitudes that are counterproductive for a person who wants to engage in a profession that helps others. We list some of these to provide a context for your own motivational assessment:

1. You believe that you have no problems in your life and therefore are in a position to help others resolve their problems.
2. You are convinced that your way is the right way and that if your clients were to accept your values, they would be happy.
3. You have very strong religious convictions.

4. You have no religious affiliation, do not believe in religion, and consider everyone who has religious convictions neurotic.
5. Your vision of helping is telling clients what they should do. For every question they raise, you are quick to provide a ready-made answer.
6. Your basic belief about humankind is that people are evil, not to be trusted, and in need of being straightened out.
7. You have made a minimal effort to expose yourself to learning situations and have avoided feedback from peers, professors, and supervisors as much as possible.
8. You cannot tolerate seeing people in pain; you want to quickly take their pain away and turn them to more pleasant thoughts.
9. You are filled with pain, yet you are unwilling to acknowledge this suffering and seek help for it; you think that your pain is being taken care of by attending to your clients' needs.
10. You consistently make your needs more important than your clients' needs.
11. You need your clients more than they need you and therefore you foster their dependency on you.
12. You are unable to enter a client's world for you can perceive reality only through your own eyes.
13. You have a very fragile ego that is easily bruised and thus you are overly sensitive to any criticisms from others.
14. You are highly defensive and have an aversion to being challenged.
15. You are unable to accept those who have different values from you.

Although these attitudes are identified as being counterproductive, we do not mean that if you have some of these attitudes you should not to enter our profession. On the contrary, we believe that the *awareness* of limitations is what is necessary, along with the *willingness* to change. Working through your own issues actually can enhance your role as a professional. Since there are many attitudinal needs of our fluency clients, clinician-counselors are encouraged to invest time in their own growth and development.

Areas of need are often understood more clearly when the theories of counseling are learned by the professional. While we do not advocate or espouse a single theory of counseling, we believe that some knowledge of the theories and the approaches that they utilize can be helpful in our understanding of clients. These theories of counseling are the second aspect of the Counseling Triangle and will be considered next.

THE COUNSELING TRIANGLE: THEORIES OF COUNSELING

Speech-language pathologists working with the client who has a fluency disorder should develop their awareness of the principles related to the theories of counseling. Knowledge of these principles helps guide the interactive process. While we are not advocating that clinician-counselors adhere to one particular theory or that they attempt to act as a psychotherapist, we do believe that a basic understanding and application of these principles can enrich the therapeutic relationship and result in more effective therapy. The theories can inform our therapy and provide a valuable means for client growth around issues that have developed because of the client's communication disorder. Knowledge of the theories enables a clinician-counselor to identify the thoughts, feelings, and behaviors of the client that need to be discussed and targeted as a goal. This aspect of fluency therapy enables one to integrate different components of theories into the rehabilitation process to expand its scope. We stress again that we are not advocating one particular theory over another and that we are not seeking to become "therapists" or "psychotherapists." We are clinician-counselors whose therapy is informed by the knowledge of current and past theories of counseling.

We will highlight four basic theories of counseling: (1) psychoanalytic therapy, (2) person-centered therapy, (3) gestalt therapy, and (4) rational emotive behavioral therapy.

1. Psychoanalytic Theory

The earliest theory of counseling emanated from the work of Freud, who provided the framework that those after him would either accept, expand, or reject. Many of those who rejected his theory, like Jung and Adler, are nevertheless also considered under the umbrella of psychoanalytic theory along with Freud.

Structural Concepts

The literature on psycholanalytic theory is extensive, and we can only highlight the basic concepts.[6,21] Freud believed that human behavior resulted from the dynamics of an interactional energy system: the id, the ego, and the superego.

The *id* consists of our basic instinctual drives. Based on the pleasure principle, it exists to provide immediate satisfaction. The id is the energizer of the personality. The *ego* has been called the "executive of the personality." It governs and controls the id and the superego and maintains relationship with the external world. The ego operates under the reality principle and adjusts according to the constraints of the environment. The *superego* embodies our personal moral standard. This aspect of the personality is absorbed from parental influences and continues throughout life. Our "shoulds," "oughts," and "musts" are part of the superego.

Freud believed that this energy system must be in balance for the person to be healthy, i.e., engaged in loving, playing, and working. This balance is the key to mental health (Figure 9.4).

Application to Fluency Therapists   When interviewing our clients, it is helpful to find out how a client's energy is being spent. In order for balance to be achieved, clients must engage in activities that allow for success, challenge, love, and play. Clinician-counselors can gain insight into a client's functioning with Freudian theory, even though they will not be using it directly as a therapeutic

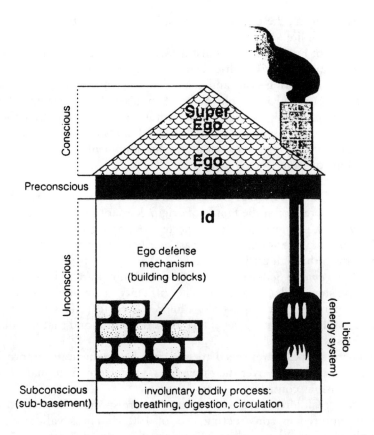

Figure 9.4 Illustration of Freud's Id-Ego-Super Ego Energy System. (Reprinted with permission from Thompson C, Rudolph L. *Counseling Children*. Pacific Grove, CA: Brooks/Cole, 1996, p. 62.)

technique. Understanding this basic structure enables one to have a deeper understanding of a client's needs and informs the creation of transfer activities. Clients dominated by the id may demonstrate behaviors that satisfy their pleasure principle. For example, when doing fluency therapy in a prison, a clinician was able to recognize that two clients appeared to be driven by the id. It therefore became an important part of their therapy to work on ego development and self-esteem. Helping clients to identify strengths and limitations accurately and to learn how to interact with the environment responsibly are ways of increasing ego functioning.

Clients who have a dominating superego often cite their "shoulds, oughts, and musts." They haven't owned up to their own need to take charge of their fluency but are at the therapy sessions because someone would like them there. Before change can happen, these clients must realize the need to take responsibility for their own speech life.

We learn from Freud that one must have a strong and balanced ego structure if one is to have a positive self-esteem. As one develops one's ego and relationships through mastering skills and demonstrating competency, self-esteem is improved. Thompson and Rudolph[6] quoted Simon's[26] observation that "Freud believed that love and work are the keys to mental health." For children, the keys to mental health are their schoolwork and their relationships with family, peers, and other significant people. Six conditions that complement the productivity and relationship equation for self-esteem are:

> *Belonging:* Children need to feel connected to their family or to a family of their own creation if the family of origin does not work out. As children grow older, they need to feel connected to a peer group.
>
> *Child Advocacy:* Children need at least one advocate who can be trusted to help them through crisis periods.
>
> *Risk Management:* Self-esteem increases as children are able to take risks and master challenging tasks. The difficulty is finding tasks that are challenging yet not impossible. Children need to believe that they are successful if they have given a task their best effort and that it is okay to take risks and fail.
>
> *Empowerment:* Children need to exercise developmentally appropriate amounts of control over their own lives. Opportunities to make choices and decisions contribute to empowerment.
>
> *Uniqueness:* Children need to feel that they are special. We need to work with children in constructing lists of 100 sentences validating their unique and positive qualities. These are "anti-suicide" lists.
>
> *Productivity:* As children get things done, they feel better. Encouragement and reinforcement of productive activity can be useful in prompting children to find intrinsic rewards in accomplishment.

We believe that these conditions for the development of a strong ego and self-concept are as important for adults as for children. While we will not be practicing psychotherapy, understanding psychoanalytic theory's personality structure definitely informs our fluency treatment.

Levels of Consciousness

Perhaps Freud's greatest contributions were his descriptions of our levels of consciousness and unconsciousness. They revolutionized our understanding of human behavior and personality. For Freud, consciousness is but a thin slice of our whole personality structure (Figure 9.5). He described consciousness as the part of our mental activity that we are aware of at any time. But he proposed that the personal unconscious comprised about 85 percent of what exists in our minds. The Unconscious is the bottom layer of the mind and contains unconscious ideas, thoughts, attitudes, and memories. This layer of the mind influences

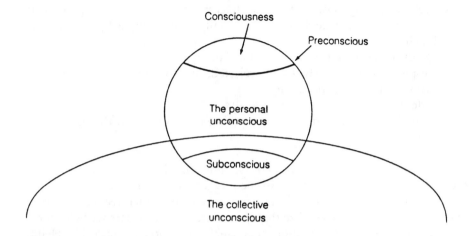

Figure 9.5 Freud's Circle of Consciousness (Reprinted with permission from Thompson C, Rudolph L. *Counseling Children*. Pacific Grove, CA: Brooks/Cole, 1996, p. 63.)

a person's behavior without their conscious unawareness. The more one brings these unconscious drives and impulses into consciousness, the less power they have to influence behavior. The Preconscious refers to material that is not immediately available to the conscious mind but that is able to be retrieved with some effort. The Subconscious refers to the involuntary processes that have been with us from birth (breathing, circulation, etc.). The Collective Unconscious was explored by Jung and refers to the inherited wisdom and insights that we share with all of humanity.

Application to Fluency Therapists   Freud's description of consciousness highlights the importance of the concepts of transference and countertransference, for there is where we can see the unconscious functioning.

Transference is the unconscious process in which clients project onto the clinician past feelings or attitudes that they have had toward significant people in their lives. Because of the client's past, a clinician may be perceived in either a positive or negative light. When transference is positive, the client may express exaggerated love, admiration, or dependency. Negative feelings include exaggerated distrust, dislike, hatred, and rejection. Hepworth and Larsen[16] cited some typical manifestations of transference reactions that we as fluency therapists and clinician-counselors should be aware of:

- Relating to the clinician in a clinging, dependent way or excessively seeking praise and reassurance
- Attempting to please by excessive compliments or praise
- Asking an inordinate number of personal questions

- Seeking special considerations, such as frequent changes in appointments
- Attempting to engage the clinician socially—for example, by inviting her to lunch
- Questioning the interest of the clinician
- Responding defensively, feeling rejected, or expecting criticism or punishment without realistic cause
- Offering personal favors or gifts
- Being late for appointments or striving to stay beyond the usual ending time

When confronting such behaviors, clinicians must first ensure that they themselves are not doing anything to encourage this behavior. After this has been ascertained, clinicians can call the attention of clients to their feelings in the here and now, helping them to realize that their patterns of transference behavior are based on unwarranted assumptions that usually have no basis in reality. Helping clients to explore these issues often has far-reaching effects in their personal lives as well as in the clinical context. In other instances, clinicians may manage transference issues by being aware of them but ignoring them. Rather than being sidetracked, clinicians keep their focus on their clients and do not permit the spotlight to shift to themselves. In either case, clinicians should know themselves, be confident about themselves, and have their own needs met outside of the clinical relationship, particularly when they are dealing with transference reactions.

Countertransference is when the clinician experiences unrealistic feelings and reactions with respect to the client that are based on past relationships. These exaggerated feelings may trigger old wounds in a clinician's life and interfere with her therapy. For example, if clinicians have not dealt with past angers in their own personalities, they may be uncomfortable when a client expresses a healthy response of anger. Hepworth and Larsen[16] identified typical ways countertransference reactions manifest themselves:

- Being unduly concerned about a client
- Having persistent fantasies about a client
- Dreading or pleasurably anticipating sessions with clients
- Consistently ending sessions early or permitting them to extend beyond designated ending points.
- Trying to impress or being unduly impressed by clients

It is important to remember that transference and countertransference are unconscious and usually happen without the knowledge of either person. Psychoanalysts use this process as an important element in their therapy. As clinician-counselors, our role is to be aware of both the possibility and the occurrence of transference and countertransference and to deal with it in a responsible way that permits growth. It is worth stressing again that clinician-counselors must continue to explore their own issues that emerge during the therapeutic relationship.

Developmental Concepts

Defense Mechanisms   These are techniques used by the ego to reduce anxiety and pressure. Such coping measures may provide short-term relief but they do not permit facing the reality of a situation. Defense mechanisms include identification, displacement, repression, projection and reaction formation, rationalization, denial, and fantasy. For our purposes, it is important to remember that defense mechanisms are the ego's attempt to handle difficult situations. They are specific, unconscious, adjustive efforts and are a part of the normal coping process. Normal defenses assist the person to grow in his/her ability to problem solve. These mechanisms are a problem only when they become a permanent part of the personality.

Dependency/Autonomy Stages   Freud initially described personality development as a succession of stages each described by a dominant way of achieving pleasure and by specific developmental tasks. All people must meet the needs of each stage if they are to move on to the next developmental stage. Erickson expanded Freud's developmental stages; both are compared in the dependence-autonomy continuum depicted in Figure 9.6. Problems in adulthood are often the results of failure to meet basic needs in childhood.

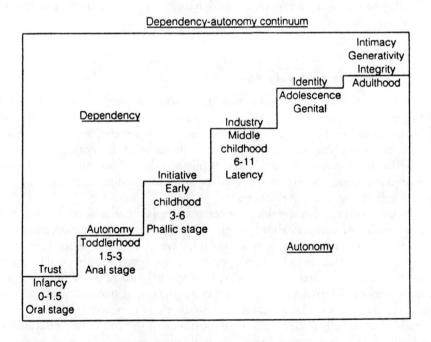

Figure 9.6   Erickson's Dependency-Autonomy Continuum (Reprinted with permission from Thompson C, Rudolph L. *Counseling Children*. Pacific Grove, CA: Brooks/Cole, 1996, p. 65.)

Application to Fluency Therapists Understanding defense mechanisms and developmental stages is important for us as clinician-counselors when dealing with all clients and parents. It must be re-emphasized that defense mechanisms are important and necessary for a client to heal. We must realize that a client or parent might not be able to "hear" about the fluency disability at the initial diagnosis. The shock of knowing about the continuous monitoring needed in fluency therapy and the inability for a cure calls forth the need to defend. Defense mechanisms are normal and they help an individual to cope with pain until they can bear it. When we see individuals in denial, it is important that we tread lightly with great understanding.

In summary, the major concepts of psychoanalytic theory as enunciated by Freud are important for clinician-counselors. But is should be remembered that others like Erickson continued to develop and refine Freud's work. Crowe[2] noted:

> These Neo-analysts—Carl Jung, Alfred Adler, Otto Rank, Erich Fromm, and Karen Horney, among others—drew liberally from Freud's basic concepts. Many of these personality theories became prominent in their own right and led to associated approaches to psychoanalysis and shorter term psychotherapy and counseling. They typically do not ascribe as much importance to sex in personality development as did Freud. They also hold different views on id-ego-superego dynamics and on the stages and temporal aspects of personality development.

2. Person-Centered Therapy

The theory that has probably had the greatest impact on the professional field of counseling is Carl Rogers' person-centered therapy.[27,28] Although some clinician-counselors might view this theory as too simplistic, we believe that it provides the underlying support to our understanding of the dynamics of a professional relationship with our clients. While we should not limit ourselves to this approach alone, Rogers has enabled us to understand the true meaning of a client-centered approach to fluency.

Person-centered therapy does not consist of specific techniques but rather is a set of beliefs and attitudes about people. Rogers believed that human beings are essentially rational, positive, self-actualizing, trustworthy, and forward moving.[27] He believed that an individual's personal growth can be enhanced by therapeutic characteristics that facilitate client awareness and responsibility for self: these are the characteristics of genuineness or congruence, unconditional positive regard and acceptance, and an accurate empathetic understanding. Finally, Rogers enabled us to fully understand the importance of the counseling relationship that facilitates change in our clients. We will consider each of these concepts in turn.

Rogers' View of Human Nature

Rogers' fundamental belief in the individual's ability to find his own answers, to become aware of the potential within, and to move toward acting in self-actualizing ways is evident in the following quotation:

> One of the most satisfying experiences I know is just fully to appreciate an individual in the same way that I appreciate a sunset. When I look at a sunset, I don't find myself saying, "Soften the orange a little on the right hand corner, and put a bit more purple along the base, and use a little more pink in the cloud color." I don't try to control a sunset. I watch it with awe as it unfolds.[27]

Person-centered therapy has continued Rogers' assertion that all people have the inherent capacity to move away from negativity and maladjustments toward psychological health. However, each person must assume the responsibility for this change in direction. The therapist is not the person who knows best. It is the therapist's role to facilitate the client's own discovery of what is best for him. Called the "humanistic approach" to counseling, it is indeed awesome to be part of the process of a person's growth and self-development. However, to do so requires a combination of skills and role adjustments. One who practices person-centered therapy must move away from the traditional understanding of the helper's primary role as educator. Education is still a component of the process, but it is the client who becomes the teacher and the one who takes responsibility for the therapy intervention. Rogers first called this process "nondirective therapy" because of the therapist's listening role. Later, he renamed it "client-centered therapy" to stress the responsibility being placed on the client, and finally "person-centered" therapy, which he hoped would expand the notion of individual therapy to a more holistic view.

Rogers' understanding of the person was partly developed in conjunction with the work of Maslow.[29,30] Maslow's research in the area of individual growth and development led to his identification of the following characteristics of self-actualizing people: "the capacity to tolerate and even welcome uncertainty in their lives, acceptance of self and others, spontaneity and creativity, a need for privacy and solitude, autonomy, the capacity for deep and intense interpersonal relationships, a genuine caring for others, a sense of humor, an inner-directedness, and an open and fresh attitude toward life."

Thompson and Rudolph[6] summarized the beliefs necessary for a person-centered counselor:

- People have worth and dignity in their own right and therefore deserve respect
- People have the capacity and right to self-direction (self-actualization) and, when given the opportunity, make wise judgments
- People can select their own values
- People can learn to make constructive use of responsibility

- People have the capacity to deal with their own feelings, thoughts, and behaviors
- People have the potential for constructive change and personal development toward a full and satisfying life (actualization)

Application to Fluency Therapists   It is our belief that a person-centered approach is an essential component of all therapy. Crowe[2] also has said that speech-language and hearing clinicians "should attempt to establish a clinical atmosphere of trust and unconditional acceptance in which a client feels comfortable externalizing anxiety and, thereby, is able to place it in an objective perspective and possibly resolve it." Clinician-counselors are encouraged to examine their own beliefs of human nature. In order to treat a client with the respect all people have a right to, one's own values must be examined. The personal prejudices or values of the clinician-counselor can interfere with the client's growth.

Clinician-counselors also need to explore their own self-actualizing efforts and look for the same in their fluency clients. Whenever a fluency client takes steps toward increased responsibility and self-actualization, it is important to be aware of and to reinforce the client's actions. A person-centered approach underlines the importance of the client's role in establishing his own goals for therapy and for carrying them out. The clinician-counselor's basic belief in the client's ability to do this determines the course of therapy and the client's ability to move toward positive, holistic, synergistic change. In the context of a warm, accepting atmosphere, fluency clients can be helped to become more autonomous, spontaneous, and confident. And as fluency clients become more aware of who they are, they learn to accept their own values instead of the values of others. Person-centered therapy includes the discussion of plans, behavioral steps to be taken, and the outcome of the steps. This approach is used throughout the therapy process.

Characteristics of a Person-Centered Therapist

As we noted above, Rogers believed that three attitudes of the person-centered counselor could facilitate the change process: congruence or genuineness, unconditional positive regard and acceptance, and accurate empathetic understanding. We will examine each of these characteristics.

Congruence or Genuineness   Rogers stressed that clinicians must be their real self in the therapy situation. It is important that clinicians authentically respect and value the client that they are working with. To do so, the clinician's inner and outer selves must be one. If the clinician is uncomfortable with what the client is saying or doing, it is important to either work through the incongruence or share it with the client. No false fronts can bring about positive change.

Being congruent might necessitate the expression of anger, frustration, liking, attraction, concern, boredom, annoyance, and a range of other feelings in the relationship. This does not mean that therapists should impulsively share all feelings, for self-disclosure must also be appropriate. Therapists must take responsibility for their own feelings and explore with the client persistent feelings that block their ability to be fully present with the client.[2]

Because therapists are human, genuineness is a process of development. As one grows in self-awareness and in experience within a therapeutic situation, one is able to become more congruent.

Unconditional Positive Regard and Acceptance   This attitude means that the clinician accepts clients as people who have self-worth, dignity, and the potential to change. Rogers described acceptance, caring, or prizing (unconditional positive regard) in the following way:

> It means that when the therapist is experiencing a positive, acceptant attitude toward whatever the client *is* at that moment, therapeutic movement or change is more likely. It involves the therapist's willingness for the client to be whatever feeling is going on at that moment—confusion, resentment, fear, anger, courage, love or pride. It is a nonpossessive caring. The therapist prizes the client in a total rather than a conditional way. This resembles the love the parent sometimes feels toward an infant. Research indicates that the more this attitude is experienced by the therapist, the greater the probability that therapy will be successfull.[31]

It is not, of course, possible to feel such an unconditional caring all of the time. A therapist who is being her real self will often admit to having very different feelings—negative feelings—toward the client. Hence it is not to be regarded as an absolute "should" that the therapist have an unconditional positive regard for the client. It is simply a fact that unless this is a reasonably frequent ingredient in the relationship, constructive change is less likely. For change to happen, clients too must feel this acceptance that enables them to share their real thoughts, feelings and behaviors.

Empathetic Understanding   In general, the person-centered counselor refrains from giving advice or providing solutions to the client's problems. They assist the client in finding his own answers. Even though clients may ask for a solution to a particular problem, they are helped to find their own answers within. To provide the answers is to imply that the clinician knows what is best for the client, which is not in keeping with person-centered therapy. One of the clinician's main tasks, however, is to understand accurately the client's feelings, thoughts and behaviors. Empathetic understanding enables the clinician to experience the world of the client from the client's perspective, without, however, becoming lost in the feelings. Rogers defined empathetic understanding in the following way:

The therapist senses accurately the feelings and personal meanings that are being experienced by the client and communicates this understanding to the client. At its best the therapist is so much inside the private world of the other that she can clarify not only the meanings of which the client is aware but even those just below the level of awareness. When she responds at such a level, the client's reaction is of this sort: "Perhaps that is what I've been trying to say. I haven't realized it, but, yes, that's how I do feel!"[27]

Therapists can learn to be more sensitive and more empathetic listeners. The process of empathetic understanding has been developed as a skill. In Chapter 8 we presented the components of the listening skills first noted by Rogers. These same skills have been included in the Counseling Triangle explored earlier in this chapter.

Application to Fluency Therapists   The development of these characteristics is an essential aspect of the clinician-counselor's personal growth and professional responsibility. We have expanded elsewhere on their importance for the clinical practice of speech-language pathologists and audiologists.[13] The major technique for empathy is active listening, which is described in Chapter 8. We believe the work of all fluency specialists would be enhanced by appropriating Rogers' person-centered approach.

The Counseling Relationship

Rogers described the relationship between the clinician and the client as the important vehicle of therapy: "If I can provide a certain type of relationship, the other person will discover within himself the capacity to use that relationship for personal growth and change, and personal development will occur. Significant personality change does not occur except in a relationship."[27] In this understanding, the counseling relationship is characterized by an equality between the clinician and the client that is the basis for the following dynamic:

- Two persons are in psychological contact.
- The first, whom we shall term the client, is in a state of incongruence, being vulnerable or anxious.
- The second person, whom we shall term the therapist, is congruent or integrated in the relationship.
- The therapist experiences unconditional positive regard for the client.
- The therapist experiences an empathetic understanding of the client's internal frame of reference and endeavors to communicate this experience to the client.The communication to the client of the therapist's empathic understanding and unconditional positive regard is to a minimal degree achieved.

If these conditions exist over time, the relationship will become the vehicle for the client's personal growth and change. It is quite possible that the clinician will also experience personal development if the relationship is strong.

Application to Fluency Therapists: As noted earlier, this relationship is basic to the practice of all therapy. Fluency clients in particular profit from the atmosphere of acceptance and personal concern. As Manning put it:

> I do not believe you can really know what to do in treatment with another person until you begin to establish a relationship with them. Establishing that relationship normally takes at least three or four sessions. Before I can make accurate and reasonable clinical decisions, I need to know how motivated the client is. I must know his story and begin to understand his situation in order to develop empathy for this person. I need to have a sense of his personality before I can probe and challenge him. Moreover, I need to get a feeling about how tough he will be when asked to apply his treatment techniques in the real world.[7]

Although we incorporate additional approaches in our therapy, the person-centered approach is the basic, relational foundation of our interaction with fluency clients. In addition to the psychoanalytic approach, we incorporate in our therapy Rogers' basic belief in the person's ability to choose his own good, his understanding of the characteristics of the counselor, and his stress on the importance of the relationship. These are the foundation for our understanding of the process of counseling, with which we may integrate other therapy approaches, several of which we consider next.

3. Gestalt Therapy

Frederick Perls has been credited with founding gestalt therapy,[32-34] according to which the most important areas to be considered are the thoughts and feelings that the client has in the moment. Perls viewed human beings as a total organism—hence the German word "gestalt," which means whole. Healthy behavior happens, according to Perls, when one is grounded in the "here and now" and responds as a total organism. Gestalt therapy teaches that when people disperse their concentration and attention among too many needs at one time, their lives become fragmented, and this fragmentation will often manifest itself physically and through our feelings rather than cognitively.

We often fool ourselves about the truth of our lives. Perls believed that healthy people may experience conflict and fragmentation, but that with a high degree of concentration and self-awareness, they can solve their problems. Thompson and Rudolph explained the process in the following way:

> The healthy person focuses sharply on one need (the figure) at a time while relegating other needs to the background. When the need is met—or the gestalt is closed and completed—it is relegated to the background, and a new need comes into focus (becomes the figure). The smoothly functioning figure-ground relationship characterizes the healthy personality. The domi-

nant need of the organism at any time becomes the foreground figure, and the other needs recede, at least temporarily, into the background.[6]

Gestalt therapy teaches that it is the need of the organism to maintain homeostasis; when a need is perceived and completed, homeostasis is restored. People who have not attended to their personal needs may be out of balance with "unfinished business." Unexpressed feelings and aborted dreams may be clamoring for their attention. This "unfinished business" may also lurk in the background to compromise a person's ability to function effectively in the present. It has been said[31] that most of Perls' doctrine can be summed up in his famous "Gestalt prayer":

> I do my thing and you do your thing.
> I am not in this world to live up to your expectations,
> And you are not in this world to live up to mine.
> You are you and I am I
> And if by chance we find each other it is beautiful.
> If not it can't be helped.

Basic Concepts of Gestalt Therapy

Here and Now Orientation   It is important for clients to gain awareness of what they are experiencing and doing *now*. The clinician calls attention to the client's posture, facial mannerisms, gestures, voice, and breathing. The client is led to fully experience the present moment through a series of "what" and "how" questions: "What are you doing now?" "How are you feeling now?" "What is going on now as you sit there trying to talk to me?" "How are you experiencing your fear?" "What are you attempting to withdraw from?" Gestaltists help the client grow in his awareness of the importance of fully experiencing the present.

Polster and Polster[35] stressed this focus of gestalt therapy and proclaimed that "power is in the present." They believed that "a most difficult truth to teach is that only the present exists now and that to stray from it distracts from the living quality of reality." For many people, the power of the present is lost as their energies are spent in feeling badly about what was and what might have been, and what may be. Perls[33] stated that such behavior leads individuals to experience anxiety. "In thinking of the future they may experience 'stage fright,' for they become filled with 'catastrophic' expectations of the bad things that will happen."

The gestalt approach does not ignore the past, but tries to understand it as somehow related to present feelings and ideas. Corey[21] explained:

> When the past seems to have a significant bearing on one's present attitudes or behavior, it is dealt with by bringing it into the present as much as possible. Thus, when clients speak about their past, the therapist asks them to bring it into the now by re-enacting it as though they were living it here and now.

This promotes a direct experiencing of the feelings rather than an abstract discussion of the situation.

Application to Fluency Therapists   In fluency therapy, we encourage our clients to carefully monitor their physiologic behaviors (Chapter 5). In addition, clients should monitor their feelings in the various situations in which they are dysfluent. Gestalt therapy helps us to recognize the movement necessary to bring the feelings of the past into the present and provides some techniques that can hasten the awareness of those feelings. But it should be cautioned that this aspect of gestalt therapy can be extremely powerful. Clinician-counselors must focus clients' awareness around the stuttering behaviors and must be willing to support them through the encounter with these often painful feelings. We know that healing often happens by going through this process, and clients feel freer after they are able to express themselves. In our experience of group therapy with fluency clients, we have found that while many are receptive to this technique, others can be quite resistant. Because of the intensity of feelings that can be uncovered by this process, we allow gestalt therapy to inform our practice, but do not pursue it in the traditional gestalt manner.

Responsibility   Gestalt therapy promotes the understanding on the part of the client that each individual, and no one else, is responsible for his life. Accepting responsibility for one's life is characteristic of a healthy personality. When one denies personal responsibility, one gives up power and control. Perls[34] cast this understanding in terms of "response-ability," by which he meant the ability to respond. Whenever a person acts, decides, or chooses, he practices response-ability. One of the ways a person keeps from exercising control over his own life is by avoidance. Because we have a tendency to avoid confronting our guilt, anxiety, fear, and grief, we often choose not to deal with them. This failure to take responsibility for these feelings block our possibilities of growth. When these emotions are not owned up to, "they become a nagging undercurrent that prevents us from being fully alive."[21] As we take more responsibility for our lives, our avoidances will decrease.

Application to Fluency Therapists   This stress on responsibility by gestalt therapy is highly valued by those who practice a synergistic approach to fluency therapy. We have highlighted it under the concept of Locus of Control. So many people who stutter consider stuttering to be "something that happens to them," or they report the feeling of being "stuck." It is enlightening for such clients to learn the language of responsibility—for example, "I am pushing my tongue against my teeth." Furthermore, the focus on avoidance behavior can be quite profitable. Many people who stutter are able to list all their avoidances with great ease while the painful feelings associated with them are kept buried inside. Only by openly acknowledging these feelings can the associated avoidance behaviors be overcome.

Use of Techniques   Gestalt uses techniques or "games" to help the client come to an increased awareness and experience of buried feelings and work through unfinished business. Although there are many games used by Gestalt therapists, we will highlight only two as outlined respectively by Thompson and Rudolph[6] and Corey.[21]

Language Games One activity is to encourage the use of the word *I* when the client uses a generalized *you*. For example: "*You* know how it is when *you* can't understand math and the teacher gets on your back," substituting "I" for "you," the message becomes, "I know how it is when I can't understand math and the teacher gets on my back." This helps children and adults to take responsibility for their own feelings, thoughts and behaviors.

In another game, substitue "what" and "how" for "why." We are often not aware of exactly why we do things, but we can become aware of what we are doing and how we are doing it.

One can also change questions into statements. This method has the effect of helping people to be more authentic and direct in expressing their thoughts and feelings. Perls believed that many questions are really disguised statements. The questions are used to prevent them from directly making declarations about themselves.

In another language game, clients are asked to fill in sentence blanks as another way of examining personal responsibility for the way that they manage their lives. For example, "Right now I am feeling _____ and I take _____ percent responsibility for how I feel." The exercise is quite an eye-opener for those clients who tend to view external causes as the total source of their good and bad feelings.

The Empty Chair Technique This technique is often used to resolve a conflict either between people or within the person. First, a person sits in one chair and acts the part of either another person or of one side of some inner conflict relating to a desirable or undesirable behavior. Then, the person moves to another chair and assumes the opposite part. It is essentially a role-playing technique in which all the parts are played by the client. This technique helps one to understand feelings and different points of view and to make better decisions. The same dynamic can be manifested as a process in which one writes to one part of the body about a feeling that then answers back. The important thing is that one tune into the feelings associated with the dialogue.

Application to Fluency Therapists Once again, we urge clinicians to exercise caution when using these techniques. Expression of feeling is essential and these games and techniques are valuable tools for doing so. However, a clinician-counselor who uses them must first have worked on her own issues and be aware of and prepared for the strength of the feelings that may be evoked. If used sensitively, these techniques can assist a fluency client to get in touch with many repressed feelings related to the experience of stuttering. It is important that some of the stutterer's shame, guilt, and embarrassment of both the past and the present be discussed. When a client can face his buried feelings, he can begin the process of letting them go. It is especially important in fluency therapy to create an atmosphere in which this might be done. Finally, the language techniques are an excellent way of helping the client assume responsibility for his fluency behavior.[36]

4. Rational-Emotive Therapy

Rational-emotive therapy (RET) departs somewhat from the other therapies we have covered in this chapter and can be considered as an example of cognitive therapy. RET stresses thinking, analyzing, and deciding. Albert Ellis,[37-41] who founded RET, found that his training as a psychotherapist was inadequate in preparing him to deal with his clients. Gradually, he began to ask his clients to do the very things they were most afraid of doing, such as risking rejection by significant others. He followed this advice in his own life and gradually developed his eclectic theory of counseling. However, Ellis acknowledged his debt to the ancient Greeks, especially the Stoic philosopher Epictetus, who is quoted as having said in the first century A.D. "Men are disturbed not by things, but by the view which they take of them."[40]

Corey[21] wrote:

> Rational-Emotive Therapy is based on the assumption that human beings are born with a potential for both rational, straight thinking and irrational, crooked thinking. People have predispositions for self-preservation, happiness, thinking and verbalizing, loving, communion with others, and growth and self-actualization. They also have the propensities for self-destruction, avoidance of thought, procrastination, endless repetition of mistakes, superstition, intolerance, perfectionism and self-blame, and avoidance of actualizing growth potentials.

Our "crooked thinking" is often learned from our environment (parents, teachers, and friends). Ellis believed that humans are often irrational, self-defeating individuals who need to be taught to be otherwise. They think crookedly about their desires and preferences and escalate them self-defeatingly into musts, shoulds, oughts, and demands. In assimilating these irrational beliefs, people become emotionally disturbed and experience anger, anxiety, depression, or other negative feelings that lead to destructive behavior.

Thompson and Rudolph[6] and Manning[7] cited Ellis' list of irrational beliefs that cause people trouble:

- It is a dire necessity for people to be loved or approved by almost everyone for virtually everything they do.
- One should be thoroughly competent, adequate, and achieving in all possible respects.
- Certain people are bad, wicked, or villainous and they should be severely blamed and punished for their sins.
- It is terrible, horrible, and catastrophic when things are not going the way one would like them to go.
- Human unhappiness is externally caused, and people have little or no ability to control their sorrows or rid themselves of their negative feelings.
- If something is or may be dangerous or fearsome, one should be occupied with and upset about it.

- It is easier to avoid facing many life difficulties and self-responsibilities than to undertake more rewarding forms of self-discipline.
- The past is all-important; because something once strongly affected one's life, it should do so indefinitely.
- People and things should be different from the way they are, and it is catastrophic if perfect solutions to the grim realities of life are not immediately found.
- Maximum human happiness can be achieved by inertia and inaction or by passively and uncommittedly enjoying oneself.
- My child is emotionally disturbed (or mentally retarded); therefore, he or she is severely handicapped and will never amount to anything.
- I cannot give my children everything they want; therefore, I am inadequate.

Strategies for the Practice of RET Ellis and Grieger[41] provided some helpful suggestions for detecting irrational beliefs: (1) Look for "awfulizing" and ask the person, "What is awful in this situation?" (2) Look for beliefs such as "I can't stand it!" and examine what it is about this situation that the person believes is unbearable. (3) Look for "musturbating" kinds of thoughts and determine what "shoulds," "oughts," or "musts" the person is telling himself about the situation. (4) Look for blaming or damning of self or others and ask, "What does the person view as damnable or unforgivable about this behavior?"

Another simple way Ellis recommends for detecting irrational beliefs is to look for them under one of three major "musterbating" belief systems: (1) I am no good unless I always do well and receive complete acceptance for my performance (I must behave perfectly and be loved and accepted by everyone). (2) You are no good unless you always act fairly and kindly toward me (you must behave in ways that please me). (3) Life is no good unless it always provides me what I want or believe I deserve (life must be the way I believe it should be). Almost all irrational beliefs are understood by Ellis to be related in some way to one or more of these three irrational beliefs.

Application to Fluency Therapists Fluency therapy built on RET has already been discussed in Chapter 7, where the three-column technique was presented. We know that no matter how hard our fluency clients work for success, if they are gripped by the fear of failure or other irrational thoughts, it will neutralize their efforts and make fluency impossible. It is important that they confront these negative, irrational thoughts explained by this cognitive theory.

Carolyn Gregory[42] has found the strength of cognitive therapy to lie in its basic premise that most emotional problems center around what you tell yourself. She listed the following unreasonable beliefs of people who stutter:

- To become a perfect fluent talker, all I *must* do is take out the stuttering blocks and leave my speech and personality just as it is. I'm perfect just as I am.

- Other people talk fast and in a continuous stream and I *must* do this.
- Other people do not dread public speaking, social gatherings, job interviews, making introductions etc. Neither *must* I hate doing these things.
- To be successful in therapy, I *must* talk perfectly without feeling a moment of tension or emitting even one of those horrible "stutter" sounds.
- I *must* never have to think about how I am talking.
- Practicing speech is a boring chore to be eliminated as soon as I talk fluently.

Gregory[42] pointed out the following techniques employed by Ellis that will help our fluency clients:

- Actively deny awfulness. Ninety-five percent of people believe in it. Deal with shame, do something embarrassing not in the realm of speech. Role-play being laughed at.
- Use coping beliefs. I'm a fallible human being—acceptable and likeable to some persons. I have some good and some bad traits. I do not need anything I want. I'd like to succeed but I don't have to. Its not bad to be rejected, because I can go on to something else.
- List the advantages and disadvantage of practicing speech, of using my modified speech, of stuttering, of phrasing, of learning voluntary disfluency. Think of 20 on each side.
- Use thought stopping. I'll only allow myself to think about this for ten minutes. For that time I'll wallow in it.
- Ask what is the worst that can happen. Feel the queasiness. Then change your thoughts and your feelings to milder disappointment or sadness—but ongoingness.
- Have clients teach RET to others. Find others who mustardize and talk them out of their irrational thoughts.
- Rate your performance but never yourself!

We, too, have found these techniques can be extremely helpful to our fluency clients. Some of our techniques have included disputing self-defeating thoughts in the following ways:

Shoulds: I *should* do. . . . I *should* be . . . It *should* happen.
Ask yourself: Is that a true rule of the whole human race?
Dispute your irrational thoughts:
   "I wish I didn't have to . . . , but. . . ."
   "It would be nice if he did, but. . . ."
   "I want that to be so, but I don't need it, so. . . ."

Awfulizing: What if. . . ? I couldn't stand it!
Ask yourself: What is the worst that could happen? How likely is that? Would you collapse or die?

Dispute your irrational thoughts:
    "That would be very unpleasant but you could stand it."
    "It might be inconvenient but I could manage."
    "I'll see what choices I can make to make it better."

Mistakes: I'm afraid I'll mess up. I'll never forgive myself.
    Ask yourself: Is there some special reason why I shouldn't
        make mistakes? All humans do. Why not me?
    Dispute your irrational thoughts:
        "Of course I made a mistake. Everyone does. Why not me?"
        "The past is over. It's okay to forget about it."
        "Now is when I can do something about it."

David Maxwell[43] studied the use of cognitive restructuring with fluency clients in which the clinician modeled revised negative thoughts. First, the client was asked by the therapist to shut his eyes, imagine himself in the classroom, and to express his thoughts about speaking as if he were talking to himself. The client verbalized the following:

Oh, Lord, here I am in class with all of these people and soon I'm going to have to talk. What if my controls don't work? What if I fall on my face—make a fool of myself ? Then they'll think I'm stupid. Maybe I ought to quietly get up and walk out of here. Maybe there won't be time to get to my report. If I stutter, will they laugh or feel pity?[43]

Serving as a model, the therapist then imitated the nonproductive content and demonstrated how to revise the negative elements comprising this internal dialogue. Specifically, the therapist modeled the following revision:

I am now in class with other students like me discussing the subject of art history. Soon I will be asked to speak on a topic that I know well. I have interesting information to share. When I speak, I plan to use, to the best of my ability, the controls that I've learned to use well in therapy. What I want to convey is the strong interest I have in my topic. I'll remember to smile, maintain eye contact with my listeners, and try to be open and friendly.[43]

The client was then asked to reverbalize several monologues until they resembled the clinician's. This cognitive strategy was found to be very successful with fluency clients.

We believe that RET is rich with applications for fluency therapy. We know that the greatest success in life occur when we recognize that we have the power to turn obstacles into opportunities. This theory provides an excellent method for empowering our clients.

THE COUNSELING TRIANGLE: THE SKILLS OF COUNSELING

These skills were thoroughly explained in Chapter 8. We believe that they allow the issues related to theory to be explored and the therapeutic response to those issues to take place.[22,44]

Active listening must be studied and practiced by the clinician-counselor. However, one must recognize that the underlying strength of this and related communication skills is the sincere interest of the therapist in the client's life and her wholehearted attempt to understand the client's world. When that happens, the clinician will be an invaluable part of the therapeutic process. Luterman[44] wrote:

> It is virtually impossible for one person to damage another by listening to him, by trying to understand what the world looks like to him, by permitting him to express what is in him, and by honestly giving him the information he needs. In this view of counseling, the clinician serves as an accepting listener. He delays his judgment and tries to accept parents (*and clients*) as they are and as they will become.

Thus, it is our belief that counseling is a multifaceted process in which the clinician-counselor has an important role. However, one must integrate each of the areas of the Counseling Triangle; understanding the current theories of counseling and finding in them issues that assist in the change process; exploring these issues within oneself; and, finally, learning the skills necessary to assist the client in reshaping his fluency disorder and his life.

SUMMARY

In this chapter, we highlighted the necessity of speech-language pathologists recognizing the importance of incorporating aspects of counseling into therapy. As clinician-counselors, we must be knowlegeable about the helping process. In addition to examining the phases of the helping process, we defined and expanded on the dimensions (the Counseling Triangle): (1) the personal development of the clinician-counselor, (2) the theories of counseling from which we draw on understanding of both counseling issues and counseling techniques (we examined four theories—psychoanalytical, person-centered, gestalt, and rational-emotive therapy), and (3) the skills of counseling (that are expanded on in Chapter 8).

REFERENCES

1. Brammer LM. Who can be a helper? *Personnel Guidance* 1977;55:303–308.
2. Crowe T. *Applications of Counseling in Speech-Language Pathology and Audiology.* Baltimore: Williams and Wilkins, 1997:ix–108.
3. Nugent F. *An Introduction to the Profession of Counseling.* Columbus, OH: Merrill, 1990:5.

4. Jones K. Counseling and the speech-language pathologist and audiologist. Presented at the annual meeting of the New York State Speech Language Hearing Association, Kimaesha Lake, NY, April 23, 1990:2.
5. Rollin WJ. *The Psychology of Communication Disorders in Individuals and Their Families.* Englewood Cliffs, NJ: Prentice Hall, 1987:4.
6. Thompson C, Rudolph L. *Counseling Children.* Pacific Grove, CA: Brooks/Cole, 1996:7–18.
7. Manning W. *Clinical Decision Making in the Diagnosis and Treatment of Fluency Disorders.* Albany, NY: Delmar, 1996:178–179.
8. Luterman D. *Counseling Persons with Communication Disorders and Their Families.* Boston: Little Brown, 1996:47.
9. American Speech Language and Hearing Association. Preferred practices patterns for the professions of speech-language pathology and audiology. *ASHA Journal,* 1993;35:3, supplement, 1–102.
10. American Speech Language and Hearing Association. Scope of practice, speech-language pathology and audiology. *ASHA Journal,* 1993;35:3, supplement, 1–102.
11. Scheuerle J. *Counseling in Speech Language Pathology and Audiology.* New York: Macmillan, 1992:22–216.
12. Kennedy E. *On Becoming a Counselor.* New York: Continuum, 1980.
13. Bloom CM, Cooperman DK. *The Clinical Interview: A Guide for Speech-Language Pathologists and Audiologists* (2nd ed). Rockville, MD: NSSLHA, 1992:61.
14. Egan G. *The Skilled Helper* (3rd ed). Monterey, CA: Brooks/Cole, 1986.
15. Carkhuff RR. *Helping and Human Relations* (Vol. 2). Amherst, MA: Human Resource Development Press, 1984.
16. Hepworth D, Larsen J. *Direct Social Work Practice.* Chicago: Dorsey Press, 1986.
17. Brammer LM. *The Helping Relationship: Process and Skills* (4th ed). Englewood Cliffs, NJ: Prentice Hall, 1988.
18. Schum RL, Cooper EB. *Counseling in Speech and Hearing Practice* (Clinical Series No. 9). Rockville, MD: NSSLHA, 1986.
19. Compton B, Galway B. *Social Work Processes* (4th ed). Belmont, CA: Wadsworth, 1989:31–306.
20. Murphy B, Dillon C. *Interviewing in Action.* Pacific Grove, CA: Brooks/Cole, 1998:252.
21. Corey G. *Theory and Practice of Counseling and Psychotherapy* (3rd ed). Monterey, CA: Brooks/Cole, 1986:102–369.
22. Ivey A. *Intentional Interviewing and Counseling* (3rd ed). Belmont, CA: Brooks/Cole, 1994.
23. Spielberg G. Graduate training in helpful relationships: Helpful or harmful? *J Humanistic Psychol,* 1980; 20:57–70.
24. Hoff B. *The Tao of Pooh.* New York: Dutton, 1982:2.
25. Corey M., Corey G. *Becoming a Helper.* Monterey, CA: Brooks/Cole, 1989:13.
26. Simon S. Six conditions for nurturing self-esteem. Presented at the American School Counselors Association Convention. Breckenridge, CA, 1998.
27. Rogers C. *On Becoming a Person.* Boston: Houghton Mifflin, 1961:90–92.
28. Rogers C. *A Way of Being.* Boston: Houghton Mifflin, 1980.
29. Maslow A. *Motivation and Personality.* New York: Harper and Row, 1970.
30. Maslow A. *The Farther Reaches of Human Nature.* New York: Viking Press, 1971.
31. Rogers C. *Carl Rogers on Personal Power.* New York: Delacorte Press, 1977.
32. Perls F. *Gestalt Therapy.* Moab, UT: Real People Press, 1969:4–30.
33. Perls F. *The Gestalt Approaches and Eyewitness to Therapy.* New York: Bantam Books, 1976.

34. Perls F. Concepts and misconceptions of gestalt therapy. *J Humanistic Psychol* 1992;32(3):50–56.
35. Polster E, Polster M. *Gestalt Therapy Integrated: Contours of Theory and Practice*. New York: Brunner/Magel, 1973:7.
36. Starkweather CW, Gootwald SR, Halfond M. *Stuttering Prevention: A Clinical Method*. Englewood Cliffs, NJ: Prentice Hall, 1990.
37. Ellis A. The theory of rationale-emotive therapy. In A Ellis, J Whitely (eds), *Theoretical and Empirical Foundations of Rationale-Emotive Therapy*. Monterey, CA: Brooks/Cole, 1979.
38. Ellis A. Reflections on rationale-emotive therapy. *J Consult Clin Psychol* 1993; 61(2):199–201.
39. Ellis A. Rationale-emotive therapy. In R Corsini (ed), *Current Psychotherapies* (3rd ed). Ithaca, NY: Peacock, 1984.
40. Ellis A. The impossibility of achieving consistently good mental health. *Amer Psychol* 1987;42:364–375.
41. Ellis A, Grieger R. *Handbook of Rationale-Emotive Therapy*. New York: Springer, 1977:10–11.
42. Gregory C. On developing a psychotherapeutic frame for work with stutterers. Stuttering Therapy: A Workshop for Specialists, Chicago, 1991:158–161.
43. Maxwell D. Cognitive and behavioral self-control strategies: Application for the clinical management of the adult stutterer. *J Fluency Disord* 1982;7:403–432.
44. Luterman D. *Counseling Persons with Communication Disorders* (3rd ed). Austin, TX: Pro-Ed, 1996:7.

10

Synergistic Model of Service Delivery

The Synergistic Model of service delivery is a combination of short-term intensive and long-term nonintensive follow-up therapy. We offer both group and individual components, and our treatment philosophy combines elements of fluency shaping and stuttering modification. These program options were described briefly in Chapter 4 and are further explained in this chapter. We have been influenced in this therapeutic decision to integrate the two approaches by our own observations as well as the investigations and reported research of many of our colleagues—Andrews and Cutler,[1] Andrews and Ingham,[2] Conture,[3] Gregory,[4] Gregory and Campbell,[5] Gregory and Hill,[6] Guitar and Peters,[7] Peters and Guitar,[8] Ryan,[9,10] Schwartz,[11,12] Sheehan,[13] Starkweather et al.,[14] Van Riper,[15] Wall and Myers,[16] and Webster.[17]

SHORT-TERM INTENSIVE THERAPY

The short-term intensive treatment usually occurs during our spring Weekend Workshop. The format of the Weekend Workshop and a schedule of a typical weekend will be described later in this chapter. For individuals who cannot attend our Weekend Workshop, there is an option for more intensive short-term treatment at our campus clinical facility. Instead of participating from Friday night until Sunday afternoon, as they would if they were to attend the Workshop, clients may elect to be scheduled for half-hour sessions four times a week for the first four to six weeks of therapy in the clinic. Although these clients miss out on the community-building and motivational benefits that always occur at the Workshop, they do benefit from this clinically intensive introduction to the fluency shaping components of the program.

LONG-TERM NONINTENSIVE TREATMENT

The long-term component of treatment takes place weekly and is usually ongoing for a period of approximately five years. Our informal research has suggested that, although fluency can be instated rather quickly, five years is the optimum period of time for maintaining fluency, for establishing a more internalized locus of control, and for developing enhanced self-esteem and assertiveness. During this long-term phase of treatment, clients are invited to participate in a weekly two-hour evening program that is divided into two separate sessions: The first is a one-hour support group meeting run by group members with consultation from graduate student clinicians and experienced speech-language pathologists; this is followed by one hour of individual therapy conducted by a graduate student with supervision, once again, from a speech-language pathologist who specializes in the treatment of stuttering. Ham[18] has written about the value of group therapy, either as a component of therapy or as the "primary therapy vehicle." Issues appropriate for group intervention, according to Ham, include "motivation, instruction, socialization, transfer, skills learning, attitude change, expansion of individual therapy, and maintenance support."

INDIVIDUAL THERAPY

Individual therapy sessions are conducted by graduate student therapists who have completed an undergraduate course in fluency disorders and who are enrolled in or who have completed a graduate-level course in fluency disorders. Lesson plans are submitted to supervisors in advance of each session and must reflect attention to the goals that have been mutually agreed upon by the student therapist and the client and that are written in a formal treatment plan at the beginning of each academic semester. Goals include the practice of fluency targets as well as a focus on the attitudinal and environmental elements described previously in this text. Although fluency shaping is emphasized during these treatment sessions, stuttering modification remains a priority in all contact with clients. Effective communication is a consistent focus throughout treatment.

Activities of treatment occur within the therapy room, on the telephone, in various campus locations, and in locations in the larger community outside the campus. Student therapists use tape recorders and videotape equipment to support individual treatment sessions. Data collection occurs during every session, beginning with the determination of a baseline for fluency in reading, monologue, and conversation at the start of each session and ending with a posttreatment measurement of each of these parameters at the session's close.

GROUP THERAPY

The support group component of our treatment model targets not only the practice of fluency enhancing controls, but also the development of self-esteem, effective communication skills, positive attitudes, and self-help strategies in preparation for dealing with the relapse that so frequently occurs in individuals who attempt to control their stuttering.[15,19] Researchers have noted that stuttering relapse occurs with a frequency ranging from more than 50 percent to up to 90 percent of the individuals (adults and teenagers) who have been "successfully" treated for stuttering.[20,21] This is a surprising statistic in view of the reported effectiveness of many stuttering treatment programs.[10,17,22]

Several hypotheses have been proposed to explain this relapse phenomenon.[23] The most typical is that the client may have assumed that the treatment he received represented a "cure" for the stuttering and did not feel the need to continue practice; therapy may have been terminated too soon and the client's fluency skills did not become well established; and the client may not have had the opportunity to change his perceptions of himself. Whatever explanations might apply in each individual case, our suspicion is that the root cause in most cases of relapse is that the client was insufficiently prepared for handling speaking situations without what we consider the necessary support systems being in place.

We have chosen very consciously to use the therapist-driven model of support for our program. In the early stages of program development, we adopted a self-help model but found that this was unsatisfactory to the clients, as they felt they needed more of a "practice" focus for meetings. We have always attempted to be responsive to the feedback of our clients and changed the nature of the support component at their request. However, in changing the focus, we did not change the philosophy of support. We believe that a support group environment should be one that fosters success in the development of positive attitudes, self-esteem, confidence, and acceptably fluent speech. This last concept is one that we encourage our clients to define for themselves. Our clients must feel comfortable with their achieved levels of fluency in order for them to be motivated to continue participating in our program.

Format for the Support Group Session

Our typical group session begins with an "ice breaker" activity that lasts for about ten minutes. During the ice breaker, group members briefly discuss topics of general interest. Although each group member is encouraged to participate in this activity, individuals may always choose to pass when it is their turn to speak. Some group members are reluctant to participate at first, but most eventually join the conversation. A different group member is responsible each week for leading the meeting and preparing the activities for that evening. Group leaders volunteer for this role, each selecting a particular meeting during the course of the semester. A schedule of meetings and group leader volunteers is then prepared by student therapists and circulated early in the semester.

Following the ice breaker, the members engage in a 20-minute speaking activity, often the discussion of a topic related to fluency or stuttering. This may be a response to a brief article that is summarized for them by the leader or a topic that may be timely (seasonal issues, holiday themes, discussion of difficult speaking situations). Student therapists generally provide materials from which the designated leader chooses the night's topic. This is a community-building activity designed to elicit the interaction and participation of all group members.

The final activity of the group meeting is a discussion of feelings connected with stuttering. The group leader for the week directs this discussion. This part of the meeting lasts for approximately 30 minutes and is usually very lively. Group members report that for some this is the first opportunity they have had to share openly their fears and triumphs with people who understand the pain of communicating in a fluent world. We are always moved by the openness and courage of group members and never fail to come away from these weekly meetings with a renewed sense of commitment to our work.

Support Groups and Self-Help

The last half of the twentieth century has seen the advent of what has become known as the "self-help movement" in the United States and Europe.[24-26] Ramig[27] reported that there are more than 500,000 support groups of various types in the United States alone, and that these groups serve more than 12 million people. Hunt[28] described the self-help movement in Britain, with a particular focus on the Association for Stammerers (AFS). He found that although the AFS has not been successful in raising the funds necessary for effective operation, it has been successful in promoting self-help principles among smaller British self-help groups of individuals who stutter. Hunt noted that "the mutual advice and support obtainable within the group setting represents their most valued feature."[28]

In addition to the AFS, there are a number of other international and American self-help groups for people who stutter. These include the National Stuttering Project (NSP), Speak Easy International Foundation, the National Council on Stuttering (NCOS), the Swedish Stammering Association, and the Canadian Association for People Who Stutter (CAPS).[21,27,29] In recent years the Internet has become a high-tech self-help network for many. The establishment of stuttering discussion groups like STUTT-L and STUT-HLP as well as the Stuttering Home Page maintained by Judy Kuster at Mankato State University have added a new dimension to the practice of self-help in that subscribers are free to explore topics of interest related to stuttering and fluency with an expanded international network of individuals.[29] For some, the fact that this is a nonverbal mode of communication allows a greater degree of freedom of expression without the fear of stuttering.

Individuals who join self-help or support groups do so for a variety of reasons. Hunt[28] suggested that these may include the desire for mutual aid and support from individuals with similar problems; the exchange of information; and the strength or political effectiveness of large groups of individuals seeking social change. Starkweather and Givens-Ackerman[29] identified the benefits of association with the self-help movement to be the experience of acceptance and support of others rather than the criticism and judgment of people in the fluent world. They went on to say that "this feeling of acceptance allows people who stutter to feel freer than they do when talking to the general public and, as a result, their speech often improves dramatically."[29] Ramig reported that, although there have been few systematic studies of the efficacy of self-help groups, clinicians and researchers tend to believe that "involvement in self-help groups for many persons who stutter is a positive and beneficial experience."[27] Our own experience suggests that support groups offer people who stutter a sense of community that has been absent from their lives. Many of our clients tell us that the support group taught them that they are not alone in their stuttering. This sentiment has been echoed many times by members of the NSP and subscribers to STUTT-L.

Cooper has endorsed the growth and development of support systems for individuals who stutter, citing the unfortunate tendency of some professionals to discourage their clients' participation in self-help groups. He suggested that "perhaps professionals experience discomfort believing that they or their colleagues have failed if former clients seek such support."[30] We have met a number of individuals who attended various behavioral treatment programs and were cautioned not to participate in self-help groups because they might ultimately begin to blend the stuttering controls they had learned in their treatment programs with the controls learned by other group members in other treatment programs, and eventually lose their fluency. We do not agree with this position.

We support our clients' interest in self-help and consider it to be an essential component of successful stuttering treatment and long-term maintenance of fluency. We agree with Johnson who wrote that after treatment "the person who stutters continues to need some support for their reality testing. In addition . . . some stuttering returns, which might shake their confidence."[31] We believe that in order for individuals who stutter to maintain what they consider acceptable fluency over time, they must form relationships with others who share their communication problem, be able to explore and express their feelings, attitudes, and beliefs in an environment of acceptance, and ultimately assume leadership roles in the community of individuals who stutter. It is for these reasons that we have organized a support group component for our treatment model. Although our group is not strictly "self-help" because we continue to remain involved in its structure and operation, we believe that it serves the purposes described earlier—namely, mutual support of individuals with similar problems, opportunities for the exchange of information, and strength in numbers when communicating with political or social agencies. In addition, we view the support group as a primary vehicle for the development of assertiveness, the enhancement of self-esteem, and the internalization of locus of control in individuals who stutter, variables that we consider essential to one's ability to maintain fluency over time.

According to Hunt, the ideal treatment program should combine "counseling with continuity of follow-up."[28] This, we contend, is a major strength of the Synergistic Approach. Our treatment model asks for a commitment to ongoing treatment in the form of support group participation that may last, optimally, for five years. Because of our support group component, we offer not only fluency instatement but ongoing counseling provided by the speech pathologist as well as peers. Hunt further wrote:

> Counseling may come from a fellow-sufferer or an older, more experienced speech therapist with a special interest. It is necessary for those who counsel stutterers, whether they be speech therapists or others, to tread a very

narrow dividing line, supporting and confirming the stutterer in the sense of his own normalcy and using this to build self-confidence, whilst at the same time promoting greater realism by enhancing the stutterer's awareness of others' perceptions of his speech patterns and coming to accept these responses, too, as "normal."[28]

Again, we believe that our Synergistic Approach allows for this kind of counseling experience. The support provided by group members and therapists takes many forms. The ongoing association of individuals who stutter allows for a sense of identification among them as well as a communicative ease, which flows from the familiarity and trust that develops. The feedback among group members is generally "on target," offered without rancor, and accepted positively. The feelings of mutual respect and trust that develop make peer counseling a successful adjunct to therapy. A fine example of the power of peer counseling was offered on the Internet by Tom Scharstein, a person who stutters and who also belongs to a chapter of the NSP. Tom shared the following experience:

> I just experienced last night what a (support group) chapter is all about. Please let me explain: A new potential member accompanied me to the meeting on Thursday night. She was hesitant at first, but came as a favor to me. I promised her she would sit next to me; not having to talk at all. . . . As we discussed the "fear of stuttering," she suddenly spoke up, and said, "What upsets me about stuttering is when people think I'm dumb . . ." as she clenched her fists in anger and the tears began to flow. . . . It seemed that possibly this was the first verbalization of this feeling. My eyes began to water . . . as everyone else's. The "moment" became tender . . . touching . . . she "reached" us. That's the beauty, the appeal, of a chapter. As we search for the "truths" within ourselves, they may suddenly appear.[32]

SUPPORT FOR INTENSIVE PROGRAMS

The decade of the 1970s saw the emerging popularity of many short-term intensive treatment programs for people who stutter. This popularity continued into the 1980s and, although less widely used today, short-term intensive treatment still has many supporters. In addition to residential summer camps like the Shady Trails Program, there were treatment-intensive opportunities like Webster's Precision Fluency Shaping Program,[33] the Geneseo College Starbuck Summer Clinics, the Australian Smooth Speech Program,[34] Boberg's Intensive Stuttering Treatment,[35] and Schwartz's Airflow Technique.[12] These programs have resulted in fluency for many individuals for some period of time, but few can claim large numbers of clients who continue to be fluent in all situations years after treatment.

Those who support intensive programs emphasize that they "allow a more focused period of intervention where external influences are minimized."[36] These proponents speak of client motivation being high during intensive treatment, with progress carefully measured and high levels of reported success.[33,37–41] When practice sessions are massed and participants have the opportunity to immerse themselves in fluency enhancing techniques, establishment of fluency can occur quickly and dramatically.

The research of Andrews and Tanner[42] suggests that short-term intensive treatment (they reported outcomes of a five-day treatment program) is less successful than more long-term intensive treatment, since the former results in temporary fluency commonly followed by relapse. They noted that intensive treatment without scheduled follow-up requires approximately 30 hours of direct therapist intervention in order for gains to be maintained over time.[42]

Hasbrouck and colleagues[43] reported on two public school applications of intensive stuttering treatment using procedures that had previously proved successful in the treatment of adults and that might serve to establish fluency quickly. In both treatment conditions, children were seen daily for a period of four weeks with no specific follow-up. The results of this study, using two slightly different program models, suggested that intensive treatment for school-age stuttering children was a practical and efficient way of delivering speech therapy services.

Cooper[30] has been highly critical of these short-term and long-term "quick-fix programs," stating that they mislead the person who stutters into thinking that he has been "cured" rather than recognizing that the intensive and in some cases residential elements of the program create an artificial environment that exerts a powerful but temporary influence over participants' behavior.

Manning[23] concurs, suggesting that although short-term intensive treatment may result in more rapid gains in fluency, the difficulty occurs when the client attempts to transfer these gains into the everyday world. The risk of failure of many short-term intensive treatment programs may relate to their lack of follow-up after the initial treatment period. Although some programs may have the option of "refresher sessions," these usually occur after the initial fluency has been lost and the client has already experienced a sense of failure. Too often, clients are not prepared for the relapse that almost certainly follows these intensive treatment experiences that may end abruptly and may have no ongoing therapist-monitored contact.

RATIONALE FOR THE SYNERGISTIC SERVICE DELIVERY MODEL

We believe that when fluency is the only goal, relapse is almost assured. Many individuals who have received stuttering treatment warn us not to teach our clients to "court the fluency god," and we have come to agree with this admonition. Fluency alone should be allowed to become the all-controlling end. It is for these reasons that we have developed the Synergistic Approach to balance the goal of establishing fluency with the attitudinal and environmental goals that are so important in assisting the client to realistically view stuttering as but one facet of life.

We use the intensive portion of our treatment program to instate fluency and to introduce the importance of attitudinal, environmental, and emotional modification. We then follow up with a long-term treatment plan that continues an emphasis on the practice of fluency skills but adds activities and exercises designed to enhance self-esteem, increase assertiveness, internalize locus of control and modify and/or manage environmental constraints. In this way we believe that we combine the best of fluency shaping and stuttering modification approaches.

WEEKEND WORKSHOP

The intensive portion of our program, as noted earlier, takes the form of what we call our "Weekend Workshop for Those Who Stutter." At the present time, given the constraints of our school calendar, we hold the Workshop only once each year, in the late winter or early spring. In 1998 we held our twenty-third annual Workshop. As our reputation has grown, the Workshop has become more popular, and during the past three years the number of clients we serve during the weekend has grown from perhaps 20 to approximately 70. Participants at first came from the local area, but we now draw participants from many east coast states, including Vermont, Massachusetts, Rhode Island, New Jersey, and Connecticut. The format of the Workshop as well as the components of the treatment program have changed over the years in response to feedback from our clients. We attempt to listen to their suggestions and incorporate them into our work, as we believe that the partnership between client and clinician is essential to successful treatment.

The specific format of each Weekend Workshop may differ as each centers around a different theme. Children and adults are grouped together for certain theme events, which has served as a powerful motivational device for both age groups. The theme concept seems to have contributed to a broad appeal for both children and adults. The adults enjoy serving as models of fluency for the younger clients and work at their fluency-enhancing skills diligently in order to demonstrate proficiency; the children, of course, are motivated by the element of friendly competition.

Themes have included the Fluency Olympics, the Super Bowl of Fluency, a Cruise to Fluency, Irish Fluency Festival, and March Madness–Shoot for Fluency. Each of these themes was developed to include activities and drills for which individual and team points were accumulated. A sample of activity/drill sheets from the March Madness weekend is provided in the Appendix. All clients at the Workshop are assigned to one of two teams. Throughout the weekend, the participants engage in various activities that earn points for their team. At the conclusion of the Workshop, the team with the greatest number of points wins the competition.

Therapists from local school districts, agencies, and private practices are invited to participate in our training program and to serve as supervisors of graduate students during the Weekend Workshop. Many of these therapists are former graduates of our program and engage in ongoing fluency therapy using the Synergistic Approach. In fact, many of our clients are referred to the Workshop by these therapists who believe that the intensive portion of the program is of great value, although they may not be able to provide this in their own work settings.

Parents and spouses are invited to meet with clinical faculty while their family members engage in practice sessions throughout the weekend. This is an excellent opportunity for the introduction of counseling techniques. Parents of new members of our program benefit from the information and insights shared by the more experienced parent group members. Spouses and significant others are introduced to the many unexpected changes and implications of a newly achieved level of fluency that occurs as a result of the Workshop.

For some the Workshop is an introduction to the treatment program while for others who have been enrolled in the program previously it serves as a refresher. Our returning clients and continuing Fluency Council members tell us that the Workshop is a very important element of their fluency maintenance. They view it as an opportunity to devote themselves to fluency-building skills for a concentrated period of time, during which they feel a renewed sense of motivation to practice. The successes that they experience during the weekend, both personal/social and fluency-related, energize them and stay with them for many weeks.

There is a Saturday night banquet, at which all program participants are encouraged to give after dinner speeches about stuttering or to perform some speaking task that provides inspiration and information for the audience members. This, too, is a highlight for many participants. Clients of all ages request an opportunity to speak before a very large audience, usually consisting of 150 to 200 people who regularly attend the dinner. Participants may elect to do group presentations and brief skits rather than speaking at the microphone, but all clients typically choose to participate in some way. For many, this is the first time they have ever chosen to speak before an audience. The sense of confidence and joy is pervasive.

The culmination of the weekend is a closing ceremony on Sunday during which each participant gives a brief talk about the weekend's experiences to an audience of other participants, family members, and students in our communication disorders program. Once again, there is a positive, upbeat, energy that pervades the assembly. The fragile fluency that has been gained during the course of the weekend is highly motivating to the participants, and this motivation must be harnessed so that more lasting fluency skills can be developed in the long-term nonintensive phase that follows.

SUMMARY

In this chapter, we have offered a description of our service delivery model that includes short-term intensive treatment followed by long-term nonintensive treatment. Our approach integrates fluency shaping with stuttering modification because we believe that fluency is not an end in itself. In order for an individual to benefit from stuttering therapy, he must go beyond the achievement of fluent speech, which often is a temporary condition, and learn self-acceptance, internalization of locus of control, increased self-esteem, and increased assertiveness, especially in communicative situations. The Synergistic Approach to fluency addresses each of these issues over the course of five years, with diminishing therapist input and increasing client independence.

We understand that we enjoy the luxury of not having to be concerned with the cost of treatment because we work in an academic setting where the fee structure is very low. But we do hope that you, the reader, will consider our philosophy of treatment and modify our Synergistic Approach to be compatible with your specific work setting requirements.

REFERENCES

1. Andrews G, Cutler J. Stuttering therapy: The relation between changes in symptom level and attitudes. *J Speech Lang Hear Disord* 1974;39:312–319.
2. Andrews G, Ingham R. Stuttering: Considerations in the evaluation of treatment. *Br J Commun Disord* 1971;6:129–138.
3. Conture EG. *Stuttering* (2nd ed). Englewood Cliffs, NJ: Prentice Hall, 1990.
4. Gregory HH. *Stuttering: Differential Evaluation and Therapy*. Austin, TX: Pro-Ed, 1986.
5. Gregory HH, Campbell JH. Stuttering in the school-age child. In DE Yoder, RD Kent (eds), *Decision Making in Speech-Language Pathology*. Toronto: B. C. Decker, 1986.
6. Gregory HH, Hill D. Stuttering therapy for children. *Semin Speech Lang* 1980;1:351–363.
7. Guitar B, Peters TJ. *Stuttering: An Integration of Contemporary Therapies*. Memphis, TN: Speech Foundation of America, 1980:16.
8. Peters TJ, Guitar B. *Stuttering: An Integrated Approach to Its Nature and Treatment*. Baltimore, MD: Williams and Wilkins, 1991.
9. Ryan BP. Stuttering therapy in a framework of operant conditioning and programmed learning. In HH Gregory (ed), *Controversies About Stuttering Therapy*. Baltimore, MD: University Park Press, 1979.
10. Ryan BP. *Programmed Therapy of Stuttering in Children and Adults*. Springfield, IL: Charles C. Thomas, 1974.
11. Schwartz MF. The core of the stuttering block. *J Speech Hear Disord* 1974;39:169–177.
12. Schwartz MF. *Stuttering Solved*. New York: McGraw-Hill, 1976.
13. Sheehan JG. *Stuttering Research and Therapy*. New York: Harper and Row, 1970.
14. Starkweather CW, Gottwald CR., Halfond M. *Stuttering Prevention: A Clinical Method*. Englewood Cliffs, NJ: Prentice Hall, 1990.
15. Van Riper C. *The Treatment of Stuttering*. Englewood Cliffs, NJ: Prentice Hall, 1973.
16. Wall MJ, Myers FL. *Clinical Management of Childhood Stuttering* (2nd ed). Austin, TX: Pro-Ed, 1995.
17. Webster RL. Empirical considerations regarding stuttering therapy. In HH Gregory (ed), *Controversies About Stuttering Therapy*. Baltimore, MD: University Park Press, 1979.
18. Ham RE. *Therapy of Stuttering*. Englewood Cliffs, NJ: Prentice Hall, 1990.

19. Perkins WH. Learning from negative outcomes in stuttering therapy: II. An epiphany of failures. *J Fluency Disord* 1983; 8:155–160.
20. Bloodstein O. *A Handbook on Stuttering* (4th ed). Chicago: National Easter Seal Society, 1987.
21. Silverman FH. Relapse following stuttering therapy. In NJ Lass (ed), *Speech and Language Advances in Basic Research and Practice*. New York: Academic Press, 1981:56–78.
22. Andrews G, Ingham R. Stuttering: An evaluation of follow-up procedures for syllable-timed speech/token system therapy. *J Commun Disord* 1972;5:307–319.
23. Manning W. *Clinical Decision Making in the Diagnosis and Treatment of Fluency Disorders*. Albany, NY: Delmar, 1996.
24. Katz AH, Bender E. *The Strength in Us: Self-Help Groups in the Modern World*. New York: Franklin Watts, 1976.
25. Kickbusch I, Hatch S. A Re-orientation of Health Care? In S Hatch, I Kickbusch (eds), *Self-Help and Health in Europe: New Approaches in Health Care*. Copenhagen: World Health Organization, 1983.
26. Richardson A, Goodman M. *Self-Help and Social Care: Mutual Aid Organizations in Practice*. London: Policy Studies Institute, 1983.
27. Ramig P. The impact of self-help groups on persons who stutter: A call for research. *J Fluency Disord* 1993;18:351–361.
28. Hunt B. Self-help for stutterers: Experience in Britain. In L Rustin, H Purser, D Rowley (eds), *Progress in the Treatment of Fluency Disorders*. London: Whurr, 1987.
29. Starkweather CW, Givens-Ackerman CR. *Stuttering*. Austin, TX: Pro-Ed, 1997: 138–139.
30. Cooper EB. Treatment of disfluency: Future trends. *J Fluency Disord* 1986;11: 317–327.
31. Johnson G. Ten commandments for long-term maintenance of acceptable self-help skills for persons who are hard-core stutterers. *J Fluency Disord* 1987;12:9–18.
32. Scharstein T. Internet posting to STUTT-L. Stuttering Research and Clinical Practice. Listserv, 1998.
33. Webster RL. Evolution of a target-based behavioral therapy for stuttering. *J Fluency Disord* 1980;5:303–320.
34. Andrew G, Neilson M, Cassar M. Informing stutterers about treatment. In L Rustin, H Purser, D Rowley (eds), *Progress in the Treatment of Fluency Disorders*. London: Whurr, 1987.
35. Boberg E. Intensive group therapy program for stutterers. *Hum Commun* 1976;1: 29–42.
36. Ward D. Outlining semi-intensive fluency therapy. *J Fluency Disord* 1992;17,4: 243–256.
37. Andrews G, Guitar B, Howie P. Meta-analysis of the effects of stuttering treatment. *J Speech Hear Disord* 1980;45:287–307.
38. Boberg E. *The Maintenance of Fluency*. New York: Elsevier, 1981.
39. Howie PM, Tanner S, Andrews G. Short- and long-term outcome in an intensive treatment program for adult stutterers. *J Speech Hear Disord* 1981;46:104–109.
40. Ingham R. Modification of maintenance and generalization during stuttering treatment. *J Speech Lang Hear Res* 1980;23:732–745.
41. Ingham RG, Andrews G, Winkler R. Stuttering: A comparative evaluation of the short-term effectiveness of four treatment techniques. *J Commun Disord* 1972;5: 91–117.

42. Andrews G, Tanner S. Stuttering: The results of five days treatment with a airflow technique. *J Speech Hear Disord* 1982;47:427–429.
43. Hasbrouck JM, Doherty J, Mehlmann MA, Nelson R, Randle B, Whitaker R. Intensive stuttering therapy in a public school setting. *Lang Speech Hear Servs Schools* 1987;18:330–343.

Appendix

CLIENT NAME: _____

I.	Warm-ups 1 minute each Reading, Monologue & Conversation with 100% accuracy	
II.	Practice Shots Talking to others with 100% accuracy 2-3 sentences = 1 point 4+ sentences = 2 points	
III.	3-point shots Talking on the phone with 100% accuracy.	
IV.	Swish Transfer activities with 100% accuracy = 2 points	
V.	Slam Dunk! Banquet Dinner- Speaking at the microphone with the group earns 3 points.	
VI.	Foul Shots Clinicians' Choice May be given for cooperation, motivation, team leadership and hard work = 1 point (client may be given up to 3 points per day).	**TOTAL=**

Student
Clinician   _____

Team Name_____

Figure A.1 March Madness—Shoot for Fluency, The College of Saint Rose, March 14–15, 1998. Standard Talking Samples (STS), striving for fluency fitness.

March Madness Fluency Score Sheet

Name_____

I. *WARM- UPS* are the use of full breath, easy onset, and movement target during reading, monologue, and conversation for 1 minute with 100% accuracy.

ACTIVITY	DAY	TIME	POINTS

TOTAL_____

Figure A.2   March Madness fluency score sheet.

March Madness Fluency Score Sheet

Name_____

II.   *PRACTICE SHOTS* are the use of full breath, easy onset, and movement targets while talking to other team members and coaches with 100% accuracy. Achieve 2-3 sentences, questions, directions, and earn 1 point. Achieve 4+ sentences, questions, directions and earn 2 points.

ACTIVITY	DAY	TIME	POINTS

TOTAL_____

Figure A.3   March Madness fluency score sheet.

March Madness Fluency Score Sheet

Name_____

III. *3-POINT SHOTS* are the use of full breath, easy onset, and movement targets while engaging in a telephone conversation with 100% accuracy. A short conversation less than 2 minutes = 1 point, a longer conversation = 2 points.

ACTIVITY	DAY	TIME	POINTS

TOTAL_____

Figure A.4   March Madness fluency score sheet.

March Madness Fluency Score Sheet

Name_____

IV. *SWISH* is the use of full breath, easy onset, and movement targets while engaging in transfer activities (e.g., role playing, videotaping , or other high level activities) with 100% accuracy. Each activity = 2 points.

ACTIVITY	DAY	TIME	POINTS

TOTAL_____

Figure A.5   March Madness fluency score sheet.

March Madness Fluency Score Sheet

Name_____

V. *SLAM DUNK* is the use of full breath, easy onset, and movement targets while speaking as a group at the microphone with 100% accuracy, during the banquet dinner. **Earn 3 points for this accomplishment!**

ACTIVITY	DAY	TIME	POINTS

TOTAL_____

Figure A.6 March Madness fluency score sheet.

March Madness Fluency Score Sheet

Name_____

VI. *FOUL SHOTS* are extra points earned by the client at the clinician's discretion. 1 point may be given for cooperation, motivation, team leadership, hard work, etc. A client may be given up to 3 points per day.

ACTIVITY	DAY	TIME	POINTS

TOTAL_____

Figure A.7   March Madness fluency score sheet.

Index